Mycotoxin Exposure and Related Diseases

Mycotoxin Exposure and Related Diseases

Special Issue Editors

Susana Viegas
Ricardo Assunção

MDPI • Basel • Beijing • Wuhan • Barcelona • Belgrade • Manchester • Tokyo • Cluj • Tianjin

Special Issue Editors
Susana Viegas
Universidade Nova de Lisboa
Portugal

Ricardo Assunção
University of Aveiro
Portugal

Editorial Office
MDPI
St. Alban-Anlage 66
4052 Basel, Switzerland

This is a reprint of articles from the Special Issue published online in the open access journal *Toxins* (ISSN 2072-6651) (available at: https://www.mdpi.com/journal/toxins/special_issues/mycotoxins_exposure_disease).

For citation purposes, cite each article independently as indicated on the article page online and as indicated below:

LastName, A.A.; LastName, B.B.; LastName, C.C. Article Title. *Journal Name* **Year**, *Article Number*, Page Range.

ISBN 978-3-03928-704-8 (Pbk)
ISBN 978-3-03928-705-5 (PDF)

Contents

About the Special Issue Editors vii

Ricardo Assunção and Susana Viegas
Mycotoxin Exposure and Related Diseases
Reprinted from: *Toxins* **2020**, *12*, 172, doi:10.3390/toxins12030172 1

Carla Martins, Duarte Torres, Carla Lopes, Daniela Correia, Ana Goios, Ricardo Assunção, Paula Alvito, Arnau Vidal, Marthe De Boevre, Sarah De Saeger and Carla Nunes
Food Consumption Data as a Tool to Estimate Exposure to Mycoestrogens
Reprinted from: *Toxins* **2020**, *12*, 118, doi:10.3390/toxins12020118 5

Bui Thi Mai Huong, Le Danh Tuyen, Henry Madsen, Leon Brimer, Henrik Friis and Anders Dalsgaard
Total Dietary Intake and Health Risks Associated with Exposure to Aflatoxin B_1, Ochratoxin A and Fuminisins of Children in Lao Cai Province, Vietnam
Reprinted from: *Toxins* **2019**, *11*, 638, doi:10.3390/toxins11110638 19

Andrea Molina, Guadalupe Chavarría, Margarita Alfaro-Cascante, Astrid Leiva and Fabio Granados-Chinchilla
Mycotoxins at the Start of the Food Chain in Costa Rica: Analysis of Six *Fusarium* Toxins and Ochratoxin A between 2013 and 2017 in Animal Feed and Aflatoxin M_1 in Dairy Products
Reprinted from: *Toxins* **2019**, *11*, 312, doi:10.3390/toxins11060312 37

Susana Viegas, Ricardo Assunção, Carla Martins, Carla Nunes, Bernd Osteresch, Magdalena Twarużek, Robert Kosicki, Jan Grajewski, Edna Ribeiro and Carla Viegas
Occupational Exposure to Mycotoxins in Swine Production: Environmental and Biological Monitoring Approaches
Reprinted from: *Toxins* **2019**, *11*, 78, doi:10.3390/toxins11020078 63

Omeralfaroug Ali, Judit Szabó-Fodor, Hedvig Fébel, Miklós Mézes, Krisztián Balogh, Róbert Glávits, Melinda Kovács, Arianna Zantomasi and András Szabó
Porcine Hepatic Response to Fumonisin B_1 in a Short Exposure Period: Fatty Acid Profile and Clinical Investigations
Reprinted from: *Toxins* **2019**, *11*, 655, doi:10.3390/toxins11110655 79

Kent M. Reed, Kristelle M. Mendoza and Roger A. Coulombe Jr.
Differential Transcriptome Responses to Aflatoxin B_1 in the Cecal Tonsil of Susceptible and Resistant Turkeys
Reprinted from: *Toxins* **2019**, *11*, 55, doi:10.3390/toxins11010055 97

Katarzyna Cieplińska, Magdalena Gajęcka, Michał Dąbrowski, Anna Rykaczewska, Sylwia Lisieska-Żołnierczyk, Maria Bulińska, Łukasz Zielonka and Maciej T. Gajęcki
Time-Dependent Changes in the Intestinal Microbiome of Gilts Exposed to Low Zearalenone Doses
Reprinted from: *Toxins* **2019**, *11*, 296, doi:10.3390/toxins11050296 117

Winnie-Pui-Pui Liew, Sabran Mohd-Redzwan and Leslie Thian Lung Than
Gut Microbiota Profiling of Aflatoxin B1-Induced Rats Treated with *Lactobacillus casei* Shirota
Reprinted from: *Toxins* **2019**, *11*, 49, doi:10.3390/toxins11010049 143

Feng'e Zhang, Mikko Juhani Lammi, Wanzhen Shao, Pan Zhang, Yanan Zhang, Haiyan Wei and Xiong Guo
Cytotoxic Properties of HT-2 Toxin in Human Chondrocytes: Could T_3 Inhibit Toxicity of HT-2?
Reprinted from: *Toxins* **2019**, *11*, 667, doi:10.3390/toxins11110667 . . . . **159**

Suvi Vartiainen, Alexandros Yiannikouris, Juha Apajalahti and Colm A. Moran
Comprehensive Evaluation of the Efficiency of Yeast Cell Wall Extract to Adsorb Ochratoxin A and Mitigate Accumulation of the Toxin in Broiler Chickens
Reprinted from: *Toxins* **2020**, *12*, 37, doi:10.3390/toxins12010037 . . . . **169**

Jin-Tao Wei, Kun-Tan Wu, Hua Sun, Mahmoud Mohamed Khalil, Jie-Fan Dai, Ying Liu, Qiang Liu, Ni-Ya Zhang, De-Sheng Qi and Lv-Hui Sun
A Novel Modified Hydrated Sodium Calcium Aluminosilicate (HSCAS) Adsorbent Can Effectively Reduce T-2 Toxin-Induced Toxicity in Growth Performance, Nutrient Digestibility, Serum Biochemistry, and Small Intestinal Morphology in Chicks
Reprinted from: *Toxins* **2019**, *11*, 199, doi:10.3390/toxins11040199 . . . . **189**

Tatevik Chalyan, Cristina Potrich, Erik Schreuder, Floris Falke, Laura Pasquardini, Cecilia Pederzolli, Rene Heideman and Lorenzo Pavesi
AFM1 Detection in Milk by Fab' Functionalized Si_3N_4 Asymmetric Mach–Zehnder Interferometric Biosensors
Reprinted from: *Toxins* **2019**, *11*, 409, doi:10.3390/toxins11070409 . . . . **199**

About the Special Issue Editors

Susana Viegas has a Ph.D. in Occupational and Environmental Health from Escola Nacional de Saúde Pública, New University of Lisbon, Portugal, and a Master in Applied Toxicology from Surrey University, United Kingdom. Professor in the Department of Occupational and Environmental Health of NOVA National School of Public Health, Public Health Research Centre, Universidade NOVA de Lisboa. Between 2015 and 2018, she worked as a co-opted member of the Risk Assessment Committee in European Chemical Agency (ECHA). Susana is a European Registered Toxicologist (ERT). Since 2019, she has been working as an expert adviser for Portuguese Environment Agency in issues related to authorizations within the scope of REACH. Her main research areas are occupational and environmental toxicology, environmental health, exposure, and risk assessment.

Ricardo Assunção completed his Ph.D. in Veterinary Sciences at the Institute for Advanced Studies and Research, University of Évora, Portugal, in 2017. His main research topics includef risk assessment of chemical contaminants, food toxicology, mycotoxins, and chemical mixtures. Ricardo Assunção post-graduated in Quality Management and Food Safety and was one of the The European Food Risk Assessment Fellowship Programme (EU-FORA) fellows, organized and supported by European Food Safety Authority (EFSA). Under EU-FORA, he was a visiting researcher at Risk-Benefit Research Group of the National Food Institute, Technical University of Denmark (DTU). Ricardo is a European Registered Toxicologist (ERT). Currently, Ricardo Assunção is developing his research at the Food and Nutrition Department of the National Institute of Health Dr. Ricardo Jorge, Lisbon, Portugal. His main research areas include risk and risk-benefit assessment of foods, food safety and public health, especially focused on the interaction between diet and health.

toxins

MDPI

Editorial

Mycotoxin Exposure and Related Diseases

Ricardo Assunção [1,2,*] and Susana Viegas [3,4,5,*]

1 Food and Nutrition Department, National Institute of Health Dr. Ricardo Jorge, Avenida Padre Cruz, 1649-016 Lisboa, Portugal
2 CESAM, Centre for Environmental and Marine Studies, University of Aveiro, Campus Universitário de Santiago, 3810-193 Aveiro, Portugal
3 NOVA National School of Public Health, Public Health Research Centre, Universidade NOVA de Lisboa, 1600-560 Lisbon, Portugal
4 Comprehensive Health Research Center (CHRC), 1150-090 Lisbon, Portugal
5 H&TRC-Health & Technology Research Center, ESTeSL-Escola Superior de Tecnologia da Saúde, Instituto Politécnico de Lisboa, 1990-096 Lisbon, Portugal
* Correspondence: ricardo.assuncao@insa.min-saude.pt (R.A.); susana.viegas@ensp.unl.pt (S.V.)

Received: 2 March 2020; Accepted: 9 March 2020; Published: 11 March 2020

Mycotoxins are considered the most frequently occurring natural contaminants in the diet of humans and animals. These toxic secondary metabolites of low molecular weight and very stable compounds are produced by different genera of filamentous fungi that infect susceptible plants throughout the world [1,2]. Considering their particular vulnerability to fungi contamination, crops represent a special concern under mycotoxins context. Most fungal strains produce more than one type of mycotoxin, therefore, co-contamination of agricultural products with multiple mycotoxins is frequently observed, and the need to consider this aspect in the risk assessment process has been emphasized [3,4].

Animals can be exposed to mycotoxins through the consumption of contaminated feed, subsequently entering into the food chain, and thus constituting a source of exposure to humans [5]. Regarding human exposure, in addition to the dietary source, the workplace environment can also represent an exposure source. Dust containing mycotoxins is released during regular tasks involving high exposure to organic dust, such as storage work, loading, handling, or milling contaminated materials (grain, waste, and feed), and other tasks such as caring for animals in animal husbandry settings [5–15].

The establishment of a disease is largely influenced by the magnitude of a given exposure. Consequently, every effort that contributes to properly characterizing the risk associated with human exposure assumes particular relevance.

The present Special Issue aims to shed light on the different perspectives of mycotoxins exposure and their implications for the establishment of a disease. The gathered studies include several important findings focusing on different perspectives and clues about the impact of human and animal exposure to mycotoxins. A broad spectrum of mycotoxins-related issues associated with mycotoxin exposure and related diseases are covered in the present Special Issue.

The detection and quantification of mycotoxins in food and feed, as an important aspect in the exposure characterization process, is focused on in two studies. An innovative detection methodology of aflatoxin M1 (AFM1) in milk using interferometric biosensors has been developed, demonstrating that viable solutions for lab-on-chip devices for food safety analyses are possible and reliable [16]. Data on the individual and combined occurrence of *Fusarium* mycotoxins and ochratoxin A (OTA) in feedstuffs in Costa Rica were collected, highlighting the implications for all stakeholders linked to the feed industry as well as the potential measures that can be considered for the management of mycotoxins in animal production [17].

The risk assessment of human exposure to mycotoxins is also considered, applying different approaches for the general population [18] or to specific populations such as children [19] or swine production workers [6]. Regarding these studies, human biomonitoring strategies, as a direct measure of internal exposure, are considered [6,18]. The exposure to mycoestrogens, namely zearalenone (ZEN) and alternariol, was estimated through data modeling, assessing the burden regarding endocrine disruption [18]. The workplace environment also represents an important exposure source to mycotoxins, namely, in swine production [6]. Exposure of children to mycotoxins in Vietnam were assessed and revealed a high risk associated with high levels of exposure and exceedance of toxicological reference levels [19]. In order to clarify the potential role of the mycotoxin HT-2 in the Kashin–Beck disease, an in vitro approach using immortalized human chondrocyte cell line, C-28/I2, is considered [20]. The study reports a potentially negative effect led by HT-2 exposure and highlights the importance of future studies to provide a better understanding of the mechanism of HT-2 toxin cytotoxicity.

In addition to the human studies, several papers examine the role of mycotoxins in the establishment and/or development of different health effects in animals [21–24]. Interference of mycotoxins exposure in the gut microbiome and immunity are evaluated in gilts, turkeys, and rats [22–24]. In pre-pubertal gilts, a minimal anticipated biological effect level (MABEL) dose of ZEN stimulated the growth of specific strains of intestinal microbiota [22]. In turkeys, the effects of aflatoxin B1 (AFB1) on the gastro-intestinal tract are investigated and show that, in addition to the hepatic transcriptome, animal resistance to this mycotoxin occurs in organ systems outside the liver [23]. In rats, and also focusing on the effects of AFB1, the findings suggest that AFB1 can alter the gut microbiota composition and that *Lactobacillus casei* Shirota can reduce the AFB1-induced dissimilarities in the gut microbiota profile [24]. Hepatoxicity associated with the exposure of piglets to fumonisin B1 (FB1) is also studied [21]. Results show that histology, cellular enzyme leakage, and hepatocellular membrane lipid fatty acid profile are affected after an exposure of 10 days to FB1.

Recognizing the potential negative impact associated to animal exposure to mycotoxins, the application of appropriate mitigation measures is also studied. The use of the yeast cell wall extract (YCWE) in chickens [25] and a novel modified hydrated sodium calcium aluminosilicate (HSCAS) in chicks [26] as adsorbents to mycotoxins are investigated. First, data showed a decrease of up to 30% in OTA deposits in the liver of broilers fed both OTA and YCWE [25]. Second, the results suggest that the modified HSCAS adsorbent can be used against T-2 toxin-induced toxicity in growth performance, nutrient digestibility, and hepatic and small intestinal injuries in chicks [26].

Altogether, and especially under an expected climate change scenario, which considers mycotoxins as an important driver of health consequences, the present Special Issue contributes with significant and impactful research that supports the anticipation of potential consequences of the exposure of humans and animals to mycotoxins, future risk assessments, and the establishment of preventive measures.

Funding: This research received no external funding.

Acknowledgments: The Editors are grateful to all of the authors who contributed with their work to this Special Issue. Special thanks go to the rigorous evaluations of all of the submitted manuscripts by the expert peer reviewers who contributed to this Special Issue. Lastly, the valuable contributions, organization, and editorial support of the MDPI management team and staff are greatly appreciated. The Editors would like to acknowledge the support of the NOVA National School of Public Health, Public Health Research Centre, Universidade NOVA de Lisboa, and are grateful to FCT/MCTES for the support to CESAM (UID/AMB/50017/2019).

Conflicts of Interest: The authors declare no conflict of interest.

References

1. Gruber-Dorninger, C.; Jenkins, T.; Schatzmayr, G. Global Mycotoxin Occurrence in Feed: A Ten-Year Survey. *Toxins* **2019**, *11*, 375. [CrossRef] [PubMed]
2. Ingenbleek, L.; Sulyok, M.; Adegboye, A.; Hossou, S.E.; Koné, A.Z.; Oyedele, A.D.; Kisito, C.S.K.J.; Dembélé, Y.K.; Eyangoh, S.; Verger, P.; et al. Regional Sub-Saharan Africa Total Diet Study in Benin, Cameroon, Mali and Nigeria Reveals the Presence of 164 Mycotoxins and Other Secondary Metabolites in Foods. *Toxins* **2019**, *11*, 54. [CrossRef] [PubMed]
3. Assunção, R.; Silva, M.J.; Alvito, P. Challenges in risk assessment of multiple mycotoxins in food. *World Mycotoxin J.* **2016**, *9*, 791–811. [CrossRef]
4. Eskola, M.; Altieri, A.; Galobart, J. Overview of the activities of the European Food Safety Authority on mycotoxins in food and feed. *World Mycotoxin J.* **2018**, *11*, 277–289. [CrossRef]
5. Viegas, S.; Assunção, R.; Twarużek, M.; Kosicki, R.; Grajewski, J.; Viegas, C. Mycotoxins feed contamination in a dairy farm—Potential implications for milk contamination and workers' exposure in a One Health approach. *J. Sci. Food Agric.* **2020**, *100*, 1118–1123. [CrossRef]
6. Viegas, S.; Assunção, R.; Martins, C.; Nunes, C.; Osteresch, B.; Twarużek, M.; Kosicki, R.; Grajewski, J.; Ribeiro, E.; Viegas, C. Occupational Exposure to Mycotoxins in Swine Production: Environmental and Biological Monitoring Approaches. *Toxins* **2019**, *11*, 78. [CrossRef]
7. Viegas, S.; Assunção, R.; Nunes, C.; Osteresch, B.; Twarużek, M.; Kosicki, R.; Grajewski, J.; Martins, C.; Alvito, P.; Almeida, A.; et al. Exposure Assessment to Mycotoxins in a Portuguese Fresh Bread Dough Company by Using a Multi-Biomarker Approach. *Toxins* **2018**, *10*, 342. [CrossRef]
8. Viegas, S.; Viegas, C.; Oppliger, A. Occupational Exposure to Mycotoxins: Current Knowledge and Prospects. *Ann. Work Expo. Health* **2018**, *62*, 923–941. [CrossRef]
9. Viegas, S.; Osteresch, B.; Almeida, A.; Cramer, B.; Humpf, H.-U.; Viegas, C. Enniatin B and ochratoxin A in the blood serum of workers from the waste management setting. *Mycotoxin Res.* **2018**, *34*, 85–90. [CrossRef]
10. Viegas, S.; Veiga, L.; Almeida, A.; dos Santos, M.; Carolino, E.; Viegas, C. Occupational Exposure to Aflatoxin B1 in a Portuguese Poultry Slaughterhouse. *Ann. Occup. Hyg.* **2016**, *60*, 176–183. [CrossRef]
11. Viegas, S.; Veiga, L.; Figueiredo, P.; Almeida, A.; Carolino, E.; Viegas, C. Assessment of Workers' Exposure to Aflatoxin B1 in a Portuguese Waste Industry. *Ann. Occup. Hyg.* **2014**, *59*, 173–181. [PubMed]
12. Viegas, S.; Veiga, L.; Figueredo, P.; Almeida, A.; Carolino, E.; Sabino, R.; Veríssimo, C.; Viegas, C. Occupational Exposure to Aflatoxin B 1 in Swine Production and Possible Contamination Sources. *J. Toxicol. Environ. Health Part A* **2013**, *76*, 944–951. [CrossRef] [PubMed]
13. Viegas, S.; Veiga, L.; Figueredo, P.; Almeida, A.; Carolino, E.; Sabino, R.; Veríssimo, C.; Viegas, C. Occupational exposure to aflatoxin B 1: The case of poultry and swine production. *World Mycotoxin J.* **2013**, *6*, 309–315. [CrossRef]
14. Viegas, S.; Veiga, L.; Malta-Vacas, J.; Sabino, R.; Figueredo, P.; Almeida, A.; Viegas, C.; Carolino, E. Occupational Exposure to Aflatoxin (AFB 1) in Poultry Production. *J. Toxicol. Environ. Health Part A* **2012**, *75*, 1330–1340. [CrossRef]
15. Viegas, C.; Monteiro, A.; Ribeiro, E.; Caetano, L.A.; Carolino, E.; Assunção, R.; Viegas, S. Organic dust exposure in veterinary clinics: A case study of a small-animal practice in Portugal. *Arch. Ind. Hyg. Toxicol.* **2018**, *69*, 309–316. [CrossRef]
16. Chalyan, T.; Potrich, C.; Schreuder, E.; Falke, F.; Pasquardini, L.; Pederzolli, C.; Heideman, R.; Pavesi, L. AFM1 Detection in Milk by Fab' Functionalized Si3N4 Asymmetric Mach–Zehnder Interferometric Biosensors. *Toxins* **2019**, *11*, 409. [CrossRef]
17. Molina, A.; Chavarría, G.; Alfaro-Cascante, M.; Leiva, A.; Granados-Chinchilla, F. Mycotoxins at the Start of the Food Chain in Costa Rica: Analysis of Six Fusarium Toxins and Ochratoxin A between 2013 and 2017 in Animal Feed and Aflatoxin M1 in Dairy Products. *Toxins* **2019**, *11*, 312. [CrossRef]
18. Martins, C.; Torres, D.; Lopes, C.; Correia, D.; Goios, A.; Assunção, R.; Alvito, P.; Vidal, A.; De Boevre, M.; De Saeger, S.; et al. Food Consumption Data as a Tool to Estimate Exposure to Mycoestrogens. *Toxins* **2020**, *12*, 118. [CrossRef]
19. Huong, B.T.M.; Tuyen, L.D.; Madsen, H.; Brimer, L.; Friis, H.; Dalsgaard, A. Total Dietary Intake and Health Risks Associated with Exposure to Aflatoxin B1, Ochratoxin A and Fuminisins of Children in Lao Cai Province, Vietnam. *Toxins* **2019**, *11*, 638. [CrossRef]

20. Zhang, F.; Lammi, M.J.; Shao, W.; Zhang, P.; Zhang, Y.; Wei, H.; Guo, X. Cytotoxic Properties of HT-2 Toxin in Human Chondrocytes: Could T3 Inhibit Toxicity of HT-2? *Toxins* **2019**, *11*, 667. [CrossRef]
21. Ali, O.; Szabó-Fodor, J.; Fébel, H.; Mézes, M.; Balogh, K.; Glávits, R.; Kovács, M.; Zantomasi, A.; Szabó, A. Porcine Hepatic Response to Fumonisin B1 in a Short Exposure Period: Fatty Acid Profile and Clinical Investigations. *Toxins* **2019**, *11*, 655. [CrossRef] [PubMed]
22. Cieplińska, K.; Gajęcka, M.; Dąbrowski, M.; Rykaczewska, A.; Lisieska-Żołnierczyk, S.; Bulińska, M.; Zielonka, Ł.; Gajęcki, M.T. Time-Dependent Changes in the Intestinal Microbiome of Gilts Exposed to Low Zearalenone Doses. *Toxins* **2019**, *11*, 296. [CrossRef] [PubMed]
23. Reed, K.; Mendoza, K.; Coulombe, R. Differential Transcriptome Responses to Aflatoxin B1 in the Cecal Tonsil of Susceptible and Resistant Turkeys. *Toxins* **2019**, *11*, 55. [CrossRef] [PubMed]
24. Liew, W.; Mohd-Redzwan, S.; Than, L. Gut Microbiota Profiling of Aflatoxin B1-Induced Rats Treated with Lactobacillus casei Shirota. *Toxins* **2019**, *11*, 49. [CrossRef]
25. Vartiainen, S.; Yiannikouris, A.; Apajalahti, J.; Moran, C.A. Comprehensive Evaluation of the Efficiency of Yeast Cell Wall Extract to Adsorb Ochratoxin A and Mitigate Accumulation of the Toxin in Broiler Chickens. *Toxins* **2020**, *12*, 37. [CrossRef]
26. Wei, J.; Wu, K.; Sun, H.; Khalil, M.M.; Dai, J.; Liu, Y.; Liu, Q.; Zhang, N.-Y.; Qi, D.-S.; Sun, L.-H. A Novel Modified Hydrated Sodium Calcium Aluminosilicate (HSCAS) Adsorbent Can Effectively Reduce T-2 Toxin-Induced Toxicity in Growth Performance, Nutrient Digestibility, Serum Biochemistry, and Small Intestinal Morphology in Chicks. *Toxins* **2019**, *11*, 199. [CrossRef]

toxins

MDPI

Article

Food Consumption Data as a Tool to Estimate Exposure to Mycoestrogens

Carla Martins [1,2,3,4,*], Duarte Torres [5,6], Carla Lopes [6,7], Daniela Correia [6,7], Ana Goios [5,6], Ricardo Assunção [1,2], Paula Alvito [1,2], Arnau Vidal [8], Marthe De Boevre [8], Sarah De Saeger [8] and Carla Nunes [3,4]

1 Food and Nutrition Department, National Institute of Health Dr. Ricardo Jorge, Avenida Padre Cruz, 1649-016 Lisboa, Portugal; ricardo.assuncao@insa.min-saude.pt (R.A.); paula.alvito@insa.min-saude.pt (P.A.)
2 CESAM, Centre for Environmental and Marine Studies, University of Aveiro, Campus Universitário de Santiago, 3810-193 Aveiro, Portugal
3 NOVA National School of Public Health, Public Health Research Centre, Universidade NOVA de Lisboa, Avenida Padre Cruz, 1600-560 Lisboa, Portugal; cnunes@ensp.unl.pt
4 Comprehensive Health Research Center (CHRC), Universidade NOVA de Lisboa, Campo Mártires da Pátria, 1169-056 Lisboa, Portugal
5 Faculty of Nutrition and Food Sciences, University of Porto, Rua Dr. Roberto Frias, 4200-465 Porto, Portugal; dupamato@fcna.up.pt (D.T.); aclgoios@gmail.com (A.G.)
6 Epidemiology Research Unit, Institute of Public Health, University of Porto, Rua das Taipas 135, 4050-091 Porto, Portugal; carlal@med.up.pt (C.L.); danielamc@med.up.pt (D.C.)
7 Department of Public Health and Forensic Sciences, and Medical Education, Faculty of Medicine, University of Porto, Alameda Prof. Hernâni Monteiro, 4200-319 Porto, Portugal
8 Centre of Excellence in Mycotoxicology and Public Health, Faculty of Pharmaceutical Sciences, Ghent University, Ottergemsesteenweg 460, B-9000 Ghent, Belgium; arnau.vidalcorominas@ugent.be (A.V.); Marthe.DeBoevre@UGent.be (M.D.B.); Sarah.DeSaeger@UGent.be (S.D.S.)
* Correspondence: carla.martins@insa.min-saude.pt; Tel.: +351-217-519-219

Received: 18 January 2020; Accepted: 7 February 2020; Published: 13 February 2020

Abstract: Zearalenone and alternariol are mycotoxins produced by *Fusarium* and *Alternaria* species, respectively, that present estrogenic activity and consequently are classified as endocrine disruptors. To estimate the exposure of the Portuguese population to these two mycotoxins at a national level, a modelling approach, based on data from 94 Portuguese volunteers, was developed considering as inputs: i) the food consumption data generated within the National Food and Physical Activity Survey; and ii) the human biomonitoring data used to assess the exposure to the referred mycotoxins. Six models of association between mycoestrogens urinary levels (zearalenone, total zearalenone and alternariol) and food items (meat, cheese, and fresh-cheese, breakfast cereals, sweets) were established. Applying the obtained models to the consumption data (n = 5811) of the general population, the median estimates of the probable daily intake revealed that a fraction of the Portuguese population might exceed the tolerable daily intake defined for zearalenone. A reference intake value for alternariol is still lacking, thus the characterization of risk due to the exposure to this mycotoxin was not possible to perform. Although the unavoidable uncertainties, these results are important contributions to understand the exposure to endocrine disruptors in Portugal and the potential Public Health consequences.

Keywords: modelling; mycotoxins; food consumption; urinary biomarkers; public health

Key Contribution: Applying data modelling, an estimate of the exposure of the Portuguese population to mycotoxins that represent a burden regarding endocrine disruption was established. The importance of the development of biomonitoring studies linked with food and health surveys, allowing the data collection in the three domains, is highlighted in this study.

1. Introduction

Mycotoxins are secondary metabolites produced by filamentous fungi and represent one of the most relevant group of food contaminants [1]. These toxins are considered ubiquitous and can affect the food chain in the different stages of production, harvest, storage, and processing [2]. They are associated with several health outcomes in humans and animals, including carcinogenic, immunotoxic, nephrotoxic, neurotoxic, teratogenic, and hepatotoxic effects [1,3]. Some mycotoxins, such as zearalenone (ZEN) and alternariol (AOH) produced by *Fusarium* and *Alternaria* species respectively, present estrogenic activity and are classified as endocrine disruptors [4–6]. According to the World Health Organization (WHO), an endocrine disruptor is a "substance that alter one or more function of the endocrine system and consequently cause adverse effects in an intact organism, its progeny and a (sub)population" [7]. Endocrine disruptors interfere with the hormones' action, disrupt homeostasis, and may alter physiology during the whole life span of an individual, from foetal development to adult growth [8].

As referred by several authors, ZEN presents a chemical structure that resembles the structure of naturally-occurring estrogens, namely 17-β-estradiol, making ZEN capable of binding to estrogen receptors (full agonist to ER-α, mixed agonist–antagonist to ER-β) [9–11]. ZEN has been implicated in the disruption of mammalian reproduction by affecting the synthesis and secretion of sex hormones such as progesterone, estradiol, and testosterone [12]. It was also reported as presenting a higher estrogenic relative potency factor than bisphenol A (BPA) [13,14]. ZEN is characterized by a fast metabolism, within 24 hours, and the excretion rates reported so far are 9.4% obtained in a human intervention study, and 36.8% obtained in an animal study [15,16]. The metabolism comprehends a phase I of reduction reactions, and a phase II of glucuronidation/sulfonation reactions [17]. Epidemiological studies also revealed the presence of zearalenone and metabolites in biological samples, confirming that human exposure to this mycotoxin is commonplace [18–23]. The consequences of human exposure to ZEN were suggested by several results. In Hungary [24], Italy [25], and Turkey [26], regions where increasing cases of early telarche and central idiopathic precocious puberty were reported, an association with ZEN and metabolites levels in biological samples was established. The latest results of Jersey Girls Study showed that girls with detectable mycoestrogen levels were significantly shorter in stature at menarche compared to girls with undetectable levels [27]. The occurrence of ZEN is mainly reported in cereals and animal products, and the ingestion of these food commodities is considered the major source of human exposure [28]. In the Regulation 1881/2006 and its amendments, the European Commission established maximum admissible levels for the occurrence of ZEN in foods. These levels were laid down for cereals and cereal-products such as bread (including small bakery wares), pastries, biscuits, cereal snacks and breakfast cereals, and cereal-based foods intended for infants and young children consumption, ranging between 20 and 400 μg kg^{-1} [29]. Based on the estrogenic effects of ZEN in pigs as the critical endpoint, the European Food Safety Authority (EFSA) recommended a tolerable daily intake (TDI) for ZEN and metabolites of 250 ng kg^{-1} bw day^{-1} [28].

Regarding AOH, very little data concerning metabolism and toxicity is available. Alternariol has been associated with genotoxic and mutagenic effects and it is considered an endocrine disruptor, being also capable of binding to estrogens' receptors (ER-β, preferentially) [30]. Recently, in a study developed by Puntscher et al. in rats, it was possible to determine an excretion rate of 8.3% for AOH, with an increase of 7% and 19% when urine and faeces samples were pre-treated with β-glucuronidase/arylsulphatase, indicating that glucuronidation and sulfonation are potentially metabolic pathways also for AOH [30]. Alternariol was recently identified and quantified in urine samples [19,31], confirming the human exposure to this mycotoxin. *Alternaria* toxins are considered important emerging risks that need to be properly assessed in food safety, yet there are no regulations for the toxins in food and feed in Europe [32]. The occurrence of AOH has been reported in fruits, vegetables and vegetable-products, cereals and cereal-products, dried fruits and nuts, sunflower seeds, wines, and infant foods [33–35]. The last assessment conducted by EFSA in 2016 concerning *Alternaria* toxins concluded there is a need for more sensitive analytical methods in order to decrease the amount of left-censored data and the uncertainty associated with risk assessment [36]. In the absence of a TDI for *Alternaria* toxins, EFSA applied the threshold for toxicological concern (TTC) approach to characterize the risk and concluded that exposure to AOH and alternariol monomethyl ether (AME) could represent a health concern [36].

Regarding the endocrine disruptive activity, the interaction between ZEN and AOH was assessed through models using Ishikawa cells and synergistic effects were observed [9].

Since food intake is considered the major source of exposure to mycotoxins, it is also important to shed a light on the food commodities that may be the determinants of this exposure. Several studies attempted to assess the association between food intake and mycotoxins' urinary biomarkers, with the majority of the studies using bivariate analysis (correlation coefficients). None reported associations for *Alternaria* toxins, namely AOH, and only one reported an association of grains and meat intake with exposure to ZEN [21]. Recently, Mitropoulou et al. [37] found a weak association between urinary ZEN concentrations and chocolate consumption using bivariate analysis, but no association were found when performing a more extensive statistical analysis and using a multivariate median regression analysis. From our knowledge, the only study thus far that has performed a deep statistical analysis to assess the influence of food consumption in mycotoxins' urinary biomarkers was performed by Turner et al. [38]. This study intended to find significant contributors for the exposure to deoxynivalenol in the UK population. The authors gathered data from urinary excretion of mycotoxins obtained from 24 h urine samples as well as food consumption data from the National Data and Nutrition Survey, and through a multivariate model reported wholemeal bread, white bread, buns/cakes, high fibre breakfast cereals, and pasta as significant contributors for exposure to deoxynivalenol [38]. Martins et al. [39] note that for mycotoxins with short half-lives, such as ZEN and AOH, it is expected to find associations between food consumption of the previous 24 h and urinary biomarkers of exposure.

A recent human biomonitoring study developed in Portugal revealed the presence of mycoestrogens in 24 h urine and first morning urine of 94 volunteers [19]. Regarding ZEN, estimates revealed that 24% of participants would surpass the established TDI [19]. Data to properly characterize the risk associated to AOH exposure were not available. These obtained results contributed to the recognition that the Portuguese population are exposed to mycoestrogens. In order to establish preventive public health measures and to anticipate potential health effects, a deeper analysis of exposure scenarios for the different age groups, regions, and sex is of utmost importance. The identification of the main food contributors through association with food consumption data could be further explored for the development of modelling tools to estimate exposure to a larger and more representative sample.

Considering the above, the recently obtained food consumption data under the National Food and Physical Activity Survey (IAN-AF) were combined with the data regarding human exposure to mycotoxins obtained through a human biomonitoring (HBM) study [19,40] aiming to: i) to develop a statistical model relating food consumption and mycotoxins exposure; and ii) to estimate the exposure to ZEN and AOH of all the participants of IAN-AF, stratified by age, sex, and region, based on the developed modelling.

2. Results and Discussion

2.1. HBM Data

2.1.1. Sociodemographic Characterization of Participants

The sociodemographic characteristics of participants are described in Table 1. Participants in the HBM study (n = 94) were similarly distributed by sex, with 51.1% of males and 48.9% of females, and were mainly from the northern region of Portugal (78.7%). Regarding the educational level, about half of the participants (51.1%) reported 9 years or less of education. Only 13.8% reported a monthly income above 1941€ and 55.3% of the participants were workers for remuneration or profit.

Participants in the IAN-AF study (n = 5811) were similarly distributed by sex, with 48.1% of males and 51.9% of females, and presented a distribution across the country with similar percentages from all regions. This group included participants from all age groups. Regarding the educational level, 44.5%

of the participants reported 10–12 years of education. Regarding the monthly income, the range of 485–1455 € was reported by almost half of the participants (49.0%). More than half of the participants (55%) were workers for remuneration or profit.

Both groups of participants presented similar sociodemographic characteristics. The group of 5811 participants was representative of the Portuguese population at regional level.

Table 1. Sociodemographic characteristics of sub-sample of participants in human biomonitoring (HBM) study ($n = 94$) and participants in National Food and Physical Activity Survey (IAN-AF) study ($n = 5811$) [40,41].

	Participants in HBM Study ($n = 94$)		**Participants in IAN-AF Study ($n = 5811$)**	
	n	%	*n*	%
Sex				
Male	48	51.1	2793	48.1
Female	46	48.9	3018	51.9
Age	-	-		
Children (0–9 years)	-	-	1327	22.8
Adolescents (10–17 years)	-	-	632	10.9
Adults (18–64 years)	81	86.2	3102	53.4
Elderly (>64 years)	13	13.8	750	12.9
Region				
North	74	78.7	989	17.0
Centre	20	21.3	1014	17.4
Lisbon Metropolitan Area	-	-	809	13.9
Alentejo	-	-	670	11.5
Algarve	-	-	766	13.2
Madeira	-	-	779	13.4
Azores	-	-	784	13.5
Educational level				
≤9 years	48	51.1	1530	26.3
10–12 years	25	26.6	2587	44.5
>12 years	21	22.3	1675	28.8
Do not know/answered	-	-	19	0.3
Working condition				
Worker for remuneration or profit	52	55.3	2119	55.0
Unemployed	14	14.9	444	11.5
Other [1]	28	29.8	1286	33.4
Do not know/answered	-	-	3	0.1
Household monthly income (€)				
<485 €	9	9.6	362	9.4
485–970 €	22	23.4	1015	26.3
971–1455 €	30	31.9	875	22.7
1456–1940 €	16	17.0	514	13.3
More than 1941 €	13	13.8	708	18.4
Do not know/answered	4	4.3	378	9.8

[1] retired, permanently disabled, student, domestic worker, performing military service or mandatory community service.

2.1.2. Mycoestrogens' Urinary Biomarkers

Martins et al. [19] reported results for the urinary biomarkers of mycoestrogens in a human biomonitoring study where 24 h urine and first morning urine (FMU) paired samples of participants from north and centre regions of Portugal were analysed. Regarding 24 h urine samples, the authors reported positive samples above the limit of detection (LOD) for ZEN (48%), ZEN-14-GlcA (16%), and AOH (29%) [19]. Regarding FMU samples, the authors reported positive samples (>LOD) for ZEN (57%), ZEN-14-GlcA (16%), α-ZEL (5%), and AOH (13%) [19]. Other known metabolites of ZEN, namely beta-zearalenol (β-ZEL), alpha-zearalanol (α-ZAL), beta-zearalanol (β-ZAL), alpha-zearalenol-glucuronide (α-ZEL-GlcA), beta-zearalenol-glucuronide (β-ZEL-GlcA), and zearalanone (ZAN), were not detected in 24 h and FMU samples [19]. If the co-exposure to both mycoestrogens is considered, 13% ($n = 12$) of participants presented urinary biomarkers for ZEN and

AOH in 24 h urine samples. This co-exposure was determined for only 5% (n = 5) of the participants when analysing the FMU samples (data not shown).

2.1.3. Food Consumption Data

As presented in Table 2, the food category with the highest reported consumption was "non-alcoholic drinks", mainly due to the consumption of water (data not shown). Regarding the remaining food groups, "fruits and vegetables" was the group presenting the highest median consumption, followed by "cereals", "dairy products", "meat, fish and eggs", and "cookies, biscuits, and sweets". The consumption reported for all food categories did not present statistically significant differences between the first and the second interview ($p > 0.05$).

2.2. Link Between Food Consumption and Exposure Levels to Mycotoxins

The results presented in Table 3 summarize the statistical links between the consumption of some food items and the ZEN and AOH urinary levels of biomarkers. The Generalized Linear Models (GLM) considered the log-transformed urinary biomarkers as dependent variables, and the food consumption data of the second interview as independent variables.

Regarding ZEN, three different models were obtained for results of ZEN's urinary biomarkers. The meat consumption was positively associated with urinary levels of ZEN-14-GlcA and total ZEN. The association between consumption of meat and exposure to ZEN was previously reported by Bandera et al. (2011) in the Jersey Girls Study [21]. When considering the results obtained for FMU samples, it was possible to develop only one model; the consumption of cheese and fresh-cheese was positively associated with urinary levels of ZEN. Despite the lactational transfer of ZEN being considered low [42], the occurrence of ZEN in milk was reported in some studies showing evidence of possible carry-over [43,44]. Humans can be indirectly exposed to ZEN through consumption of animal products that have themselves been exposed [45], and these results are corroborated by previous reports of feed contamination in Portugal. Almeida et al. [46] reported 45% of feed samples (cows, ewes, goats) contaminated with ZEN, in low levels and below the recommended value of 500 µg/kg, and if considering specifically feed for cows the percentage of positive samples reported was 54.4% [46]. In a more recent review, Abrunhosa et al. reported a total of 25% of feed samples were contaminated by ZEN [47]. Cereal-based foods are well recognized as important determinants of exposure to ZEN and are thus regulated regarding the occurrence of ZEN [29]. Nevertheless, the need for a deeper knowledge on the occurrence of ZEN in foods from animal origins is also recognized by EFSA and Agence nationale de sécurité sanitaire de l'alimentation, de l'environnement et du travail (ANSES) (former Agence française de sécurité sanitaire des aliments (AFSSA)) in several reports [28,48,49] and should be properly addressed for a better risk estimation. Data generated under the present study, where animal products were found to be important contributors for the human exposure to ZEN, corroborate the importance of an extended assessment of the presence of ZEN in these products.

Positive and significant associations were found between the consumption of breakfast cereals and AOH urinary levels in 24 h urine samples. These results are consistent with the occurrence data reported so far for AOH. Cereals and cereal-products are one of the food commodities often contaminated with *Alternaria* toxins, including AOH [36,50]. The model obtained for first morning urines and food consumption revealed a positive association for meat and sweets. There are no reported data for the occurrence of AOH in animal products such as meat; on the contrary, there are available data reporting the occurrence of AOH in sweets [36]. Nevertheless, results obtained for this model should be considered carefully due to the lack of support from occurrence data. The food group of vegetables and fruits, which is frequently reported as being contaminated with *Alternaria* toxins, was not found as a determinant for the urinary levels of AOH [34,36].

Table 2. Food consumption reported in edible grams per day (g/day) by the two groups of IAN-AF: $n = 94$ and $n = 5811$. [41].

	1st Interview (g/day)						2nd Interview (g/day)					
	n = 94			*n* = 5811			*n* = 94			*n* = 5811		
	Median	IQR	P95	Median	IQR	P95	Median	IQR	P95	Median	IQR	P95
Fruits and vegetables	297.4	186.2–528.7	699.1	272.6	159.4–408.0	662.7	311.9	177.9–465.8	783.9	263.4	153.7–393.2	655.4
Dairy products	193.0	27.6–384.7	744.8	272.8	118.9–462.1	794.7	222.8	100.9–326.3	528.4	268.8	109.0–460.1	789.7
Cereals	287.5	186.8–393.6	661.8	264.4	169.1–379.2	623.9	278.1	179.8–416.7	720.0	256.1	167.6–366.4	606.2
Meat, fish, and eggs	188.7	117.8–284.4	535.9	133.7	69.5–220.8	391.1	165.9	94.5–275.3	457.2	134.2	68.9–221.7	405.5
Cookies, biscuits, and sweets	39.6	10.4–121.8	209.3	29.0	6.0–101.2	240.0	38.9	9.5–102.5	259.4	28.0	6.0–100.0	242.4
Non-alcoholic drinks	1273.0	726.2–1822.8	2884.3	899.1	412.1–1551.0	2351.6	1183.1	742.0–1811.8	2548.7	866.1	410.0–1514.2	2329.4
Alcoholic drinks	8.3	0.0–251.1	921.9	0.0	0.0–27.7	582.2	7.6	0.0–238.4	979.9	0.0	0.0–25.3	591.3

IQR = Interquartile range; P95 = Percentile 95.

Table 3. Effect of consumption of food categories and the urinary levels of AOH, ZEN and ZEN-14-GlcA.

Mycotoxin	Urine Sample	Model	Urinary Biomarker	Food Category	Regression Coefficients	*p* Value	*R*	Omnibus
ZEN	24 h U	1	ZEN-14-GlcA (µg/g crea)	Meat	0.001	0.033	0.220	0.033
		2	Total ZEN (µg/g crea)	Meat	0.001	0.045	0.217	0.047
	FMU	3	ZEN (µg/g crea)	Cheese, Fresh-cheese	0.004	0.029	0.256	0.031
AOH	24 h U	4	AOH (µg/g crea)	Breakfast Cereals	0.010	0.019	0.153	0.021
		5	AOH (µg/day)	Breakfast Cereals	0.009	0.022	0.197	0.023
	FMU	6	AOH (µg/g crea)	Meat	0.001	0.020	0.285	0.011
				Sweets	0.002	0.003		

R = Spearman' Correlation coefficient; Omnibus = Adjustment of model; AOH = Alternariol; ZEN = Zearalenone; ZEN-14-GlcA = Zearalenone-14-Glucuronide; Total ZEN = Sum of ZEN, ZEN-14-GlcA and α-ZEL considering the mass ration between the parent compound and the metabolites; FMU = First Morning Urine; 24 h U = 24 h urine.

2.3. Estimation of Exposure of Portuguese Population by Sex, Age Group and Region to Mycoestrogens

Data collected under the IAN-AF and the models developed in the present study (detailed in Section 2.2) allowed the estimation of exposure to mycoestrogens for a representative sample of the Portuguese population (n = 5811) stratified by region, sex, and age groups.

The usual exposure for the 5811 participants was estimated using SPADE software (Statistical Program to Assess Dietary Exposure, R package SPADE.RIVM), a tool developed by RIVM [51]. Results are presented in Table 4.

Table 4. Estimated usual exposure to mycoestrogens of 5811 participants of IAN-AF, weighted for the Portuguese population distribution.

	Distribution					Reference Intake	
	P25	*Median*	*Mean*	*P75*	*P95*	*RVI*	*% ≥ RVI*
Total ZEN							
Exposure (μg/g crea)	0.587	0.648	0.655	0.714	0.823	-	-
PDI (μg/kg bw/day)	0.217	0.240	0.242	**0.265**	**0.305**	0.250	38.6%
AOH							
Exposure (μg/g crea)	0.322	0.582	0.621	0.742	1.053	-	-
PDI (μg/kg bw/day)	0.146	0.253	0.268	0.318	0.439	-	-

PDI = Probable Daily Intake; AOH = Alternariol; Total ZEN = Sum of ZEN, ZEN-14-GlcA and α-ZEL considering the mass ration between the parent compound and the metabolites; RVI = Reference Value for Intake, 0.250 μg/kg bw/day for ZEN (group TDI). Highlighted values reveal PDI > RVI. P25 = Percentile 25; P75 = Percentile 75; P95 = Percentile 95.

Regarding ZEN, the median estimate of PDI applying modelling was 0.240 μg/kg bw/day. The estimation of the percentage of participants that would exceed the tolerable daily intake for total ZEN (38.6%) was similar to the percentage determined by Martins et al. (24%) [19], with considerably lower estimates of intake for the high percentiles of exposure [19]. Regarding AOH, the median estimate for PDI applying modelling was 0.253 μg/kg bw/day. As there are no reference values for the intake, it is not possible to compare this exposure to a reference value [36]. A recent exposure assessment performed by EFSA [32] using occurrence and consumption data estimated an overall lower intake for AOH [32].

Results for the estimated exposure of 5811 participants, stratified by sex, age, and region, and the percentage of participants from each category that exceeded the TDI established for ZEN are presented in Table 5.

Regarding sex, males presented the highest exposure for ZEN and AOH, and this pattern was obtained not only for the estimated exposure (urinary levels), but also for the estimated PDI where the body weight and urinary volume were also considered. With the exception of exposure to AOH (urinary levels), all the exposure parameters presented statistically significant differences between males and females ($p < 0.05$). Regarding the exposure to ZEN, it was estimated that 22.5% and 15.0% of males and females, respectively, may exceed the TDI of 0.250 μg/kg bw/day. Regarding age categories, children and adolescents presented higher estimates than the remaining age groups for exposure to AOH. These results are probably due to higher consumption of breakfast cereals (data not shown) than other age groups, and to a lower proportion body weight/food consumption. For ZEN, children and adolescents did not present in general the highest estimates for exposure and PDI; however, the children age group was where a higher percentage of participants exceeded the TDI (58.2). Recently, Gratz et al. [52] estimated through a human biomonitoring study that 5% of the participants (children 2–6 years) may exceed the TDI for ZEN. Regarding the geographical distribution of exposure, and although all estimates for exposure and PDI presented statistically significant differences among the different considered categories, the estimated results followed a similar pattern for the seven regions of Portugal. The estimated PDI to AOH was higher for Algarve and Madeira. Regarding exposure to ZEN, Algarve and Lisbon Metropolitan Area presented the highest PDI estimates. This pattern of exposure, with relevant percentages of population exceeding the TDI, raises a potential health concern due to the health effects attributed to ZEN exposure, such as liver toxicity, reproductive toxicity, genotoxicity, and immunotoxicity [53].

Table 5. Estimated exposure to mycoestrogens of 5811 participants of IAN-AF, stratified by sex, age, and region.

	Distribution Exposure (µg/g crea); PDI (µg/kg bw/day)				Reference Intake
	Median	*Mean*	*P75*	*P95*	*% ≥ RVI*
AOH					
Sex *					
Male	0.445; 0.127	0.873; 0.294	0.445; 0.254	2.270; 0.656	-
Female	0.445; 0.127	0.670; 0.230	0.445; 0.254	1.401; 0.581	-
Age **					
Children (0–9 years)	0.445; 0.254	0.651; 0.340	0.465; 0.254	1.339; 0.614	-
Adolescents (10–17 years)	0.445; 0.191	1.206; 0.396	1.339; 0.387	4.036; 1.349	-
Adults (18–64 years)	0.445; 0.127	0.779; 0.224	0.445; 0.127	1.529; 0.442	-
Elderly (>64 years)	0.445; 0.127	0.558; 0.160	0.445; 0.127	1.003; 0.290	-
Region **					
North	0.445; 0.127	0.696; 0.239	0.445; 0.254	1.339; 0.431	-
Centre	0.445; 0.127	0.631; 0.213	0.445; 0.254	1.339; 0.515	-
Lisbon Metropolitan Area	0.445; 0.127	0.828; 0.281	0.445; 0.254	2.270; 0.656	-
Alentejo	0.445; 0.127	0.674; 0.231	0.445; 0.254	1.367; 0.607	-
Algarve	0.445; 0.127	0.870;0.286	0.445; 0.254	2.270; 1.080	-
Madeira	0.445; 0.127	0.715; 0.249	0.445; 0.254	1.763; 0.619	-
Azores	0.445; 0.127	1.001; 0.343	0.586; 0.254	2.270; 0.952	-
Total ZEN					
Sex *					
Male	0.607; 0.185	0.682; 0.203	0.741; 0.250	1.107; 0.316	22.5
Female	0.567; 0.158	0.606; 0.180	0.644; 0.218	0.839; 0.290	15.0
Age **					
Children (0–9 years)	0.533; 0.255	0.561; 0.263	0.586; 0.280	0.728; 0.330	58.2
Adolescents (10–17 years)	0.622; 0.178	0.688; 0.194	0.741; 0.218	1.038; 0.308	13.6
Adults (18–64 years)	0.611; 0.153	0.678; 0.170	0.739; 0.185	1.065; 0.265	6.7
Elderly (>64 years)	0.558; 0.140	0.606; 0.152	0.646; 0.163	0.867; 0.218	2.4
Region **					
North	0.519; 0.175	0.643; 0.194	0.696; 0.250	0.989; 0.300	20.2
Centre	0.584; 0.168	0.636; 0.188	0.692; 0.225	0.918; 0.299	17.8
Lisbon Metropolitan Area	0.587; 0.173	0.653; 0.194	0.706; 0.250	1.024; 0.313	18.8
Alentejo	0.586; 0.173	0.649; 0.191	0.711; 0.245	1.032; 0.299	17.3
Algarve	0.586; 0.170	0.665; 0.196	0.694; 0.250	1.079; 0.315	19.3
Madeira	0.565; 0.160	0.613; 0.184	0.647; 0.223	0.871; 0.295	17.9
Azores	0.577; 0.170	0.643; 0.193	0.695; 0.250	0.959; 0.310	18.8

* Mann-Whitney test ($p < 0.05$); AOH exposure did not present significant differences regarding sex; **: Kruskal-Wallis test ($p < 0.05$); significant differences were found for all the categories of age and region, and for exposure and probable daily intake predicted. Reference Value for Intake (RVI) = 0.250 µg/kg bw/day for ZEN (group TDI).

Results obtained under this study are the first estimates of exposure to AOH and ZEN for a representative sampling of the Portuguese population. For ZEN, and since there is an established TDI, it was possible to estimate the percentage of participants that may exceed the reference intake value, and whose exposure could potentially represent a health concern.

This study gathered data from different datasets: dataset of IAN-AF of 5811 participants (food consumption and sociodemographic data) and dataset of IAN-AF of 94 participants (food consumption, sociodemographic data, and paired urine samples), complemented with the dataset obtained by Martins et al. [19]. Data used in this study for modelling was obtained at the individual level (food consumption data, mycotoxin's urinary biomarkers, body weight) and included urine samples collected through a standardized protocol for the entire survey. The sample collection was performed in parallel with the second interview, thus contributing for the quality of estimated data.

Nevertheless, the interpretation of these estimates should be considered carefully since they are also affected by a degree of uncertainty. Left-censored data of urinary biomarkers was replaced by a multiple imputation method which keeps variability in the low levels of distribution but not exemption from uncertainty. The estimations of exposure and PDI are based on modelled data, and a fixed value for daily urinary volume was assumed (48 mL/kg for participants ≤ 5 years, 36 mL/kg for participants > 5 years and ≤ 11 years, and 24 mL/kg for participants ≥12 years) [54]. Additionally, these estimates considered only the food consumption variables that remained significant in the statistical models, leaving aside other possible sources of exposure. In this specific study, the generated models considered ZEN exposure through meat consumption, however, other food groups, e.g., cereal-based products, are traditionally considered as the main sources of ZEN exposure. This fact supports the need to consider a future review of legislation and for example inclusion of animal products as a possible source of ZEN exposure. Even considering the uncertainty associated with modelling and results obtained with this approach, data presented herewith indicates for the first time a potential health concern for the Portuguese population since a percentage of participants (38.6%) are estimated to surpass the tolerable daily intake for ZEN. The over-exposure of children is again demonstrated when compared to other age groups, meaning that this is an issue requiring further assessments. It should be reinforced that ZEN is considered more potent than BPA, one of the endocrine disruptors that raise more concern [13,14].

Despite the uncertainties referred, these results are important contributors in a public health perspective. They highlight the importance of properly and periodically assessing the exposure of the Portuguese population to mycotoxins, with the development of epidemiological studies including collection of blood paired with urine samples for a broader view on exposure, and consequently a more accurate risk characterization. These assessments will make possible the continuous identification of vulnerable population groups and the evaluation of time trends regarding exposure. If needed, and using the precautionary principle, the implementation of control strategies for the contamination levels of food products should be put in place, as well as the establishment of health-based guidance values for intake for emerging mycotoxins as AOH [55].

3. Conclusions

The estrogenic effects of ZEN and AOH represent a potential threat from public health and economic perspectives. Through mathematical modelling of HBM and food consumption data, it was possible to estimate the exposure of the Portuguese population to ZEN and AOH for a representative sampling of the Portuguese population stratified by age, sex, and region. These estimates revealed that the Portuguese population is exposed to ZEN in concentrations that are very close to the tolerable daily intake, and to AOH in concentrations higher than the ones determined in a previous study. There is also a contribution for a deeper knowledge of the potential exposure to endocrine disruptors in Portugal, with more data generated for these two mycoestrogens.

The importance of the development of biomonitoring studies linked with food and health surveys is highlighted in this study, since a more complete analysis has become possible. The acquisition of data from participants in these three domains opens the possibility of designing tailored public health interventions aiming to reduce exposure levels and the potential associated toxic effects.

4. Materials and Methods

4.1. Participants

For the National Food, Nutrition, and Physical Activity Survey (IAN-AF), sampling was performed in two stages: first, based on the random selection of primary health care units, stratified by the seven Nomenclature of Territorial Units for Statistics (NUTS II; weighted by the number of individuals registered in each health unit); and second, based on the random selection of registered individuals in each health unit, according to sex and age groups [40]. From these, a convenience sample of 94 participants was recruited to participate in the biological sample collection for human biomonitoring studies. First morning urines and 24 h urine paired samples were collected on the previous and the day itself of the second interview and following a standardized protocol, in the conditions previously described by Martins et al. [19]. Ethical approval was obtained from the National Commission for Data Protection (Authorization number 4940/2015) and the Ethical Committee of the Institute of Public Health of the University of Porto (Decision number CE). All participants provided their written informed consent according to the Ethical Principles for Medical Research involving human subjects expressed in the Declaration of Helsinki and the national legislation. Data collection was performed under pseudo-anonymization, and all documents with identification data were treated and stored in a different dataset [40].

Considering the sampling strategy presented above, in the present study two groups of participants were considered. The first group, used to model food consumption and exposure to ZEN and AOH, included the 94 participants from whom we had HBM data (obtained through measurement of mycotoxins in urine samples as reported by Martins et al. [19]) and reported consumption data. The second group, for whom we estimated their exposure to ZEN and AOH using the modelling tools generated in this study, includes 5811 participants that reported consumption data.

4.2. *Food and Sociodemographic Questionnaires*

Participants performed two non-consecutive 24 h recalls, 8–15 days apart from each other, and an attempt was made to schedule the second interview for a day different from the first interview (n = 5811). The interview-based dietary assessment performed using computer-assisted personal interview (CAPI) (eAT24 software, SilicoLife, Braga, Portugal) allowed us to obtain a detailed description and quantification of foods, recipes, and food supplements consumed in the course of the preceding day. All foods, including beverages and composite dishes/recipes consumed during the previous 24 h period, were quantified as eaten. Several methods were used to assist participants in quantifying the food consumption such as: photo method, household measure method, weight or volume method, and standard unit method. Food categories comprised three levels of aggregation [40,56]. For the present study, seven food categories in the 1st and 2nd levels of aggregation were considered for the modelling approach: "fruits and vegetables" (fruits, vegetables, pulses, nuts, and oilseeds), "dairy products" (milk, cheese, yoghurt, milk cream), "cereals" (pasta, rice and other grains, flours and bakery powders, breakfast cereals and bars), "meat, fish, and eggs"(meat, fish, eggs), "cookies, biscuits, and sweets" (sweets, cakes, cookies, and biscuits), "non-alcoholic drinks" (tea, coffee, and water), and "alcoholic drinks" (wine, beer, and other drinks).

The questionnaires included sociodemographic data. Sex and age (calculated using the first interview date and birth date) were automatically imported from datasets obtained from the National Health Registries and checked during the first contact with the participants. Information on marital status, number of completed years of education, professional situation, household structure, and household monthly income was collected in a format of closed questions [40,56].

4.3. *Exposure Data to ZEN and AOH Using HBM Data*

ZEN and AOH urinary biomarkers were used to estimate the exposure of the Portuguese population, taking into account the results obtained by Martins et al. [19]. Data regarding urinary biomarkers were obtained for 24 h urine and first morning urine paired samples using a QuEChERS-based procedure (Quick, Easy, Cheap, Effective, Rugged, Safe) for sample preparation followed by identification and quantification by liquid chromatography with mass spectrometry detection (LC-MS/MS). The analytical method was previously optimized by Vidal et al. [57] and is described in detail by Martins et al. [19].

The probable daily intake (PDI) was estimated considering the following excretion rates: 9.4% for ZEN [15] and 8.3% for AOH [30]. Regarding the left-censored data obtained for urinary biomarkers results, a multiple imputation procedure was applied based on 20 simulations and with a maximum of 100,000 for cases and parameters [19]. This procedure allowed us to keep variability within the results below the limit of detection (LOD) [58]. The complete dataset was used for the modelling approach

4.4. Modelling Approach for the Food Consumption and HBM Data

Data obtained by Martins et al. [19] for urinary levels of ZEN, ZEN-14-GlcA, Total ZEN (Sum of ZEN, ZEN-14-GlcA and α-ZEL considering the mass ratio between the parent compound and the metabolites), and AOH, expressed as volume weighted concentrations (μg/L), creatinine (crea) adjusted concentrations (μg/g crea), and daily excretion (μg/day) were used for the modelling approach. These data were compared with food consumption data (1st and 2nd level of aggregation, in a total of 30 variables) obtained with food questionnaires. Both variables (biomarkers and food consumption) were compared as continuous variables by bivariate analysis (Spearman's correlation coefficient) ($n = 94$). Considering that significant associations between food consumption of last 24 h and urinary biomarkers are expected for mycotoxins with short half-lives [39], only consumption data from the second interview was considered for this modelling.

Food consumption variables associated with urinary biomarkers concentration ($p < 0.2$) were retained for the multivariate analysis. For the multivariate analysis, the Generalized Linear Model was chosen due to the non-normality of urinary biomarkers' distributions. For the model, food consumption variables were considered as independent variables, and urinary biomarkers levels were considered as dependent variables. Three types of Generalized Linear Model (GLM) were tested i) linear distribution; ii) gamma distribution; and iii) linear distribution with dependent variable log transformed. Variables were retained and considered to contribute significantly to the GLM if $p < 0.1$. The criteria considered for assessing the adjustment of models were the Spearman correlation coefficient and Omnibus test. Residuals analysis was performed.

The models developed were used to derive HBM and PDI data for the group of 5811 participants of IAN-AF study. For estimation of usual exposure, the models were applied to consumption data of both interviews using SPADE software (Statistical Program to Assess Dietary Exposure, implemented in R software as package SPADE.RIVM) [51], and an overall analysis considering the weights for the Portuguese population was performed, presenting mean, median, and percentiles 75 and 95 for HBM (μg/g creatinine) and PDI (μg/kg bw/day). For estimation of exposure stratified by sex (male; female), age (children 0–9 years; adolescents 10–17 years; adults 18–64 years; elderly >64 years), and region (north, centre, Lisbon Metropolitan Area, Alentejo, Algarve, Madeira, Azores), a descriptive and inferential analysis was performed, presenting mean, median, and percentiles 75 and 95, and the results for Mann-Whitney and Kruskal Wallis non-parametric tests.

The estimates of PDI were performed considering the derived HBM data and the individual body weight. For daily urinary volume the following values were considered: 48 mL/kg for participants ≤ 5 years, 36 mL/kg for participants > 5 years and ≤ 11 years, and 24 mL/kg for participants ≥ 12 years [54].

Normality of distributions was verified by Kolmogorov-Smirnov test. Statistical analysis was performed with SPSS v.24 (manufacturer, city, abbreviation of state (if it has), country) and R software.

Author Contributions: Conceptualization, C.M. and C.N.; Data curation, C.M.; Formal analysis, C.M., D.C., and C.N.; Funding acquisition, C.M., D.T., C.L., R.A., P.A., M.D.B., and S.D.S.; Investigation, C.M. and C.N.; Methodology, C.M. and C.N.; Resources, C.M., D.T., C.L., A.G., R.A., P.A., A.V., M.D.B., and S.D.S.; Validation, C.M. and C.N.; Writing – original draft, C.M.; Writing – review and editing, C.M., D.T., C.L., D.C., A.G., R.A., P.A., A.V., M.D.B., S.D.S., and C.N. All authors have read and agreed to the published version of the manuscript.

Funding: Thanks are due to FCT/MCTES for the financial support to CESAM (UID/AMB/50017/2019), through national funds. This research was also supported by the project MYTOX-SOUTH, Ghent University Global Minds program, and the IAN-AF survey funded by the EEA Grants Program, Public Health Initiatives (PT06-000088SI3).

Acknowledgments: The authors thank all the volunteers who participated in the study.

Conflicts of Interest: The authors declare no conflict of interest. The funders had no role in the design of the study; in the collection, analyses, or interpretation of data; in the writing of the manuscript; or in the decision to publish the results.

References

1. Bennett, J.W.; Klich, M. Mycotoxins. *Clin. Microbiol. Rev.* **2003**, *16*, 497–516. [CrossRef]
2. Vettorazzi, A.; López de Cerain, A. Mycotoxins as Food Carcinogens. In *Environmental Mycology in Public Health*; Elsevier: Amsterdam, The Netherlands, 2016; pp. 261–298. ISBN 9780124114715.
3. Eskola, M.; Kos, G.; Elliott, C.T.; Hajšlová, J.; Mayar, S.; Krska, R. Worldwide contamination of food-crops with mycotoxins: Validity of the widely cited 'FAO estimate' of 25%. *Crit. Rev. Food Sci. Nutr.* **2019**, 1–17. [CrossRef] [PubMed]
4. El Khoury, D.; Fayjaloun, S.; Nassar, M.; Sahakian, J.; Aad, P.Y. Updates on the Effect of Mycotoxins on Male Reproductive Efficiency in Mammals. *Toxins* **2019**, *11*, 515. [CrossRef] [PubMed]
5. Frizzell, C.; Ndossi, D.; Verhaegen, S.; Dahl, E.; Eriksen, G.; Sørlie, M.; Ropstad, E.; Muller, M.; Elliott, C.T.; Connolly, L. Endocrine disrupting effects of zearalenone, alpha- and beta-zearalenol at the level of nuclear receptor binding and steroidogenesis. *Toxicol. Lett.* **2011**, *206*, 210–217. [CrossRef] [PubMed]
6. Frizzell, C.; Ndossi, D.; Kalayou, S.; Eriksen, G.S.; Verhaegen, S.; Sørlie, M.; Elliott, C.T.; Ropstad, E.; Connolly, L. An in vitro investigation of endocrine disrupting effects of the mycotoxin alternariol. *Toxicol. Appl. Pharmacol.* **2013**, *271*, 64–71. [CrossRef]
7. UNEP; WHO. *State of the Science of Endocrine Disrupting Chemicals - 2012*; WHO: Geneva, Switzerland, 2012.
8. Gore, A.C.; Chappell, V.A.; Fenton, S.E.; Flaws, J.A.; Nadal, A.; Prins, G.S.; Toppari, J.; Zoeller, R.T. EDC-2: The Endocrine Society's Second Scientific Statement on Endocrine-Disrupting Chemicals. *Endocr. Rev.* **2015**, *36*, E1–E150. [CrossRef]
9. Vejdovszky, K.; Hahn, K.; Braun, D.; Warth, B.; Marko, D. Synergistic estrogenic effects of Fusarium and Alternaria mycotoxins in vitro. *Arch. Toxicol.* **2017**, *91*, 1447–1460. [CrossRef]
10. Rogowska, A.; Pomastowski, P.; Sagandykova, G.; Buszewski, B. Zearalenone and its metabolites: Effect on human health, metabolism and neutralisation methods. *Toxicon* **2019**, *162*, 46–56. [CrossRef]
11. Metzler, M.; Pfeiffer, E.; Hildebrand, A. Zearalenone and its metabolites as endocrine disrupting chemicals. *World Mycotoxin J.* **2010**, *3*, 385–401. [CrossRef]
12. Zheng, W.; Feng, N.; Wang, Y.; Noll, L.; Xu, S.; Liu, X.X.; Lu, N.; Zou, H.; Gu, J.; Yuan, Y.; et al. Effects of zearalenone and its derivatives on the synthesis and secretion of mammalian sex steroid hormones: A review. *Food Chem. Toxicol.* **2019**, *126*, 262–276. [CrossRef]
13. Olsen, C.M.; Meussen-Elholm, E.T.M.; Hongslo, J.K.; Stenersen, J.; Tollefsen, K.-E. Estrogenic effects of environmental chemicals: An interspecies comparison. *Comp. Biochem. Physiol. Part C Toxicol. Pharmacol.* **2005**, *141*, 267–274. [CrossRef] [PubMed]
14. Li, Y.; Burns, K.A.; Arao, Y.; Luh, C.J.; Korach, K.S. Differential Estrogenic Actions of Endocrine-Disrupting Chemicals Bisphenol A, Bisphenol AF, and Zearalenone through Estrogen Receptor α and β in Vitro. *Environ. Health Perspect.* **2012**, *120*, 1029–1035. [CrossRef] [PubMed]
15. Warth, B.; Sulyok, M.; Berthiller, F.; Schuhmacher, R.; Krska, R. New insights into the human metabolism of the Fusarium mycotoxins deoxynivalenol and zearalenone. *Toxicol. Lett.* **2013**, *220*, 88–94. [CrossRef] [PubMed]
16. Gambacorta, S.; Solfrizzo, H.; Visconti, A.; Powers, S.; Cossalter, A.M.; Pinton, P.; Oswald, I.P. Validation study on urinary biomarkers of exposure for aflatoxin B 1, ochratoxin A, fumonisin B 1, deoxynivalenol and zearalenone in piglets. *World Mycotoxin J.* **2013**, *6*, 299–308. [CrossRef]
17. Slobodchikova, I.; Sivakumar, R.; Rahman, M.S.; Vuckovic, D. Characterization of Phase I and Glucuronide Phase II Metabolites of 17 Mycotoxins Using Liquid Chromatography—High-Resolution Mass Spectrometry. *Toxins* **2019**, *11*, 433. [CrossRef] [PubMed]
18. Ali, N.; Degen, G.H. Urinary biomarkers of exposure to the mycoestrogen zearalenone and its modified forms in German adults. *Arch. Toxicol.* **2018**, *92*, 2691–2700. [CrossRef]
19. Martins, C.; Vidal, A.; De Boevre, M.; De Saeger, S.; Nunes, C.; Torres, D.; Goios, A.; Lopes, C.; Assunção, R.; Alvito, P. Exposure assessment of Portuguese population to multiple mycotoxins: The human biomonitoring approach. *Int. J. Hyg. Environ. Health* **2019**, *222*, 913–925. [CrossRef]
20. Solfrizzo, M.; Gambacorta, L.; Visconti, A. Assessment of multi-mycotoxin exposure in southern Italy by urinary multi-biomarker determination. *Toxins* **2014**, *6*, 523–538. [CrossRef]

21. Bandera, E.V.; Chandran, U.; Buckley, B.; Lin, Y.; Isukapalli, S.; Marshall, I.; King, M.; Zarbl, H. Urinary mycoestrogens, body size and breast development in New Jersey girls. *Sci. Total Environ.* **2011**, *409*, 5221–5227. [CrossRef]
22. Franco, L.T.; Petta, T.; Rottinghaus, G.E.; Bordin, K.; Gomes, G.A.; Alvito, P.; Assunção, R.; Oliveira, C.A.F. Assessment of mycotoxin exposure and risk characterization using occurrence data in foods and urinary biomarkers in Brazil. *Food Chem. Toxicol.* **2019**, *128*, 21–34. [CrossRef]
23. Fan, K.; Xu, J.; Jiang, K.; Liu, X.; Meng, J.; Di Mavungu, J.D.; Guo, W.; Zhang, Z.; Jing, J.; Li, H.; et al. Determination of multiple mycotoxins in paired plasma and urine samples to assess human exposure in Nanjing, China. *Environ. Pollut.* **2019**, *248*, 865–873. [CrossRef] [PubMed]
24. Szuets, P.; Mesterhazy, A.; Falkay, G.Y.; Bartok, T. Early telarche symptoms in children and their relations to zearalenon contamination in foodstuffs. *Cereal Res. Commun.* **1997**, *25*, 429–436. [CrossRef]
25. Massart, F.; Meucci, V.; Saggese, G.; Soldani, G. High Growth Rate of Girls with Precocious Puberty Exposed to Estrogenic Mycotoxins. *J. Pediatr.* **2008**, *152*, 690–695. [CrossRef]
26. Asci, A.; Durmaz, E.; Erkekoglu, P.; Pasli, D.; Bircan, I.; Kocer-Gumusel, B. Urinary zearalenone levels in girls with premature thelarche and idiopathic central precocious puberty. *Minerva Pediatr.* **2014**, *66*, 571–578.
27. Rivera-Núñez, Z.; Barrett, E.S.; Szamreta, E.A.; Shapses, S.A.; Qin, B.; Lin, Y.; Zarbl, H.; Buckley, B.; Bandera, E.V. Urinary mycoestrogens and age and height at menarche in New Jersey girls. *Environ. Health* **2019**, *18*, 24. [CrossRef]
28. EFSA. Appropriateness to set a group health-based guidance value for zearalenone and its modified forms. *EFSA J.* **2016**, *14*, e04425.
29. European Commission. Commission Regulation (EC) No 1881/2006 of 19 December 2006 setting maximum levels for certain contaminants in foodstuffs. *Off. J. Eur. Union* **2006**, *L 364/5*.
30. Puntscher, H.; Hankele, S.; Tillmann, K.; Attakpah, E.; Braun, D.; Kütt, M.L.; Del Favero, G.; Aichinger, G.; Pahlke, G.; Höger, H.; et al. First insights into Alternaria multi-toxin in vivo metabolism. *Toxicol. Lett.* **2019**, *301*, 168–178. [CrossRef]
31. Šarkanj, B.; Ezekiel, C.N.; Turner, P.C.; Abia, W.A.; Rychlik, M.; Krska, R.; Sulyok, M.; Warth, B. Ultra-sensitive, stable isotope assisted quantification of multiple urinary mycotoxin exposure biomarkers. *Anal. Chim. Acta* **2018**, *1019*, 84–92. [CrossRef]
32. Crudo, F.; Varga, E.; Aichinger, G.; Galaverna, G.; Marko, D.; Dall'Asta, C.; Dellafiora, L. Co-Occurrence and Combinatory Effects of Alternaria Mycotoxins and other Xenobiotics of Food Origin: Current Scenario and Future Perspectives. *Toxins* **2019**, *11*, 640. [CrossRef]
33. Ostry, V. Alternaria mycotoxins: An overview of chemical characterization, producers, toxicity, analysis and occurrence in foodstuffs. *World Mycotoxin J.* **2008**, *1*, 175–188. [CrossRef]
34. Aichinger, G.; Krüger, F.; Puntscher, H.; Preindl, K.; Warth, B.; Marko, D. Naturally occurring mixtures of Alternaria toxins: Anti-estrogenic and genotoxic effects in vitro. *Arch. Toxicol.* **2019**, *93*, 3021–3031. [CrossRef] [PubMed]
35. Gotthardt, M.; Asam, S.; Gunkel, K.; Moghaddam, A.F.; Baumann, E.; Kietz, R.; Rychlik, M. Quantitation of Six Alternaria Toxins in Infant Foods Applying Stable Isotope Labeled Standards. *Front. Microbiol.* **2019**, *10*. [CrossRef] [PubMed]
36. Arcella, D.; Eskola, M.; Gómez Ruiz, J.A. Dietary exposure assessment to Alternaria toxins in the European population. *EFSA J.* **2016**, *14*, e04654.
37. Mitropoulou, A.; Gambacorta, L.; Lemming, E.W.; Solfrizzo, M.; Olsen, M. Extended evaluation of urinary multi-biomarker analyses of mycotoxins in Swedish adults and children. *World Mycotoxin J.* **2018**, *11*, 647–659. [CrossRef]
38. Turner, P.C.; Rothwell, J.A.; White, K.L.M.; Gong, Y.; Cade, J.E.; Wild, C.P. Urinary deoxynivalenol is correlated with cereal intake in individuals from the United kingdom. *Environ. Health Perspect.* **2008**, *116*, 21–25. [CrossRef]
39. Martins, C.; Assunção, R.; Nunes, C.; Torres, D.; Alvito, P. Are Data from Mycotoxins' Urinary Biomarkers and Food Surveys Linked? A Review Underneath Risk Assessment. *Food Rev. Int.* **2020**, 1–26. [CrossRef]
40. Lopes, C.; Torres, D.; Oliveira, A.; Severo, M.; Guiomar, S.; Alarcão, V.; Ramos, E.; Rodrigues, S.; Vilela, S.; Oliveira, L.; et al. National Food, Nutrition, and Physical Activity Survey of the Portuguese General Population (2015–2016): Protocol for Design and Development. *JMIR Res. Protoc.* **2018**, *7*, e42. [CrossRef]

41. Lopes, C.; Torres, D.; Oliveira, A.; Severo, M.; Alarcão, V.; Guiomar, S.; Mota, J.; Teixeira, P.; Rodrigues, S.; Lobato, L.; et al. *Bases de Dados do IAN-AF 2015-2016 [ficheiro de dados]*; IAN-AF Consortiu: Porto, Portugal, 2018.
42. Maragos, C. Zearalenone occurrence and human exposure. *World Mycotoxin J.* **2010**, *3*, 369–383. [CrossRef]
43. Becker-Algeri, T.A.; Castagnaro, D.; Bortoli, K.; Souza, C.; Drunkler, D.A.; Badiale-Furlong, E. Mycotoxins in Bovine Milk and Dairy Products: A Review. *J. Food Sci.* **2016**, *81*, R544–R552. [CrossRef]
44. Huang, L.C.; Zheng, N.; Zheng, B.Q.; Wen, F.; Cheng, J.B.; Han, R.W.; Xu, X.M.; Li, S.L.; Wang, J.Q. Simultaneous determination of aflatoxin M1, ochratoxin A, zearalenone and α-zearalenol in milk by UHPLC–MS/MS. *Food Chem.* **2014**, *146*, 242–249. [CrossRef]
45. Maragos, C.M.; Busman, M. Rapid and advanced tools for mycotoxin analysis: A review. *Food Addit. Contam. Part A. Chem. Anal. Control. Expo. Risk Assess.* **2010**, *27*, 688–700. [CrossRef] [PubMed]
46. Almeida, I.F.M.; Guerra, M.M.; Martins, H.M.L.; Costa, J.M.G.; Bernardo, F.M.A. Aflatoxin B1 and zearalenone in dairy feeds in Portugal, 2009–2011. *Mycotoxin Res.* **2013**, *29*, 131–133. [CrossRef] [PubMed]
47. Abrunhosa, L.; Morales, H.; Soares, C.; Calado, T.; Vila-Chã, A.S.; Pereira, M.; Venâncio, A. A Review of Mycotoxins in Food and Feed Products in Portugal and Estimation of Probable Daily Intakes. *Crit. Rev. Food Sci. Nutr.* **2016**, *56*, 249–265. [CrossRef] [PubMed]
48. AFSSA. *Risk Assessment for Mycotoxins in Human and Animal Food Chains*; AFSSA: Maisons-Alfort, France, 2006.
49. AFSSA. *Évaluation des Risques liés à la Présence de Mycotoxines dans les Chaînes Alimentaires Humaine et Animale*; AFSSA: Maisons-Alfort, France, 2009.
50. Scott, P.M.; Zhao, W.; Feng, S.; Lau, B.P.Y. Alternaria toxins alternariol and alternariol monomethyl ether in grain foods in Canada. *Mycotoxin Res.* **2012**, *28*, 261–266. [CrossRef] [PubMed]
51. Dekkers, A.L.; Verkaik-Kloosterman, J.; van Rossum, C.T.; Ocké, M.C. SPADE, a New Statistical Program to Estimate Habitual Dietary Intake from Multiple Food Sources and Dietary Supplements. *J. Nutr.* **2014**, *144*, 2083–2091. [CrossRef]
52. Gratz, S.W.; Currie, V.; Duncan, G.; Jackson, D. Multimycotoxin Exposure Assessment in UK Children Using Urinary Biomarkers—A Pilot Survey. *J. Agric. Food Chem.* **2020**, *68*, 351–357. [CrossRef]
53. Rai, A.; Das, M.; Tripathi, A. Occurrence and toxicity of a fusarium mycotoxin, zearalenone. *Crit. Rev. Food Sci. Nutr.* **2019**, 1–20. [CrossRef]
54. Hazinski, M.F. *Nursing Care of Critically Ill Child*; Mosby-Year Book: Maryland Heights, MO, USA, 1992; ISBN 9780801653124.
55. Eskola, M.; Elliott, C.T.; Hajšlová, J.; Steiner, D.; Krska, R. Towards a dietary-exposome assessment of chemicals in food: An update on the chronic health risks for the European consumer. *Crit. Rev. Food Sci. Nutr.* **2019**, 1–22. [CrossRef]
56. Lopes, C.; Torres, D.; Oliveira, A.; Severo, M.; Alarcão, V.; Guiomar, S.; Mota, J.; Teixeira, P.; Rodrigues, S.; Lobato, L.; et al. *O Inquérito Alimentar Nacional e de Atividade Física, IAN-AF 2015–2016*; Universidade do Porto: Porto, Portugal, 2017.
57. Vidal, A.; Claeys, L.; Mengelers, M.; Vanhoorne, V.; Vervaet, C.; Huybrechts, B.; De Saeger, S.; De Boevre, M. Humans significantly metabolize and excrete the mycotoxin deoxynivalenol and its modified form deoxynivalenol-3-glucoside within 24 hours. *Sci. Rep.* **2018**, *8*, 5255. [CrossRef]
58. Chen, H.; Quandt, S.A.; Grzywacz, J.G.; Arcury, T.A. A Bayesian multiple imputation method for handling longitudinal pesticide data with values below the limit of detection. *Environmetrics* **2013**, *24*, 132–142. [CrossRef] [PubMed]

toxins

MDPI

Article

Total Dietary Intake and Health Risks Associated with Exposure to Aflatoxin B_1, Ochratoxin A and Fuminisins of Children in Lao Cai Province, Vietnam

Bui Thi Mai Huong [1,2], Le Danh Tuyen [2], Henry Madsen [1], Leon Brimer [1], Henrik Friis [3] and Anders Dalsgaard [1,4,*]

[1] Department of Veterinary and Animal Disease, Faculty of Health and Medical Sciences, University of Copenhagen, DK- 1870 Frederiksberg C, DK-1870 Copenhagen, Denmark; buithimaihuong@dinhduong.org.vn (B.T.M.H.); hmad@sund.ku.dk (H.M.); lbr@sund.ku.dk (L.B.)

[2] National Institute of Nutrition, 48 Tang Bat Ho Street, Hanoi, Hanoi 100000, Vietnam; Ledanhtuyen@dinhduong.org.vn

[3] Department of Nutrition, Exercise and Sports, Faculty of Sciences, University of Copenhagen, Frederiksberg C, DK-1958 Copenhagen, Denmark; hfr@life.ku.dk

[4] School of Chemical and Biomedical Engineering, Nanyang Technological University, Singapore 639798, Singapore

* Correspondence: adal@sund.ku.dk

Received: 6 October 2019; Accepted: 31 October 2019; Published: 2 November 2019

Abstract: The health burden of foodborne mycotoxins is considerable, but particularly for children due to their lower detoxification capacity, rapid growth and high intake of food in proportion to their weight. Through a Total Dietary Study approach, the objective was to estimate the dietary exposure and health risk caused by mycotoxins for children under 5 years living in the Lao Cai province in northern Vietnam. A total of 40 composite food samples representing 1008 individual food samples were processed and analyzed by ELISA for aflatoxin B_1, ochratoxin A and fumonisins. Results showed that dietary exposure to aflatoxin B_1, ochratoxin A and total fumonisins were 118.7 ng/kgbw/day, 52.6 ng/kg bw/day and 1250.0 ng/kg bw/day, respectively. Using a prevalence of hepatitis of 1%, the risk of liver cancer related to exposure of aflatoxin B_1 was 12.1 cases/100,000 individual/year. Age-adjusted margin of exposure (MOE) of renal cancer associated with ochratoxin A was 127, while MOE of liver cancer associated with fumonisins was 542. Antropometric data show that 50.4% (60/119) of children were stunted, i.e. height/length for age z-scores (HAZ) below −2, and 3.4% (4/119) of children were classified as wasted, i.e. weight for height z-scores (WHZ) below −2. A significant negative relationship between dietary exposure to individual or mixture of mycotoxins and growth of children was observed indicating that the high mycotoxin intake contributed to stunning in the children studied.

Keywords: risk assessment; total diet study; aflatoxin B_1; ochratoxin A; fumonisins; children; Vietnam

Key Contribution: Exposure to mycotoxins are high and exceeds toxicological reference levels in children under five in Lao Cai province, Vietnam. Risk assessments showed a high risk for liver cancer due to the consumption of aflatoxin B1 contaminated foods and high exposure to mycotoxins was associated with impaired child growth when adjusted for age, gender and dietary intake.

1. Introduction

Children are especially vulnerable to foodborne hazards due to their higher dietary exposure per kg body weight and differences in physiology compared to adults. Due to significant postnatal development of different organ systems during childhood, children up to four years of age are more sensitive to some neurotoxic, endocrine and immunological effects [1]. Dietary exposure to mycotoxins is associated with various health disorders and recognized as a major food safety hazard [2]. Among pathogenic mycotoxins, Aflatoxin B_1, ochratoxin A and fumonisins are common and potent ones which can contaminate various types of foods [3]. The International Agency for Research of Cancer (IARC) [4,5] has classified aflatoxin B_1 and mixtures of total aflatoxins into group 1: "Carcinogenic for humans". Aflatoxins are documented causes of human liver cancer and impaired child growth, as well as an immunosuppressant [6]. The IARC has reported fumonisins as Group 2B as "Possible carcinogenic to humans" [5,7], based on evidence showing that fumonisins act as a promoter of liver and kidney tumors in rodents. Ochratoxin A has been evaluated to be carcinogenic in the kidney of some animal species, in addition to causing numerous other specific toxic effects, such as hepatotoxicity, teratogenicity and immune-suppressivity, in different animals [8–10]. Ochratoxin A is also classified into Group 2B as possibly carcinogenic to humans by the IARC [11].

Increased risk of liver cancer has been reported in people co- exposed to aflatoxins and hepatitis B virus (HBV) [3]. Thirty times higher risk of developing liver cancer was observed among individuals who experienced both exposures compared to those exposed to the mycotoxins only [12]. Vietnam is endemic for hepatitis B, with a prevalence of 7 to 24% among adults depending on age and geographic region. Of those, about 10 to 12% of pregnant women are chronically infected with hepatitis B. Hence, mother-to-child transmission is an important factor contributing to the high levels of chronic hepatitis B infection in Vietnam [13]. Newborn infants who become infected with hepatitis B virus show no symptoms, yet have a 90% chance of developing a chronic, life-long infection. By increasing the cover rate of vaccination, Vietnamese authorities expect to reduce the rate of chronic hepatitis B infection among children from 18% in 2003 to below 1% in 2017 [14].

Child malnutrition, including both energy- and nutrient deficiencies, is caused by multiple factors and are harmful to their health, growth, development, and burden of infectious diseases. Stunting remains common in Vietnam despite general economic development, particularly in areas with large populations of ethnic minority people such as the Central Highlands, Northern Midlands and mountainous regions [15]. About 25% of children younger than five years old in Vietnam are considered stunted [16]. The stunting rate among children in rural areas is twice as high as that in urban areas, while the level of stunting is approximately three times higher among Vietnamese children from the poorest households to which ethnic minority groups belong [15]. The Lao Cai province in the North West mountainous area of Vietnam is inhabited by 25 ethnic groups and has one of the highest prevalence's of stunted children younger than five years of age countrywide. Based on nutrition profiles of the year 2014, 35% of the children younger than five years of age were stunted, 20% was underweight and wasting was seen among 6% of the children [16].

Chronic exposure to mycotoxins is increasingly seen as a threat to child health. Therefore, it is important to assess and predict the negative health implications of exposure to different mycotoxins. Exposure assessment, as one part of risk assessment, integrates mycotoxin contamination in food with consumption data and is used to identify which mycotoxins compromise food safety and health hazards [17]. Exposure data collected by so-called total dietary study (TDS) approaches consider and include all different foods consumed in the whole diet. Risk characterizations for the mycotoxins associated with cancer risk are available. Thus, the FAO/WHO Joint Expert Committee on Food Additives (JECFA) estimates the cancer risk for a certain population using the incidence of the hepatitis B virus (HBsAg+ individuals) and the carcinogenic potency of aflatoxins, which has been defined for HBV carriers and non-carriers [12]. The European Food Safety Authority (EFSA) and JECFA recommended to use the margin of exposure (MOE) approach to evaluate compounds that are both carcinogenic and genotoxic [18,19]. The MOE is the ratio between a toxicological threshold obtained from animal studies and the estimated human exposure [18]. A small margin of exposure suggests a higher risk than a larger margin of exposure. Hence, risk managers can use this information for priority setting [15].

Using the TDS approach, this study aimed at estimating the dietary exposure to aflatoxin B_1, ochratoxin A and total fumonisins and the associated health risks among children younger than five years old in Lao Cai province, Vietnam.

2. Results and Discussion

2.1. Food and Nutrient Intake

Children were generally fed the same dishes as the rest of the family. Complementary foods were composed mainly of commodities from locally available food products (Table 1).

Table 1. Food groups and food preparation procedures in households in Lao Cai province, Vietnam.

	Food Groups [a]	Food Items	Food Preparation [b]
1	Rice and products	Rice Sticky rice Rice noodle	Boiled Boiled Boiled
2	Wheat and products	Noodle	Boiled
3	Tubes, root and products	Vicermine Shrimp chip	Boiled Deep fried
4	Beans and products	Black bean Mung bean Soybean milk Soy bean	Stewed Stewed Ready to eat Stewed
5	Tofu	Tofu	Boiled
6	Oily seeds	Peanut	Stir fried
7	Vegetables	Bamboo shot, fermented	Boiled
8	Sugar, confectionary	Biscuit Wafers Cookies Sesame candy Nugget/peanut candy	Ready to eat Ready to eat Ready to eat Ready to eat Ready to eat
9	Oil, fat	Pork, fat Cooking oil	Fried
10	Meat and products	Dry pork meat Pork pie, fried Pork pie, boiled Pork rib, boneless Pigeon Beef Dog meat Chicken Pork, lean Pork Pork liver	Ready to eat Ready to eat Ready to eat Stewed Stewed Stir fried Boiled Boiled Boiled, stir fried Boiled, stir fried Stir fried
11	Egg and milk	Egg, chicken Egg, duck Condensed Milk Milk powder Milk	Boiled, fried Boiled, fried Ready to eat Ready to eat Ready to eat
12	Fish	Dried fish Fish, fresh water	Stir fried Boiled
13	Other aquaculture products	Dried shrimp Shrimp	Boiled Stir fried

[a] Food groups were categorized according to a previous national survey [16]. [b] Food items were prepared as practiced by households in the Lao Cai province.

Common foods were rice, groundnuts, banana, beans, meat, powder milk, eggs and vegetables. The daily food-, energy- and nutrient intake are summarized in Table 2. The estimated daily mean energy intake was 870 (range 218–1713) kcal and mean protein intake was 28 (8–67) g. Daily intake of essential micronutrients such as vitamin A, iron and zinc were 99 (0–1044) mcg, 4.8 (1.0–9.5) mg and 3.7 (1.1–6.5) mg, respectively. The latter three intakes were lower than the national recommended daily intake [20].

Table 2. Food and nutrient intake amongst children in Lao Cai.

	Mean	Range
Food Intake (g per child per day)		
Rice and products	196	49–313
Wheat and products	11	0–93
Tubes, root and products	3	0–100
Bean and products	11	0–293
Tofu	4	0–63
Oily seed	2	0–29
Vegetable leaf	50	0–149
Vegetable tube	12	0–157
Fruit	22	0–225
Confectionary	15	0–215
Seasoning	0	0–4
Oil, fat	2	0–12
Meat and products	30	0–110
Egg and milk	38	0–281
Fish	6	0–31
Other aquaculture products	2	0–55
Other spices	0	0–4
Dietary Composition (per child per day)		
Energy (kcal)	871	218–171
Protein (g) total	28	8–67
Protein from animal sources (g)	10	0–50
Non-animal protein (g)	18	4–33
Protein (eggs and milk) (g)	3	0–17
Protein from meat (g)	6	0–45
Carbohydrate (g)	152	37–258
Fat (g)	17	2–57
Vegetable fat/oil (g)	7	1–48
Fiber (g)	2.5	0.4–6.9
Ash (g)	3.5	0.9–7.2
Total vitamin A [a] (mcg)	99.0	0–1044.0
Animal source vitamin A [a] (mcg)	90.0	0–1044.0
Non-animal vitamin A [a] (mcg)	9.0	0–145.0
Carotenoid (mcg)	2353.0	0–8576.0
Vitamin C (mg)	33.1	0.0–170.3
Thiamin (mg)	0.4	0.1–1.0
Riboflavin (mg)	0.3	0.0–1.1
Niacin (mg)	5.1	1.2–13.2
Vitamin D (mcg)	0.4	0.0–4.7
Folic acid (mcg)	0.0	0.0–0.0
Folate (mcg)	94.5	8.6–308.3
Vitamin B12 (mcg)	0.6	0.0–4.2
Calcium (mg)	181.8	27.8–707.9
Sodium (mg)	167	8–1087
Potassium (mg)	784.9	176.1–1716.6
Magnesium (mg)	69.5	11.7–177.4
Zinc (mg)	3.7	1.1–6.7
Phosphorous (mg)	361	73–905
Iron (mg)	4.8	1.0–9.5
Iron from meat/fish/poultry (mg)	0.5	0.0–3.4

[a] Retinol equivalent.

Forty mothers and caregivers attended five focus group discussions to talk about how they fed their children and handled food for children and family. The main reasons for stopping breast feeding after 3 to 6 months of birth were that the mothers had to go back to work; some had to stay in the field for a week or more during harvest time. Mothers who did not stay in the field overnight also did not breast feed their child, because they were not aware about the advantage of breast feeding or simply followed the traditional weaning practice.

2.2. Mycotoxins in Food Samples

Aflatoxin B_1 was found in 87.5% of composite food samples except the tofu products group (Table 3). The highest contamination was detected in egg and milk products (5326 ng/kg), followed by oily seed (4086 ng/kg), then meat and meat products (4077 ng/kg) (Table 3). In rice, the aflatoxin B_1 concentration was 2998 ng/kg. Rice products were consumed in large amounts (Table 2). There have been a few surveys of mycotoxins in foods in Vietnam, including small sample sizes; however, they indicated that aflatoxins are common in maize kernel and maize flour [21,22]. In Lao Cai, it was reported that 25% of self-supplied cereal samples collected in households were contaminated with aflatoxins [23].

Among 40 composite samples analyzed, ochratoxin A was found in 20 samples (49.5%), with the highest concentration (9683 ng/kg, range 9208–10158 ng/kg) found in bean products. Lower ochratoxin A concentrations were shown in the food groups of animal original such as aquaculture products (4850 ng/kg), egg and milk products (3164; 2930–3402 ng/kg), meat products (2685; 2339–3030 ng/kg) and fish products (2245; 1770–2720 ng/kg) (Table 3). In contrast, the concentration of ochratoxin A in all staple cereal samples (rice products, wheat products, other cereal and tube, roof products) was below the detection limit.

Only one black bean and one milk composite sample were found to be contaminated by fumonisins. Among 25 cereal samples collected in various locations of Vietnam, Trung found that eight samples (32%) were contaminated with fumonisins with concentrations ranging from 400 to 3300 ng/g [22]. We have previously reported fumonisins in 8.1% of rice and 23.5% of maize in households supplying their own cereals in Lao Cai province [23].

2.3. Growth Indicators and Their Correlates

The overall proportions of stunted children (HAZ < −2) were 50.4% (60/119), 3.4% (4/119) of the children were classified as wasted (WHZ < −2). Mean HAZ was −1.94 (range: −3.31–2.50), mean WHZ was −0.57 (range: −3.33–3.27). Some of the z-scores are summarized in Table 4 listed by age group and gender together with selected nutritional intake measures and estimated intake of mycotoxins. Differences between boys and girls were minor, while the older age group had lower z-scores than the younger group. A significant difference of vitamin A daily intake ($p < 0.05$) was observed between the two age groups of boys only.

In the principal component analysis (PCA) analysis of the dietary variables, the first seven principal components explained 89.1% of the variation in dietary intake with the 7th component having an eigenvalue of 1.04. The loadings (only those above 0.3 are shown) of the included food intake variables on the seven rotated components are shown in Table 5. Loadings are correlations between the original dietary variables and the principal components. Many variables loaded slightly on the unrotated component 1, which likely represents the amount of food eaten, i.e., carbohydrate, non-animal protein and total energy intake loaded most strongly on the rotated component 1. Zinc intake was another factor loading on component 1 (Table 5). High loadings on components 2 to 5 were mainly various vitamin and mineral variables, while for component 6, vegetable fat/oil, vitamin A from non-animal sources, the fiber content and fat from animals were important (Table 5). On component 7, the most important variables were protein from meat and iron derived from meat (Table 5). The seven principal component scores were used as potential correlates in the growth indicator analyses.

Table 3. Aflatoxin B_1 and ochratoxin A contents (ng/kg) in food groups included in the total dietary study.

Food Group [a]	Number of Composite Samples	Aflatoxin B_1			Ochratoxin A		
		Number of Test Results < LOD	Concentration (ng/kg) [b]		Number of Test Results < LOD	Concentration (ng/kg) [b]	
			MB	LB-UB		MB	LB-UB
Rice and products	3	1	2989	2400–3020	3	950	0–1900
Wheat and products	1	0	1000	1000	1	950	0–1900
Tubes, root and products	2	1	2171	1670–2670	2	950	0–190
Beans and products	4	1	2864	2610–3110	2	9683	9210–10,160
Tofu	1	1	1000	0–2000	1	950	0–1900
Oily seeds	1	0	4086	4086	1	950	0–1900
Vegetables	1	0	3470	3470	1	950	0–1900
Sugar/confectionary	5	0	4033	4033	4	1173	410–1930
Oil, fat	2	0	3382	3382	1	1462	980–1940
Meat and products	11	1	4077	3990–4170	4	2685	2340–3032
Egg and milk	4	0	5326	5325	1	3164	2930–3400
Fish	2	1	2301	1800–2800	1	2245	1770–2720
Other aquaculture products	3	0	2518	1850–3180	0	4850	4850
Total	40	6			20		

[a] Food groups were categorized according to a previous national survey [16]. [b] Medium bound (MB) figures (ND = LOD/2) were used as mean values. Lower bound (LB) and upper bound (UB) figures. LOD, limit of detection.

Table 4. Anthropometric measurements, selected dietary intake and mycotoxin exposure (mean and range) by age group and gender.

		Boy		Girl		*p*-Value
		n	Mean and Range	*n*	Mean and Range	
Anthropometric Measurement						
Length/height for age Z- score	13–23 months	6	−0.34 (−0.76–0.65)	8	1.01 (−2.36–2.50)	n.s.
	24–59 months	58	−2.22 (−3.19–1.52)	47	−2.29 (−3.31–1.60)	n.s.
	p-value		<0.01		<0.001	
Weight for length/height Z- score	13–23 months	6	−0.49 (−1.05–0.37)	8	0.27 (−1.00–2.00)	n.s.
	24–59 months	58	−0.66 (−2.33–1.13)	47	−0.61 (−2.41–3.27)	n.s.
	p-value		n.s.		<0.05	
% Length/height for age Z- score < −2 (%)	13–23 months	6	0	8	12.5	n.s.
	24–59 months	58	53.4	47	59.6	n.s.
	p-value		<0.05		<0.05	
Dietary Intake						
Energy intake(kcal/day)	13–23 months	6	790 (434–1097)	9	742 (367–1164)	n.s.
	24–59 months	58	901 (218–1436)	47	868 (378–1713)	n.s.
	p-value		n.s.		n.s.	
Protein intake (g/day)	13–23 months	6	24 (11–49)	9	22 (9–38)	n.s.
	24-59 months	58	29 (8–67)	47	28 (9–48)	n.s.
	p-value		n.s.		n.s.	
Vitamin A intake (mcg/day)	13–23 months	6	15.5 (0.0–60.9)	9	47.1 (0.0–160.9)	n.s.
	24–59 months	58	95.3 (0.0–629.8)	47	124.1 (0.0–1043.7)	n.s.
	p-value		<0.05		n.s.	
Iron intake (mg/day)	13–23 months	6	5.6 (3.7–8.3)	9	4.6 (1.9–6.5)	n.s.
	24–59 months	58	4.8 (1.1–9.5)	47	4.7 (1.6–9.4)	n.s.
	p-value		n.s.		n.s.	
Zinc intake (mg/day)	13–23 months	6	3.7 (2.6–5.7)	9	3.6 (1.1–4.8)	n.s.
	24-59 months	58	3.8 (1.1–6.7)	47	3.75 (1.5–6.5)	n.s.
	p-value		n.s.		n.s.	
Mycotoxin Exposure						
Aflatoxin B1 (ng/kg bw/day)	13–23 months	6	135.9 (87.2–170.3)	8	100.5 (49.1–156.6)	n.s.
	24–59 months	58	123.5 (28.4–247.3)	47	121.6 (40.2–246.3)	n.s.
	p-value		n.s.		n.s.	
Fumonisins (ng/kg bw/day)	13–23 months	6	3.6 (2.1–4.6)	8	2.7 (1.6–4.0)	n.s.
	24–59 months	58	3.5 (0.8–7.5)	47	3.5 (1.3–7.1)	n.s.
	p-value		n.s.		n.s.	
Ochratoxin A (ng/kg bw/day)	13–23 months	6	43.2 (20.4–82.1)	8	31.3 (17.6–47.2)	n.s.
	24–59 months	58	54.8 (11.0–344.7)	47	57.2 (13.7–239.5)	n.s.
	p-value		n.s.		n.s.	

n.s.: not significant.

Mycotoxin exposure estimates showed a skewed distribution, and scores were therefore $\log_n$-transformed. Pairwise correlations between exposures to the three toxins were high, i.e., correlation coefficients varied from 0.85 to 0.98 (results now shown). This could obviously result in problems of collinearity in regression models where the three toxins were used as simultaneous correlates. Hence, we performed a principal component analysis on $\log_n$(exposure) of the three toxins. The first principal component accounted for 94.3% of the total variation in mycotoxin exposure and all three toxins loaded similarly on the first component. The principal component scores for the first component were used as a correlate in further analysis of correlation between toxins and the growth indicators.

Table 5. Correlations (loadings) between dietary variables and the rotated principal components (Comp 1 to 7). Only loadings above 0.3 are shown. Factors not loading on the first seven components are not shown.

Variable Label	Principal Component Score						
	Comp 1	Comp 2	Comp 3	Comp 4	Comp 5	Comp 6	Comp 7
Energy (Kcal)	0.38						
Non-animal protein sources (g)	0.39						
Carbohydrate by difference (g)	0.51						
Zinc (mg)	0.33						
Riboflavin (mg)		0.31					
Vitamin D (mcg)		0.44					
Calcium (mg)		0.38					
Sodium (mg)		0.40					
Poly-unsaturated fatty acid (g)			0.50				
Mono- saturated fatty acid (g)			0.62				
Animal source vitamin A (mcg)				0.55			
Vitamin B12 (mcg)				0.48			
Cholesterol (g)				0.50			
Carotenoid (mcg)					0.58		
Vitamin C (mg)					0.44		
Folate (mcg)					0.48		
Vegetable Fat/oil (g)						0.57	
Fiber (dietary fiber) (g)						0.32	
Fat (g)						0.33	
Non-animal source vitamin A						0.57	
Protein from meat (mg)							0.58
Niacin (mg)							0.31
Iron from fish, poultry and other meat product (mg)							0.64

We tested a number of potential correlates of HAZ and WHZ scores one by one (for each score adjusting for age in months and gender) and jointly in multivariable analyses where age, gender and energy consumption was forced into the model (data not shown). The HAZ and WHZ scores declined with increase in age in a linear manner (Table 4). None of the mycotoxins or the combined principal component score was significantly correlated with HAZ or WHZ when tested alone together with age and gender (data not shown).

In the final analysis, we decided to model for each toxin separately and the combined score from PCA. Age and gender were considered potential correlates and were included in any model. We tried four different models (Y = growth indicator and T = toxins, individual or combined; the factors included in brackets were forced into the model): (1) Y = b1×age + b2×gender + b3×T + const.; (2) Y = b1×age + b2×gender + b3×T + b4×Energy + const.; (3) Y = (b1×age + b2×gender + b3×T + b4×Energy) + b5×VitA + b6×Zn + b7×Fe + const; and (4) Y = (b1×age + b2×gender + b3×T + b4×PC1) + b5×PC2 + ... + b10×PC7 + const. Results are summarized in Table 6. None of the toxins were significantly correlated with the growth indicators when adjusting for age and gender. When adjustments were also made for total energy (model 2), all toxins showed a significant correlation with HAZ but not with WHZ. This was also the case when adding vitamin A, total protein, iron and zinc (model 3). When adjusting for dietary intake using the principal component scores, all three toxins showed a negative correlation with HAZ, while only aflatoxin B_1 and fumonisin were negatively correlated with WHZ (Table 6).

Table 6. Multivariable analyses of potential correlates of HAZ and WHZ tested adjusting for age and gender using four different models.

Model	Factors Adjusted for (Forced into Model)	Other Potential Correlates	Log_n (Aflatoxin B_1 Exposure)	Log_n (Fuminosin Exposure)	Log_n (Ochratoxin A Exposure)	Combined (Based on PCA Score)
			HAZ			
1	Age (months) + gender	None	0.21 (−0.40–0.81)	0.11 (−0.54–0.75)	−0.07 (−0.48–0.35)	0.02 (−0.13–0.17)
2	Age (months) + gender + total energy	None	−1.13 (−1.81—0.45) **	−1.52 (−2.24—0.80) ***	−0.76 (−1.18—0.35) ***	−0.32 (−0.49—0.16) ***
3	Age (months) + gender + total energy	Vitamin A; total protein; iron; zinc	−2.19 (−2.80—1.58) ***	−2.62 (−3.24—1.99) ***	−1.24 (−1.62—0.86) ***	−0.58 (−0.72—0.43) ***
4	Age (months) + gender + PC1	PC2 to PC7 [a]	−2.66 (−3.40—1.92) ***	−2.99 (−3.71—2.27) ***	−0.96 (−1.31—0.61) ***	−0.66 (−0.83—0.48) ***
			WHZ			
1	Age (months) + gender	None	−0.16 (−0.56–0.25)	−0.14 (−0.57–0.28)	0.01 (−0.26–0.29)	−0.02 (−0.12–0.08)
2	Age (months) + gender + total energy	None	−0.26 (−0.78–0.26)	−0.26 (−0.82–0.30)	0.0145 (−0.30–0.33)	−0.04 (−0.17–0.09)
3	Age (months) + gender + total energy	Vitamin A; total protein; iron; zinc	−0.534 (−1.07–0.00) *	−0.50 (−1.07–0.084)	−0.08 (−0.40–0.24)	−0.09 (−0.22–0.04)
4	Age (months) + gender + PC1	PC2 to PC7	−1.50 (−2.17—0.83) ***	−1.26 (−1.95—0.56) ***	−0.41 (−0.81–0.00)	−0.27 (−0.44—0.11) **

* p-value < 0.05, ** p-value < 0.01, *** p-value < 0.001. [a] Principal component scores (PC1-PC7) were used as potential correlates of growth indicators. PC1 is a measure of total food intake.

Children such as the ones studied in the Lao Cai province are constantly exposed to numerous mycotoxins in the food chain. There are several studies linking aflatoxin intake to growth impairment in children. A dose-response relationship between high aflatoxin levels in the blood and low WAZ ($p = 0.005$) and HAZ scores ($p = 0.001$) were found in a cross-sectional study in Togo and Benin [24]. A study in the Gambia found an association between high exposure to aflatoxin in utero and low weight ($p = 0.012$) and length gains ($p = 0.044$) in the first year of life [25]. A strong negative correlation between blood aflatoxin levels and child growth (stunting) was reported in a longitudinal study of 200 children between 16 and 37 months of age. Fumonisin exposure was pointed out to be a possible factor in slowed child growth as levels of urinomarker of fumonisin B_1 concentration were negatively associated with growth [26].

2.4. Risk Assessment for Mycotoxin Exposure

2.4.1. Aflatoxin B_1

Using the data of contamination level and daily intake of each food group, mean dietary exposure of aflatoxin B_1 was estimated at 118.7 ng/kgbw/day (range 104.9–124.2 ng/kgbw/day) resulting in a risk of hepatocellular carcinomas (HCC) of 12.1 cases/100,000 individual/year (range 10.7–12.7 cases/100,000 individual/year). The rice product group was found to be the main source of aflatoxin B_1 exposure (52.2 ng/kg bw/day), therefore contributed with the highest risk (5.3 cases/100,000 individual/year) of HCC in comparison to other food groups (Table 7). Our previous study in Lao Cai on risks for HCC when consuming self-supplied staple cereals showed that the dietary exposure to aflatoxins and risk of HCC were 33.7 ng/kg bw/day and 2.7 cases/100,000 individual/year, respectively [23].

In line with the above risk estimation, MOEs of aflatoxin B_1 of all food groups are far lower than 10,000 (range from 3 to 532), resulting in a combined MOE of total aflatoxin B_1 daily intake as low as 1.4, which is of major public health concern. This is supported by evidence of increased susceptibility to cancer from early-life exposure, particularly for chemicals acting through a genetoxic mode of action like aflatoxins [1]. The high dietary intake exposure of aflatoxins found in the present study together with HBV and HCV infections is likely to represent increased risks of children to liver cancer much more than for adults.

Table 7. Dietary exposure to aflatoxin B_1 and ochratoxin A and risk of liver and renal cancer.

Food Groups [a]	Aflatoxin B_1						Ochratoxin A			
	Exposure (ng/kg bw [b]/day)		HCC Risk [d] (cases/100,000 Population)		MOE^e_{HCC}	MOE^f_{HCC} Adjusted	Exposure (ng/kg bw/day)		MOE^e_{RC}	MOE^f_{RC} Adjusted
	MB[c]	LB-UB[c]	MB	LB-UB			MB	LB-UB		
Rice and products	52.2	41.2–52.8	5.3	4.2–5.4	3	1	14.2	0–1900	1478	468
Wheat and products	1.0	0–1.9	0.1	0–0.2	183	58	0.9	0–1900	>10,000	7384
Tubes, roof and products	0.7	0.5–0.8	0.1	0–0.1	261	83	0.3	0–1900	>10,000	>10,000
Beans and products	3.9	3.6–4.1	0.4	0.4	44	14	9.8	9208–10,158	2142	678
Tofu	0.3	0–0.6	0.0	0–0.1	532	168	0.3	0–1900	>10,000	>10,000
Oily seeds	0.6	0.6	0.1	0.1	287	91	0.1	0–1900	>10,000	>10,000
Vegetables	18.9	18.9	2.0	2	9	3	5.2	0–1900	4,038	1278
Sugar/confectionary	6.8	5.5	0.7	0.7	25	10	1.6	413–1933	>10,000	4153
Oil, fat	0.5	0.5	0.1	0.1	347	110	0.2	987–1937	>10,000	>10,000
Meat and products	13.8	13.5–14.0	1.4	1.4	12	4	7.1	1339–3030	2957	936
Egg and milk	18.0	18	1.9	1.9	9	3	10.7	2927–3401	1962	621
Fish	1.3	1.0–1.6	0.1	0.2	133	42	1.2	1770–2720	>10,000	5538
Other aquaculture products	0.4	0.3–0.6	0.0	0–0.1	384	122	0.9	4850	>10,000	7384
Total	118.7	104.9–124.2	12.1	10.7–12.7	1.4	0.5	52.6	29.7–77.0	400	127

[a] Food groups were categorized followed those applied in data of National Survey in the year 2010 [16]. [b] Mean body weight (bw) of children was 11.3 kg. [c] Medium bound (MB) figures (ND = LOD/2) were used for mean. Lower bound (LB) and upper bound (UB) figures (ND = 0, ND = LOD) were used for range. [d] Children risk of hepatitis carcinogen is calculated on the assumption of HbsAg + prevalence 2% [14] and mean exposure. [e] MOE, Margin of exposure, based on the calculated as a ratio of benchmark dose lower limit 10% lower bound of AFB_1 (170 ng/kw bw/day [6]) or OTA (21 µg/kg bw/day [27]) and MB of exposure. HCC, hepatocellular cancer; RC, renal cancer. [f] MOEs adjusted by age-dependent adjustment factors for children aged 2–16 (ADAF = 3.16) [28].

2.4.2. Ochratoxin A

An amount of 52.6 ng/kg bw/day was estimated as the average ochratoxin A exposure, while 77.0 ng/kg bw/day was the highest exposure value (Table 7). The mean and high dietary exposure levels of ochratoxin A were, respectively, equivalent to 261% and 413% of PTDI (14 ng/kg bw/day) [29]. It should be noted that the ochratoxin A exposure level in our study was based on average food intake of children only, which means that the actual exposure dose with the 95th percentile might be much higher. Among the few reports on exposure of children to ochratoxin A, children aged 4 to 6 years were found to be the age group with the highest ochratoxin exposure in the Czech Republic [30]. Results from a French total diet study showed that the estimated average intake of ochratoxin A in children was 4.1 ng/kg bw/day with the 95th percentile exposure being 7.8 ng/kg bw/day [31]. Ochratoxin A contamination of raw pork and meat products is detected quite commonly in Europe [32–34]. Mycotoxins in meat originate mainly from contaminated feed. In our study, the food groups contributing the most to ochratoxin A exposure were rice products (14.2 ng/kg bw/day) followed by egg and milk products (10.7 ng/kg bw/day) and beans (9.8 ng/kg bw/day). Thus, a MOE of less than 10,000 was observed for the five food groups. Taking into account the ochratoxin A exposure level of food groups, MOE of the total daily intake was 400, which represents a real risk for renal cancer in the study population.

2.4.3. Fumonisins

Although fumonisins contamination was the least common of the mycotoxins studied; still, an average and highest exposure dose of 1250 and 1929 ng/kg bw/day, equal to 63% and 96% of PTDI (2000 ng/kg bw/day), respectively, were observed, using a hepato-carcinogen benchmark dose lower limit 10% ($BMDL_{10}$) of 150 μg/kg bw/day [35]. Assuming that the contamination level of fumonisin B_1 is 70% of that of total determined fumonisins [17], the MOE of fumonisin B_1 in total daily intake was 1713, indicating a health risk for the children due to consumption of large portions of various food items containing low levels of fumonisins.

2.4.4. Aged Adjusted MOEs of the Mycotoxins

Cancer risk assessment methods currently assume that children and adults are equally susceptible to exposure to chemicals. However, research indicates that individuals exposed to mycotoxins at a young age are at higher risk developing cancer than adults [36]. Consequently, a modifying factor may need to be applied to our cancer-risk estimates to ensure risks are not underestimated. The US EPA calculated age-dependent adjustment factors (ADAFs) to account for that children are more susceptible to carcinogens [28]. These factors, which apply to carcinogens with a genotoxic mode of action, are as follows: ADAF is 10 for children <2 years of age; ADAF is 3.16 for children aged 2 to <16 years; and there should be no adjustment (ADAF = 1) for children ≥16 years of age. The MOEs adjusted by ADFA of aflatoxin B1 and ochratoxin A in total daily intake were calculated and are shown in Table 7, while the one of fumonisin B_1 was 542.

2.4.5. Combined Exposure to All Three Mycotoxins

Co-occurrence of mycotoxins is common worldwide [37]. A study in Tanzania showed that in three geographically distant villages, 82% (n = 148) of children aged 12 to 22 months were exposed to both aflatoxin and fumonisins [26]. Studies in Asian countries show that aflatoxin and fumonisin are commonly found together in foods [37]. In our study, frequency histograms of the mycotoxins showed a skewed distribution and scores were therefore log-transformed. Pairwise correlations between the three toxins were high, i.e., correlation coefficients from 0.8457 to 0.9772 document a frequent co-exposure to the mycotoxins studied. We know too little about the toxicity associated with exposure to multiple mycotoxins, e.g., additive, synergistic or antagonistic toxic effects.

3. Conclusions

We estimated exposure to aflatoxin B1, ochratoxin A and fumonisins among children in the Lao Cai province using a total dietary study (TDS) approach. Exposures to all three mycotoxins were high and exceeded toxicological reference levels. Risk assessments showed a high risk for liver cancer due to the consumption of aflatoxin B_1 contaminated foods and lower risks for liver cancer due to fumonisin exposure and renal cancer due to ochratoxin A exposure. Furthermore, high exposure to mycotoxins was associated with impaired child growth when adjusted for age, gender and dietary intake. Though the mechanisms are not clear, stunning and the associated compromised immunity together with high mycotoxin exposure are likely to further negatively impact child development. Locally adapted post-harvest interventions that effectively reduce mycotoxin development in stable cereals are needed.

4. Materials and Methods

4.1. Study Area

The study took place in and covered the entire Lao Cai province, which consists of nine sub-regions; Lao Cai city itself, together with eights districts (Figure 1).

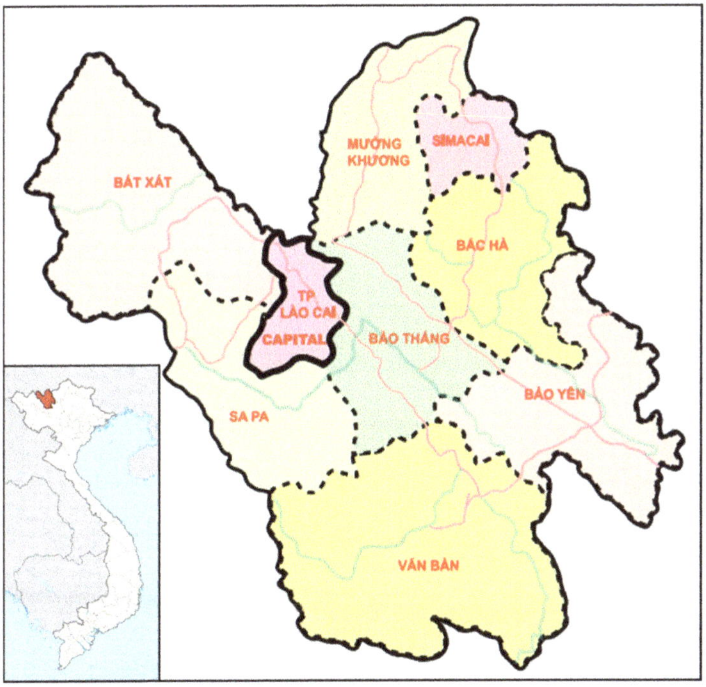

Figure 1. Map of nine districts of the Lao Cai province.

4.2. Anthropometric Measurement

An anthropometric study was conducted in the Ta Phoi and Hop Thanh communes, Lao Cai district, where the inhabitants represented five ethnic groups, i.e., Dao, Giay, Xapho, Tay and Kinh. From a list of 300 households, all 119 children aged 13 to 59 months were selected. Children were weighed and measured once while wearing light-weight clothing following WHO's instructions [38]. Children younger than 24 months of age were laid horizontally and weighed using a children scale.

Their length was also measured using a measuring tape. Children aged 24 to 59 months were weighed barefoot using an electronic scale. The height of these children was measured using a stadiometer while standing straight on a horizontal surface with their heels together and eyes straight forward.

4.3. *Daily Food Intake Surveillance*

The food consumed by the children studied was estimated based on information collected from 24 h recall food intake interviews conducted on three consecutive days combined with actual weighing of the reported consumptions [39]. The mother or grandmother was interviewed on the types of dishes consumed during the last day, including information about all ingredients used for food preparation. Supporting tools, such as spoon, table spoon, bowl and cups, were used to activate the household member's memory and to allow subsequent weighing of the foods. Accordingly, available foods were weighted for confirming amount stated by household members using a Tanita electronic scale, (Tokyo, Japan).

For collecting further information about feeding practices of children, five focus group discussions were carried out with mothers or caregivers. Eight to 10 mothers belonging to the same ethical group were invited to discuss about breast feeding, complementary feeding, food safety practice and taking care of sick children.

4.4. *Mycotoxins Exposure Risk Assessment*

The guidance for Total Dietary Study (TSD) approach issued by EFSA, WHO and FAO [40] was employed to assess dietary exposure of the aflatoxin B_1, ochratoxin A and fumonisins of children younger than 5 years old.

4.4.1. Food Sample Collection and Analysis

Data collected in the daily food intake surveillance came up with a list containing 89 food items. Of these, 40 were selected for the TDS (Table 1). The selection was made on the basis that these food items were most commonly consumed and probably could be contaminated with one or more of the three mycotoxins analyzed. In each of the nine sub-regions, three retail markets were selected. Choosing one retailer at each market made up a total of 27 retailers. At each of the 27 retailers, three independent samples of about 100 g size were collected for each of the 40 pre-selected food items. Thus, 1080 individual foods samples were collected (40 food items × 9 sub-regions × 3 retail markets).

For each of the 40 composite food items, samples taken were compounded in the following way. The three 100 g samples from a given retailer were mixed, and from the 300 g of the resulting mixed sample a 100 g sub-sample were taken. The nine sub-samples of 100 g, representing each of the nine sub-regions, were then mixed, to give a sample of 900 g representing the province. Three hundred grams of this sample was taken for preparation and cooking according to the most common local cooking practices. The means of preparation and cooking complied with the EFSA/FAO/WHO guidance in kitchen preparation [40]. In total, this procedure resulted in 40 composite cooked samples each representing one food item as "averaged" over the whole of the province. Each of these 40 food item samples were analyzed for the three mycotoxins mentioned above as describe in the following.

4.4.2. Mycotoxin Contamination Analysis

ELISA-based methods with aflatoxin B_1, ochratoxin A and fumonisin B_1 as standards and commercially available detection kits (AgraQuant®, Romer Labs, Inc., Newark, DE, USA) were used for aflatoxin B_1 (COKAQ 8000, limit of detection is 2 ng/g), ochratoxin A (COKAQ 2000, limit of detection is 1.9 ng/g), and fumonisins (COKAQ 3000, limit of detection is 0.2 μg/g) analyses according to the manufacturer's instructions and as reported previously [23]. Briefly, for each sample, one extract was produced then duplicate determinations of the toxin were performed. Standard curves were plotted using standard aflatoxin B_1, ochratoxin A and fumonisin B_1. The concentration of aflatoxin B_1, ochratoxin A and fumonisins were calculated on a dry weight basis according to the specifications of the manufacturer. The sample moisture content was measured by drying 10.0 g in an oven at 105 °C for 17 h [41].

4.4.3. Mycotoxins Exposure

The deterministic (or single point) approach was adopted to estimate the dietary mycotoxin exposure [39]. According to these recommendations, half of the limit of detection (LOD) was used for all results of aflatoxin B_1 less than LOD, since concentration of the mycotoxin was below LOD in less than 60% of samples. In contrast, since the contamination level of ochratoxin A and fumonisins in more than 60% of samples were lower than LOD, then two estimates using zero (lower bound) and LOD (upper bound) for all results less than LOD were applied.

The chronic daily exposure to each of the mycotoxins was calculated based on the mycotoxin contamination level of each TDS food group (ng/kg food) and the daily intake (kg food/day) of this food group using an 11.3 kg mean of body weight of children.

4.4.4. Risk Characterization

As recommended by EFSA and JEFCA, the MOEs of all three mycotoxins were calculated [18,19]. The MOE was given by the ratio between the benchmark dose level that caused a 10% increase in cancer incidence in animal ($BMDL_{10}$) and the total intake (MOE = $BMDL_{10}$/total intake) [18]. For estimation of MOE, BMLD 10 of developing hepatocellular carcinoma HCC (170 ng/kg bw/day and 150 μg/kg bw/day; 95% lower confidence limit) were applied for aflatoxin B_1 [6] and fumonisins [35], respectively. For ochratoxin A, a MOE based on the lowest BMDL10 associated with an increase in renal cancer (21 μg/kg bw/day) by exposure to ochratoxin A was determined [27]. MOE values lower than 10,000 may indicate a public health concern [18].

The mycotoxin of most concern is aflatoxin B_1, which has been reported to increase liver cancer among people infected with hepatitis virus. Risk assessment for aflatoxin B_1 was performed based on the dietary exposure to aflatoxin B_1 and its potency using the prevalence of individuals being hepatitis B surface antigen- (HbsAg) positive and having a primary liver cancer potency of 0.3 cancers per year per 100,000 population per ng aflatoxin B_1/kg body weight (kg bw)/day and the negative individuals set to have 0.01 cancers per year per 100,000 population per ng AFB_1/kg bw/day [12,42]. In this study, we assumed that 1% of children younger than five years old were HbsAg-positive [14].

4.5. Data Analysis

The WHO standards were used to determine the nutritional status of children, i.e., weight for age (WAZ), height (length) for age (HAZ or LAZ) and weight for height (WHZ) z-scores [20]. Descriptive statistics for these growth indicators, selected variables on dietary intake and mycotoxin exposure were summarized by gender and age group (13–23 months versus 24–59 months). The two age groups, however, were represented with very different sample sizes and in subsequent analyses age in months was used. Linearity of the associations between various outcome variables and age in month was tested by polynomial regression [43].

The dietary variables could all be potential correlates of the growth indicators. Correlation coefficients between pairs of dietary variables ranged from −0.14 to 0.94. The 50, 75 and 90 percentile of all possible pairwise correlations among the dietary variables (n = 528) were 0.38, 0.61 and 0.76, respectively. Therefore, we conducted a Principal Component Analysis (PCA) on these variables. The number of components retained was based on a scree plot, the retained components were then submitted to a varimax rotation [44] and the factor scores were used as predictors in the regression analysis.

Correlates of the growth indicators were tested using multiple linear regression, where age (months) and gender were entered as well. Regression models were either specified by us or using a backwards stepwise regression procedure (p for removal = 0.051; p for entry = 0.050), but with some factors (see results) forced into the model. Mycotoxin species were tested individually as correlates of the growth indicators, and since these toxins were all correlated, they were also tested as a combined score based on the principal component score.

4.6. Ethical clearance

Mother or caregivers of all 119 subjects gave their informed consent for their attendance before they participated in the study. The study was conducted in accordance with the Declaration of Helsinki, and the protocol was approved by the Ethics Committee of the National Institute of Nutrition, Hanoi, Vietnam (ID 6 VDD 2009, dated 8 September 2009).

Author Contributions: Conceptualization, B.T.M.H., A.D. and L.B.; Methodology, B.T.M.H., L.D.T., H.M. and H.F.; Validation, B.T.M.H. and H.M.; Formal analysis, B.T.M.H., H.M., L.D.T., L.B., H.F. and A.D.; Investigation, B.T.M.H.; Resources, B.T.M.H. and A.D.; Writing—original draft preparation, B.T.M.H. and A.D.; Writing—review and editing, B.T.M.H., L.D.T., H.M., L.B., H.F. and A.D.; Visualization, B.T.M.H.; Supervision, H.M., L.B. and A.D.; Project Administration, A.D.; Funding acquisition, A.D.

Funding: This research was funded by the Danish International Development Assistance (Danida) through the project SANIVAT "Water supply, sanitation, hygiene promotion and health in Vietnam" (www.sanivat.com.vn; 104.DAN.8.L.711).

Acknowledgments: The authors thank Nguyen Thi Anh Tuyet, Ha Thi Tuong Van and Bui Thi Kim Ngan for their support in the field and laboratory.

Conflicts of Interest: The authors declare no conflict of interest. The sponsors have no role in the choice of research project; design of the study; in the collection, analyses or interpretation of data; in the writing of the manuscript; or in the decision to publish the results.

References

1. Boon, P.E.; Bakker, M.I.; Van Klaveren, J.D.; Van Rossum, C.T.M. *RIVM Report 350070002/2009: Risk Assessment of the Dietary Exposure to Contaminants and Pesticide Residues in Young Children in the Netherlands*; RIVM National Institute for Public Health and the Environment: Bilthoven, The Netherlands, 2009.
2. World Health Organization (WHO). *Food Safety. Fact Sheet N 399*; World Health Organization: Geneva, Switzerland, 2015.
3. Wu, F.; Groopman, J.D.; Pestka, J.J. Public health impacts of foodborne mycotoxins. *Annu. Rev. Food Sci. Technol.* **2014**, *5*, 351–372. [CrossRef] [PubMed]
4. International Agency for Research on Cancer (IARC). Aflatoxins: B1, B2, G1, G2, M1. In *Some Naturally Occurring Substances: Food Items and Constituents, Heterocyclic Aromatic Amines and Mycotoxins, Aflatoxins*; IARC: Lyon, France, 1993; Volume 56, pp. 245–396.
5. International Agency for Research on Cancer (IARC). Aflatoxins. In *Some Traditional Herbal Medicines, Some Mycotoxins, Naphthalene and Styrene*; IARC: Lyon, France, 2002; Volume 82, pp. 301–366.
6. EFSA. Opinion of the Scientific Panel on Contaminants in the Food Chain on a request from the Commission related to the potential increase of consumer health risk by a possible increase of the existing maximum levels for aflatoxin in almonds, hazenuts, and pistachios and derived products. *EFSA J.* **2007**, *446*, 1–127.
7. International Agency for Research on Cancer (IARC). Toxins derived from Fusarium moniliforme: Fumonisins B1 and B2 and fusarin. In *Some Naturally Occurring Substances: Food Items and Constituents, Heterocyclic Aromatic Amines and Mycotoxins*; IARC: Lyon, France, 1993; Volume 56, pp. 445–466.
8. Mally, A. Ochratoxin A and mitotic disruption: Mode of action analysis of renal tumor formation by ochratoxin A. *Toxicol. Sci.* **2012**, *127*, 315–330. [CrossRef] [PubMed]
9. Mantle, P.G.; Nagy, J.M. Binding of ochratoxin A to a urinary globulin: A new concept to account for gender difference in rat nephrocarcinogenic responses. *Int. J. Mol. Sci.* **2008**, *9*, 719–735. [CrossRef] [PubMed]
10. Heussner, A.H.; Lewis, E.H.B. Comparative ochratoxin toxicity: A review of the available data. *Toxins* **2015**, *7*, 4253–4282. [CrossRef]
11. International Agency for Research on Cancer (IARC). Ochratoxin A. In *Some Naturally Occurring Substances: Food Items and Constituents, Heterocyclic Aromatic Amines and Mycotoxins, Ochratoxin*; IARC: Lyon, France, 1993; Volume 56, pp. 489–521.
12. World Health Organization (WHO). *Safety Evaluation of Certain Food Additives and Contaminants: Aflatoxins*; WHO Food Additives Series 40; WHO: Geneva, Switzerland, 1998; pp. 359–468.

13. Lia, X.; Wiesen, E.; Diorditsab, S.; Todac, K.; Duong, H.; Nguyen, L.H.; Nguyen, V.C.; Nguyen, T.H. Impact of adverse events following immunization in Viet Nam in 2013 on chronic hepatitis B infection. *Vaccine* **2016**, *34*, 869–873. [CrossRef]
14. World Health Organization Western Pacific Representative Office (WHOWPRO). Frequently Asked Questions: Hepatitis B and Hepatitis B Vaccine. Last updated: 09 August 2013. Available online: http://www.wpro.who.int/vietnam/topics/hepatitis/faqhepatitis/en/ (accessed on 28 July 2019).
15. UNICEF. *Unicef Annual Report*; UNICEF: Hanoi, Vietnam, 2014.
16. National Institute of Nutrition (NIN). *National Surveillance on Nutrition, 2009*; National Institute of Nutrition, Medical Publishing House: Hanoi, Vietnam, 2011; pp. 1–248.
17. International Agency for Research on Cancer (IARC). *IARC Working Group Reports: Mycotoxin Control in Low- and Middle-Income Countries*; Wild, C.P., Miller, J.D., Groopman, J.D., Eds.; International Agency for Research on Cancer (IARC): Lyon, France, 2015.
18. European Food Safety Authority (EFSA). Statement on the applicability of the Margin of Exposure approach for the safety assessment of impurities which are both genotoxic and carcinogenic in substances added to food/feed. *EFSA J.* **2012**, *10*, 2578.
19. FAO; WHO. *Evaluation of Certain Food Contaminants. Sixty-Fourth Report of the Joint FAO/WHO Expert Committee on Food Additives*; WHO Technical Report Series, No. 930; World Health Organization: Geneva, Switzerland, 2006; Available online: http://hqlibdoc.who.int/trs/WHO_TRS_930_eng.pdf (accessed on 10 August 2019).
20. National Institute of Nutrition (NIN). *Daily Nutrient Intake Recommendation for Vietnamese*; Medical Publishing House: Hanoi, Vietnam, 2016.
21. Wang, D.S.; Liang, Y.X.; Nguyen, T.C.; Le, D.D.; Tanaka, T.; Ueno, Y. Natural co-occurrence of fusarium toxins and aflatoxin B1 in corn for feed in North Vietnam. *Nat. Toxins* **1995**, *3*, 445–449. [CrossRef]
22. Trung, T. Mycotoxins in maize in Vietnam. *World Mycotoxin J.* **2008**, *1*, 87–94. [CrossRef]
23. Huong, B.T.M.; Tuyen, L.D.; Do, T.T.; Madsen, H.; Brimer, L.; Dalsgaard, A. Aflatoxins and fumonisins in rice and maize staple cereals in Northern Vietnam and dietary exposure in different ethnic groups. *Food Control.* **2016**, *70*, 191–200. [CrossRef]
24. Gong, Y.; Cardwell, K.; Hounsa, A.; Egal, S.; Turner, P.C.; Hall, A.J.; Wild, C.P. Dietary aflatoxin exposure and impaired growth in young children from Benin and Togo: Cross sectional study. *BMJ* **2008**, *325*, 20. [CrossRef] [PubMed]
25. Turner, P.C.; Collinson, A.C.; Cheung, Y.B.; Gong, Y.; Hall, A.J.; Prentice, A.M.; Wild, C.P. Aflatoxin exposure in utero causes growth faltering in Gambian infants, 2007. *Int. J. Epidemiol.* **2007**, *36*, 1119–1125. [CrossRef] [PubMed]
26. Shirima, C.P.; Kimanya, M.E.; Kinabo, J.L.; Michael, N.; Routledge, M.N.; Srey, G.; Wild, C.P.; Gong, Y.Y. Dietary exposure to aflatoxin and fumonisin among Tanzanian children as determined using biomarkers of exposure. *Mol. Nutr. Food Res.* **2013**, *57*, 1874–1881. [CrossRef]
27. European Food Safety Authority (EFSA). Opinion of the scientific panel on contaminants in the food chain on a request from the commission related to Ochratoxin A. *EFSA J.* **2006**, *365*, 1–56.
28. United States Environmental Pollution Assessment (US EPA). *Guidelines for Carcinogen Risk Assessment (PDF)*; 630-P-03-001F; United States Environmental Pollution Assessment (US EPA): Washington, DC, USA, 2005; 166p.
29. JECFA. Ochratoxin A (addendum). In *Safety Evaluation of Certain Food Additives and Contaminants. Prepared by the Sixty-Eighth Meeting of the Joint FAO/WHO Expert Committee on Food Additives, 2007*; WHO food additive series; Food and Agriculture Organization of the United Nations (FAO); World Health Organization (WHO): Geneva, Switzerland, 2008; Volume 357, pp. 429–454.
30. Ostry, V.; Malir, F.; Dofkova, M.; Skarkova, J.; Pfohl-Leszkowicz., A.; Ruprich, J. Ochratoxin A dietary exposure of ten population groups in the Czech Republic: Comparison with data over the world. *Toxins* **2015**, *7*, 3608–3635. [CrossRef]
31. Leblanc, J.C.; Tard, A.; Volatier, J.L.; Verger, P. Estimated dietary exposure to principal food mycotoxins from the first French total diet study. *Food Addit. Contam.* **2005**, *22*, 652–672. [CrossRef]
32. Bintvihok, A.; Thiengnin, S.; Doi, K.; Kumagai, S. Residues of aflatoxins in the liver, muscle and eggs of domestic fowls. *J. Vet. Med. Sci.* **2002**, *64*, 1037–1039. [CrossRef]
33. Herzallah, S.M. Determination of aflatoxins in eggs, milk, meat and meat products using HPLC fluorescent and UV detectors. *Food Chem.* **2009**, *114*, 1141–1146. [CrossRef]

34. Pleadin, J.; Staver, M.M.; Vahčić, N.; Kovačević, D.; Milone, S.; Saftić, L.; Scortichini, G. Survey of aflatoxin B1 and ochratoxin A occurrence in traditional meat products coming from Croatian households and markets. *Food Control* **2015**, *52*, 71–77. [CrossRef]
35. Bondy, G.; Mehta, R.; Caldwell, D.; Coady, L.; Armstrong, A.; Savard, M.; Miller, J.D.; Chomyshyn, E.; Bronson, R.; Zitomer, N.; et al. Effects of long term exposure to the mycotoxin fumonisin B1 in p53 heterozygous and p53 homozygous transgenic mice. *Food Chem. Toxicol.* **2012**, *50*, 3604–3613. [CrossRef]
36. Murdoch, D.J.; Krewski, D.; Wargo, J. Cancer risk assessment with intermittent exposure. *Risk Anal.* **1992**, *12*, 569–577. [CrossRef] [PubMed]
37. Smith, M.C.; Madec, S.; Coton, E.; Hymery, N. Natural co-occurrence of mycotoxins in foods and feeds and their in vitro combined toxicological effects. *Toxins* **2016**, *8*, 94. [CrossRef] [PubMed]
38. World Health Organization (WHO). *Training Course on Child Growth Assessment*; WHO: Geneva, Switzerland, 2008.
39. European Food Safety Authority (EFSA). Guidance of EFSA General principles for the collection of national food consumption data in the view of a Pan-European dietary survey. *EFSA J.* **2009**, *7*, 1435. [CrossRef]
40. EFSA; FAO; WHO. Joint guidance of EFSA, FAO AND WHO. Towards a harmonised total diet study approach: A guidance document. *EFSA J.* **2011**, *9*, 2450. [CrossRef]
41. Miren, C.; Sonia, M.; Vicente, S.R. Distribution of fumonisins and aflatoxins in corn fractions during industrial cornflake processing. *Int. J. Food Microbiol.* **2008**, *123*, 81–87.
42. Liu, Y.; Wu, F. Global burden of aflatoxin-induced hepatocellular carcinoma: A risk assessment. *Environ. Health Perspect.* **2010**, *118*, 818–824. [CrossRef] [PubMed]
43. Zar, J.H. *Biostatistical Analysis*, 4th ed.; Pearson Publishing House: Upper Saddle River, NJ, USA, 1999.
44. Jolliffe, I. *Principal Component Analysis*; (Springer Series in Statistics); Springer: Berlin, Germany, 2013.

toxins

MDPI

Article

Mycotoxins at the Start of the Food Chain in Costa Rica: Analysis of Six *Fusarium* Toxins and Ochratoxin A between 2013 and 2017 in Animal Feed and Aflatoxin M_1 in Dairy Products

Andrea Molina [1,2], Guadalupe Chavarría [1], Margarita Alfaro-Cascante [1], Astrid Leiva [1] and Fabio Granados-Chinchilla [1,*]

1. Centro de Investigación en Nutrición Animal (CINA), Universidad de Costa Rica, Ciudad Universitaria Rodrigo, San José 11501-2060, Costa Rica; andrea.molina@ucr.ac.cr (A.M.); molinaucr@gmail.com (G.C.); alfarocascante@gmail.com (M.A.-C.); astrid.leiva@ucr.ac.cr (A.L.)
2. Escuela de Zootecnia, Universidad de Costa Rica, Ciudad Universitaria Rodrigo, San José 11501-2060, Costa Rica

* Correspondence: fabio.granados@ucr.ac.cr; Tel.: +506-2511-2028; Fax: +506-2234-2415

Received: 2 March 2019; Accepted: 17 April 2019; Published: 31 May 2019

Abstract: Mycotoxins are secondary metabolites, produced by fungi of genera *Aspergillus*, *Penicillium* and *Fusarium* (among others), which produce adverse health effects on humans and animals (carcinogenic, teratogenic and immunosuppressive). In addition, mycotoxins negatively affect the productive parameters of livestock (e.g., weight, food consumption, and food conversion). Epidemiological studies are considered necessary to assist stakeholders with the process of decision-making regarding the control of mycotoxins in processing environments. This study addressed the prevalence in feed ingredients and compound feed of eight different types of toxins, including metabolites produced by *Fusarium* spp. (Deoxynivalenol/3-acetyldeoxynivalenol, T-2/HT-2 toxins, zearalenone and fumonisins) and two additional toxins (i.e., ochratoxin A (OTA) and aflatoxin M_1 (AFM_1)) from different fungal species, for over a period of five years. On the subject of *Fusarium* toxins, higher prevalences were observed for fumonisins (n = 80/113, 70.8%) and DON (n = 212/363, 58.4%), whereas, for OTA, a prevalence of 40.56% was found (n = 146/360). In the case of raw material, mycotoxin contamination exceeding recommended values were observed in cornmeal for HT-2 toxin (n = 3/24, 12.5%), T-2 toxin (n = 3/61, 4.9%), and ZEA (n = 2/45, 4.4%). In contrast, many compound feed samples exceeded recommended values; in dairy cattle feed toxins such as DON (n = 5/147, 3.4%), ZEA (n = 6/150, 4.0%), T-2 toxin (n = 10/171, 5.9%), and HT-2 toxin (n = 13/132, 9.8%) were observed in high amounts. OTA was the most common compound accompanying *Fusarium* toxins (i.e., 16.67% of co-occurrence with ZEA). This study also provided epidemiological data for AFM_1 in liquid milk. The outcomes unveiled a high prevalence of contamination (i.e., 29.6–71.1%) and several samples exceeding the regulatory threshold. Statistical analysis exposed no significant climate effect connected to the prevalence of diverse types of mycotoxins.

Keywords: *Fusarium* mycotoxins co-contamination; ochratoxin A; feed prevalence and safety; HPLC analysis

Key Contribution: This study generated essential epidemiological and toxicological evidence about the individual and combined occurrence of *Fusarium* mycotoxins and ochratoxin A in feedstuffs in Costa Rica. These findings portray imperative implications for all stakeholders linked to the feed industry as well as supplies for improving the management of mycotoxins in animal production.

1. Introduction

Mycotoxins are toxic fungal metabolites that can be found in feed ingredients and compound feeds [1,2]. Due to their compositions, they are detrimental to animal and human health [3–8]. Currently, more than 400 different types of mycotoxins have been identified [9]. However, *Fusarium* toxins are among the most commonly monitored as they are acknowledged to present serious health concerns [7,10]. Under certain conditions, some fungi can produce several toxins simultaneously [11–13].

In feed production, ca. 60% of the formulation consists of cornmeal, soybean meal, and their derivates [14,15]. In Costa Rica, cereal production represents 38% of the agricultural sector imports [16], where its main suppliers are the United States and Brazil with 84% and 15% contribution, respectively [17]. In this regard, corn imports have increased from 738,539.97 to 781,903.54 metric tons from 2015 to 2017 [18]. On the other hand, soybean imports have risen to 309,897.97 metric tons per year, even though 83% of the soybean meal used as a feedstuff comes from national production [18]. Furthermore, only 38% of the products destined for animal consumption are from national origin, representing a total feed production of 1,238,243 metric tons in 2017. Approximately 45%, 27%, 20%, and 4% of this production is intended to be destined to poultry, higher ruminants, swine, and pets (i.e., cats and dogs), respectively [18]. That is, import and export of animal feed and feed ingredients play an essential part in the co-occurrence of various types of mycotoxins in the finished feed [19,20]. Hence, co-occurrence could be a far more certain and prevalent issue in real mycotoxin feed analysis [11,12,20–23].

Mycotoxin metabolites retain toxicity and thus must be surveilled [24,25]. Mycotoxins and their metabolites have several implications for animal and human health. Some are identified/classified as teratogenic, genotoxic, carcinogenic, and immunotoxic. The ingestion of contaminated feed affects animal health and may reduce productivity in animals, generating economic losses [26]. Some mycotoxins ingested and metabolized by productive animals could be accumulated in different organs and tissues reaching the food chain through meat, milk, or eggs [24,27,28]. In Costa Rica, during 2018, consumption of these commodities was estimated in 58.7 kg (i.e., 14.3, 15.4, and 29 kg year^{-1} for cattle, pork, and chicken, respectively), 215 L, and 218 units per capita, individually [18].

In this regard, epidemiological information tends to be more comprehensive when exploring data from several toxins simultaneously [29]. Accurate mycotoxin data about their presence in feeds are paramount for stakeholders' decision-making process towards the risk management in their manipulation [30]. Numerous reports have explicitly documented the incidence of mycotoxins in feeds, especially in Europe [11,31,32], USA [33], Asia [31], and China [34]. Nowadays, there are insufficient reports oriented to describe the incidence of mycotoxins in feed in Costa Rica. The emphasis has been made towards the investigation of aflatoxins [35,36].

Herein, the prevalent data from feed and feed ingredient samples of eight different toxins, mainly produced by *Fusarium* spp. (deoxynivalenol/3-acetyldexoynivalenol (DON/3-ADON), T-2/HT-2 toxins, zearalenone (ZEA) and fumonisins (FB_1 and FB_2)), but also ochratoxin A (OTA), during five years are provided. Finally, in the same period, we analyzed the behavior of AFM_1 in liquid milk.

2. Results

2.1. *Fusarium* Toxins Present in Animal Feed

The highest prevalence of *Fusarium* toxins during the analyzed period (2012–2017) was observed for fumonisin and DON in 70.8% (n = 80/113) and 58.4% (n = 212/363) of the cases, respectively. For FB_1 + FB_2 the prevalence ranged from 27.8% (n = 5/18) in 2013 to 85.2% (n = 23/27) in 2014, with a maximum concentration of 53,580 μg kg^{-1} observed in 2015. The prevalence for DON ranged from 42.0% (n = 40/94) in 2016 to 79.3% (n = 69/87) in 2014, with a maximum concentration of 151,060 μg kg^{-1} presented in 2013 (Table 1). Lower prevalences of 21.2% (n = 45/212) and 36.1% (n = 97/269) with a maximum mycotoxin level of 16,100 μg kg^{-1} (in 2015) and 12,500 μg kg^{-1} (in 2014) were observed for 3-acetyldeoxynivalenol and HT-2, respectively (Table 1). Concentration-wise and among periods, ZEA and T-2 toxin increased meaningfully in 2017 and 2013, respectively. For HT-2, OTA, DON, 3-ADON, FB_1, FB_2, and FB_1 + FB_2, no differences were observed.

Table 1. Mycotoxin presence and concentration in animal feedstuff commercialized in Costa Rica.

Year	Sample Numbers, *n*						Prevalence (%) (Samples over the Limit of Detection)	Average ± Standard Deviation [b]	Median [b]
		Concentration Range, μg kg^{-1} [a]					Concentration, μg kg^{-1}		
		x < LoD	x < 250	250 ≤ x < 500	500 ≤ x < 1000	x ≥ 1000			
					Zearalenone				
2013	47	19	27	1	0	0	59.6	30 ± 80	10
2014	57	8	49	0	0	0	86.0	15 ± 15	11
2015	62	44	18	0	0	0	29.0	33 ± 62	7
2016	99	79	12	6	2	0	20.0	180 ± 225	44
2017	61	35	8	9	3	6	42.6	1055 ± 1587	392
Total	335	194	114	16	5	6	42.1	236 ± 784	18
					3-acetyldeoxynivalenol				
2015	67	53	7	3	2	2	20.9	1602± 4238	251
2016	91	74	7	0	3	7	18.7	1691 ± 2757	594
2017	54	40	7	3	3	1	25.9	400 ± 398	275
					Deoxynivalenol				
Total	212	167	21	6	8	10	21.2	1261 ± 2909	295
2013	40	11	0	7	10	12	72.5	10,439 ± 29,521	830
2014	87	18	15	32	10	12	79.3	966 ± 2442	372
2015	81	44	9	11	10	7	45.7	703 ± 916	467
2016	94	54	13	7	7	11	42.5	1150 ± 1888	355
2017	61	24	10	13	8	6	60.7	4147 ± 18,710	400
Total	363	151	47	70	45	48	58.4	2822 ± 13,805	439
		x < LoD	5 < x	10 ≤ x < 25	25 ≤ x < 50	x ≥ 50			
					Ochratoxin A				
2013	49	41	8	0	0	0	16.3	2 ± 2	2
2014	101	59	42	0	0	0	41.6	1 ± 2	1
2015	64	15	49	0	0	0	76.7	11 ± 23	1
2016	95	68	26	0	0	1	28.4	90 ± 346	3
2017	50	30	20	0	0	0	40.0	32 ± 63	5
Total	360	214	145	0	0	0	40.6	25 ± 152	1

Table 1. *Cont.*

Year	Sample Numbers, n						Prevalence (%) (Samples over the Limit of Detection)	Average ± Standard Deviation [b]	Median [b]
		Concentration Range, µg kg^{-1} [a]					Concentration, µg kg^{-1}		
		x < LoD	x < 250	250 ≤ x < 500	500 ≤ x < 1000	x ≥ 1000			
					T-2 toxin				
2013	48	23	12	8	1	4	52.1	406 ± 467	273
2014	126	49	56	15	6	0	61.1	171 ± 227	61
2015	91	66	24	0	1	0	27.5	39 ± 130	9
2016	93	77	15	0	0	1	17.2	180 ± 509	15
2017	47	36	11	0	0	0	23.4	20 ± 18	13
Total	406	251	119	23	8	5	47.0	177 ± 317	47
					HT-2 toxin				
2014	47	17	16	6	4	4	63.8	1113 ± 2661	217
2015	86	66	14	3	2	1	23.2	257 ± 399	151
2016	92	56	29	3	1	3	39.1	199 ± 359	53
2017	44	33	10	1	0	0	25.0	108 ± 71	103
Total	269	172	66	13	7	8	36.1	463 ± 1495	115
		x < LoD	x < 1250	1250 ≤ x < 2500	2500 ≤ x < 5000	x ≥ 5000			
					Fumonisin B_1				
2013	31	29	1	0	1	0	6.4	1691 ± 2117	1670
2014	35	27	3	1	2	2	22.9	3814 ± 3793	3625
2015	24	10	6	2	1	5	58.3	4551 ± 5774	3865
2016	88	54	13	5	4	12	38.6	3468.48 ± 7159	740
2017	59	43	11	2	3	0	27.1	203.64 ± 48	230
Total	237	163	34	10	11	19	31.2	3390 ± 5505	3110
					Fumonisin B_2				
2014	8	0	4	0	0	4	100.0	2794 ± 2252	2830
2015	11	1	3	2	2	3	90.9	6635 ± 9404	2010
2016	33	21	10	0	0	2	36.4	9931 ± 18,380	1793
2017	29	24	5	0	0	0	17.2	866 ± 1131	175
Total	81	46	22	2	2	9	43.2	6353 ± 13,559	1560

[a] Ranges based on guidance values for mycotoxins in animal feeds within the European Union (Commission Recommendations 2006/576/EC and 2013/165/EU). [37,38]. [b] Values are calculated based on the number of samples above limit of detection.

2.2. Mycotoxin Prevalence in Feed Ingredients

In the matter of feed ingredients, cornmeal exceeded guideline values for HT-2 toxin (n = 3/24, 12.5%), T-2 toxin (n = 3/61, 4.9%), and ZEA (n = 2/45, 4.4%) (Table 2). In a soybean meal, merely HT-2 toxin (n = 1/6, 16.7%) was detected in this situation, and just one sample of wheat had an excessive amount of DON (n = 1/8, 12.5%) (Table 2). With reference to other raw materials, of less inclusion, such as rice byproducts, palm oil byproducts, of the citrus industry, as well as forages, silages, and hays (treated as a whole group), there are no regulatory guidelines to establish an acceptance parameter. However, it is interesting to notice that, in the groups described above, they share as a common feature a high prevalence of DON (i.e., 66.7%) (Table 2).

Table 2. Mycotoxin contamination levels for feed ingredients. [a]

Average ± Standard Deviation	Median	Sample Numbers above Guidance Value, n	Prevalence, % (Sample Totals Analyzed by Toxin) [c]
Concentration, μg kg^{-1}			
		Corn and Byproducts	
		Deoxynivalenol (12,000 μg kg^{-1}) [b]	
650 ± 346	440	0	61.1 (36)
		Fumonisin B_1 (60,000 μg kg^{-1} sum FB_1/FB_2) [b]	
18,280 ± 16,016	3230	0	35.9 (39)
		HT-2 toxin (500 μg kg^{-1} sum T-2/HT-2) [b]	
493 ± 927	84	3	62.6 (24)
		Ochratoxin A (250 μg kg^{-1}) [b]	
18 ± 45	1	0	25.6 (39)
		T-2 toxin	
195 ± 256	53	3	55.7 (61)
		Zearalenone (3000 μg kg^{-1}) [b]	
314 ± 895	15	2	71.1 (45)
		Soybean Meal (there is no recommended Guidelines) [b]	
		Deoxynivalenol	
188 ± 69	200	Not applicable	60.0 (5)
		Fumonisin B_1	
3045 ± 1096	3045	Not applicable	100.0 (2)
		HT-2 toxin	
5013 ± 6542	2140	Not applicable	50.0 (6)
		T-2 toxin	
120 ± 141	50	Not applicable	61.5 (13)
		Wheat and Byproducts	
		Deoxynivalenol (8000 μg kg^{-1}) [b]	
20,290 ± 52,867	890	1	100.0 (8)
		Fumonisin B_1 (60,000 μg kg^{-1} sum FB_1/FB_2) [b]	
2050 ± 2234	576	0	50.0 (4)
		HT-2 toxin (500 μg kg^{-1} sum T-2/HT-2) [b]	
44 ± 50	65	0	66.7 (3)

Table 2. *Cont.*

Average ± Standard Deviation	Median	Sample Numbers above Guidance Value, n	Prevalence, % (Sample Totals Analyzed by Toxin) [c]
Wheat and Byproducts			
Ochratoxin A (250 μg kg^{-1}) [b]			
2 ± 2	1	0	50.0 (4)
T-2 toxin			
64 ± 61	54	0	75.0 (8)
Zearalenone (2000 μg kg^{-1}) [b]			
12 ± 14	5	0	28.6 (7)
Rice and Byproducts			
3-acetyldeoxynivalenol (there is no recommended guideline) [c]			
351 ± 79	351	Not applicable	50.0 (4)
Deoxynivalenol (8000 μg kg^{-1}) [b]			
890 ± 400	1101	0	60.0 (5)
Palm Oil and Byproducts (there is no recommended guidelines) [b]			
Deoxynivalenol			
400 ± 359	286	Not applicable	55.6 (18)
T-2 toxin			
330 ± 625	58	Not applicable	61.5 (13)
Zearalenone			
19 ± 18	13	Not applicable	30.0 (10)
Fruit Pulps and Peels (there is no recommended guidelines) [b]			
3-acetyldeoxynivalenol			
2204 ± 2394	2104	Not applicable	40.0 (10)
Deoxynivalenol			
21,249 ± 41,315	2160	Not applicable	50.0 (14)
Fumonisin B_1			
16,564 ± 18,916	7010	Not applicable	34.7 (32)
Fumonisin B_2			
10,100 ± 13,096	16,564	Not applicable	50.0 (4)
Ochratoxin A			
4 ± 7	1	Not applicable	50.0 (12)
T-2 toxin			
330 ± 464	50	Not applicable	13.3 (15)
Zearalenone			
43 ± 31	21	Not applicable	11.8 (17)
Forages, Silages, and Hay (there is no recommended guidelines) [b]			
3-acetyldeoxynivalenol			
476 ± 431	335	Not applicable	54.5 (22)
Deoxynivalenol			
655 ± 514	410	Not applicable	66.7 (30)

Table 2. *Cont.*

Average ± Standard Deviation	Median	Sample Numbers above Guidance Value, n	Prevalence, % (Sample Totals Analyzed by Toxin) [c]
		Fumonisin B_1	
11,883 ± 6917	7740	Not applicable	9.4 (32)
		Fumonisin B_2	
3985 ± 5310	1020	Not applicable	22.2 (9)
		HT-2 toxin	
124 ± 132	126	Not applicable	25.0 (16)
		Ochratoxin A	
15 ± 30	2	Not applicable	54.5 (22)
		T-2 toxin	
119 ± 177	25	Not applicable	30.4 (23)
		Zearalenone	
314 ± 724	27	Not applicable	37.5 (24)
		Others (there is no recommended guidelines) [b]	
		Deoxynivalenol	
610 ± 519	567	Not applicable	38.5 (13)
		Fumonisin B_1	
4931 ± 5994	693	Not applicable	66.7 (3)
		HT-2 toxin	
193 ± 136	197	Not applicable	75.0 (12)
		Ochratoxin A	
1 ± 3	1	Not applicable	56.3 (64)
		T-2 toxin	
6 ± 3	6	Not applicable	38.5 (13)
		Zearalenone	
9 ± 5	9	Not applicable	18.2 (11)

[a] Toxins detected only once for a specific matrix type were not included. [b] Data in parentheses indicate the permitted maximum or recommended toxin concentrations according to EU Commission Recommendations (2006/576/EC) [37] and (2013/165/EU) [34]. [c] Prevalence is calculated based on the number of samples above limit of detection.

2.3. Mycotoxin Prevalence in Compound Feed

Among compound feeds, beef cattle feed presented only a few samples above the guideline level (specifically, T-2 and HT-2 toxin, n = 2/63, 3.2%). Dairy cattle feed presented the highest number of samples that surpassed the recommended levels of mycotoxins (n = 34/105, 32.4%), specifically DON (n = 5/147, 3.4%), ZEA (n = 6/150, 4.0%), T-2 toxin (n = 10/171, 5.8%) and HT-2 (n = 13/132, 9.8%) (Table 3). Poultry feed presented only 10 samples exceeding the guidelines, for DON (n = 2/14, 14.3%), FB_1 (n = 1/7, 14.3%), HT-2 toxin (n = 1/15, 6.7%), and OTA (n = 1/9, 11.1%). Cat and dog food also showed values above legal thresholds for fumonisins (n = 6/13, 46.1%), with a maximum of 18,910 μg kg^{-1} (Table 3). The second highest prevalence was observed connected with swine feed (n = 14/71, 19.7%) with the mycotoxins ZEA (n = 2/18, 11.2%), FB_1 (n = 2/9, 22.2%), and DON (n = 6/17, 35.3%) infringing the respective recommended guidelines (Table 2). Fish feed also exceeded thresholds for DON (n = 2/16, 12.5%). Finally, in horse feed, Fumonisin B_2 was found (n = 1/26, 3.8%) (Table 3).

Table 3. Mycotoxin contamination levels for compound animal feed. [a]

Average ± Standard Deviation	Median	Sample Numbers above Recommended Guidance Value, n	Prevalence, % (Sample Totals Analyzed by Toxin) [d]
Concentration, μg kg^{-1}			
Beef Cattle Feed			
3-acetyldeoxynivalenol (there is no recommended guideline) [c]			
166 ± 159	77	Not applicable	42.9 (7)
Deoxinivalenol (5000 μg kg^{-1}) [c]			
988 ± 1371	530	0	70.0 (10)
Fumonisin B_1 (50,000 μg kg^{-1} sum FB_1/FB_2) [c]			
8912 ± 13,416	3305	0	88.9 (9)
Fumonisin B_2			
4020 ± 4921	134	0	66.7 (3)
HT-2 toxin (250 μg kg^{-1} sum T-2/HT-2 [c]			
442 ± 736	20	1	37.5 (8)
T-2 toxin			
128 ± 126	110	1	30.0 (10)
Ochratoxin A (there is no recommended guideline) [c]			
19 ± 22	12	Not applicable	44.4 (9)
Zearalenone (500 μg kg^{-1}) [c]			
269 ± 216	157	0	57.1 (7)
Ingredients [b†]: cornmeal (no restriction), soybean meal (no restriction), DDGG (12–15 g/100 g), palm kernel meal (max 10–15 g/100 g), wheat middlings (max 10–20 g/100 g), rice bran and polishings (max 10–20 g/100 g), soybean hulls (max 10 g/100 g), citrus pulp (10 g/100 g).			
Dairy cattle Feed (Adults and Heifers)			
3-acetyldeoxynivalenol (there is no recommended guideline) [c]			
1843 ± 4135	218	Not applicable	19.0 (105)
Deoxynivalenol (5000 μg kg^{-1}) [c]			
1578 ± 4613	338	5	55.1 (147)
Fumonisin B_1 (50,000 μg kg^{-1} sum FB_1/FB_2 [c]			
6171 ± 7908	1480	0	44.4 (144)
Fumonisin B_2			
3838 ± 5913	2310	0	43.2 (44)
HT-2 toxin (250 μg kg^{-1} sum T-2/HT-2 [c]			
207 ± 282	106	13	35.6 (132)
Ochratoxin A (there is no recommended guideline [c]			
55 ± 259	1	Not applicable	35.0 (140)
T-2 toxin			
184 ± 351	40	10	27.5 (171)
Zearalenone (500 μg kg^{-1} [c]			
215 ± 810	16	6	44.0 (150)
Ingredients [b†]: cornmeal (no restriction), soybean meal (no restriction), DDGG (12–15 g/100 g), palm kernel meal (max 10–15 g/100 g), wheat middlings (max 10–20 g/100 g), rice bran and polishings (max 10–20 g/100 g), soybean hulls (max 10 g/100 g), citrus pulp (10 g/100 g).			

Table 3. *Cont.*

Average ± Standard Deviation	Median	Sample Numbers above Recommended Guidance Value, n	Prevalence, % (Sample Totals Analyzed by Toxin) [d]
Concentration, µg kg^{-1}			
		Poultry Feed	
		Deoxynivalenol (5000 µg kg^{-1}) [c]	
1550 ± 2327	405	2	71.4 (14)
		Fumonisin B_1 (20,000 µg kg^{-1} sum FB_1/FB_2) [c]	
17,147 ± 33,569	3860	1	70.0 (10)
		Fumonisin B_2	
436 ± 467	835	0	80.0 (5)
		HT-2 toxin (250 µg kg^{-1} sum T-2/HT-2) [c]	
353 ± 284	208	1	33.3 (15)
		Ochratoxin A (100 µg kg^{-1}) [c]	
31 ± 48	11	1	44.4 (9)
		T-2 toxin	
316 ± 462	67	5	51.7 (29)
		Zearalenone (there is no recommended guideline) [c]	
75 ± 117	28	Not applicable	50.0 (10)
Ingredients [b†]: corn meal (no restriction), soybean meal (no restriction), DDGG (max 10–15 g/100 g), palm kernel meal (3–3.5 g/100 g), wheat middlings (max 3–3.5 g/100 g), rice bran and polishings (max 3–3.5 g/100 g), soybean hulls (max 3–3.5 g/100 g).			
		Pet Food (Cat and Dog Dry Food)	
		Deoxynivalenol (2000 µg kg^{-1}) [c]	
940 ± 1317	470	0	50.0 (14)
		Fumonisin B1 (5000 µg kg^{-1} sum FB1/FB2) [c]	
143,560 ± 479,783	3570	6	93.3 (15)
Ingredients [b†]: cornmeal (max 50 g/100 g), DDGG (max 25 g/100 g), palm kernel meal, wheat middlings (max 20 g/100 g), rice meal and bran (max 20 g/100 g).			
		Swine Feed (Lactating and Gestating Sows and Pig Grower)	
		Deoxynivalenol (900 µg kg^{-1}) [c]	
6302 ± 14,932	590	6	76.5 (17)
		Fumonisin B_1 (5000 µg kg^{-1} sum FB_1/FB_2) [c]	
20,042 ± 35,978	3124	2	55.6 (9)
		Fumonisin B_2	
376 ± 472	376	0	40.0 (5)
		HT-2 toxin (250 µg kg^{-1} sum T-2/HT-2) [c]	
3409 ± 4738	3409	1	28.6 (7)
		T-2 toxin	
183 ± 187	88	3	46.7 (15)
		Zearalenone (100 µg kg^{-1}) [c]	
518 ± 1327	37	2	44.4 (18)
Ingredients [b†]: cornmeal (no restriction), soybean meal (no restriction), DDGG (max 10 g/100 g), palm kernel meal (max 10 g/100 g), wheat middlings (max 20–25 g/100 g), rice bran and polishing (max 20–25 g/100 g), soybean hulls (no restriction).			

Table 3. *Cont.*

Average ± Standard Deviation	Median	Sample Numbers above Recommended Guidance Value, n	Prevalence, % (Sample Totals Analyzed by Toxin) [d]
		Fish Feed	
		Deoxynivalenol (500 μg kg^{-1}) [c]	
570 ± 318	635	2	25.0 (16)
		Fumonisin B_1 (10,000 μg kg^{-1} sum FB_1/FB_2) [c]	
10,851 ± 10,781	1565	2	52.4 (21)
		Ochratoxin A (there is no recommended guideline) [c]	
3 ± 5	1	Not applicable	66.7 (24)
	T-2 toxin		
4 ± 4	3	0	35.0 (20)
		Zearalenone (there is no recommended guideline) [c]	
84 ± 122	35	Not applicable	25.0 (16)
Ingredients[b†]: cornmeal (max 15 g/100 g), soybean meal (max 75 g/100 g), DDGG, palm kernel meal (max 30 g/100 g), wheat middlings (max 20 g/100 g), rice meal and bran (max 15 g/100 g), soybean hulls.			
		Horse Feed	
		Deoxynivalenol (5000 μg kg^{-1}) [c]	
740 ± 295	580	0	50.0 (6)
		Fumonisin B_2	
3355 ± 2623	3355	1	66.7 (3)
		HT-2 toxin (250 μg kg^{-1} sum T-2/HT-2) [c]	
52 ± 26	52	0	40.0 (5)
		Ochratoxin A (there is no recommended guideline) [c]	
95.36 ± 47.43	95	Not applicable	33.3 (6)
		T-2 toxin	
49 ± 60	49	0	33.3 (6)
Ingredientsb†: cornmeal (max 45 g/100 g), soybean meal (max 13 g/100 g), DDGG (max 20 g/100 g), palm kernel meal, wheat middlings (max 25 g/100 g), rice bran, soybean hulls (max 20 g/100 g).			

[a] Toxins detected only once for a specific matrix type were not included. [b] Plant-derived constituents according to guaranteed labels. Data in parentheses indicate maximum inclusion recommended for each ingredient during feed formulation. † Data compiled from [15,39–42]. [c] Data in parentheses indicate maximum permitted or recommended toxin concentrations according to EU Commission Recommendations (2006/576/EC) [37] and (2013/165/EU) [38]. [d] Prevalence is calculated considering the number of samples above limit of detection.

2.4. Geographical Distribution and Climate Influence for Fusarium Toxins Present in Animal Feed

Geographical and national toxin hotspot distribution was similar for those toxins produced by *Fusarium* species (Figure 1A–G). A completely different profile was observed when studying OTA and AFM_1. Interestingly, only 3-ADON and HT-2 toxins prevailed during the rainy season. For other toxins, there were no differences in the levels of contamination between the dry season and the rainy season (Table 4). As expected, the co-occurrence of two different toxins was the most common situation (i.e., n = 141/279, 50.5%) (Table 5). Therefore, as the number of simultaneous toxins increased, co-occurrence was less likely to be found (Table 5). In the case of the parent compound–metabolite comparison, the most common combination was the pair T-2/HT-2 toxin with (n = 66/155) 42.6% of prevalence, followed by FB_1/FB_2 (n = 23/137, 16.8%) and DON/3-ADON (n = 18/177, 10.2%) (Table 5).

Table 4. Seasonal prevalence and behavior per toxin.

		Concentration, mg kg^{-1}	
Season [a]	**Positive Samples, *n* (Prevalence, %)**	**Average ± SD**	**Maximum**
	3-ADON		
Rainy Season	36/145 (24.8)	2 ± 3	16
	DON		
Dry Season	57/101 (56.4)	3 ± 7	52
Rainy Season	130/229 (56.8)	17 ± 161	1830
	FB_1		
Dry Season	29/97 (29.9)	7 ± 12	40
Rainy Season	111/226 (49.1)	7 ± 13	77
	FB_2		
Dry Season	9/21 (42.9)	4 ± 8	23
Rainy Season	25/56 (44.6)	3 ± 4	19
	HT-2 toxin		
Rainy Season	96/180 (53.3)	1 ± 2	11
	T-2 toxin		
Dry Season	54/145 (37.2)	< 1	2
Rainy Season	94/248 (37.9)	< 1	1
	OTA, μg kg^{-1}		
Dry Season	31/112 (27.7)	7 ± 24	137
Rainy Season	88/204 (43.1)	37 ± 193	1810
	ZEA		
Dry Season	46/94 (48.9)	1 ± 1	6
Rainy Season	90/228 (39.5)	1 ± 6	4
	Overall Months with Higher Levels and Prevalence		
3-ADON	April and May	DON	No clear distribution
FB_1	June, July, and September	FB_2	April, June, and September
HT-2 toxin	October and November	T-2 toxin	No clear distribution
OTA	May and September	ZEA	May, July, and October

[a] Dry season and rainy season defined as per mean precipitation, the former exemplified by the months between December and April where $x < 80$ mm rain.

Table 5. Mycotoxin co-occurrence in the sample totals.

Number of Toxins Simultaneously Present	**2**	**3**	**4**	**5**	**6**	**7**
Samples, *n* (Incidence, %)	141/279 [a] (50.54)	81/279 (29.0)	36/279 (12.9)	17/279 (6.1)	1/279 (0.4)	3/279 (1.1)
Toxin/Metabolite	Sample Numbers with the toxin present, *n*		Co-occurrence, *n*		Incidence, %	
DON/3-ADON	177		18		10.2	
FB_1/FB_2	137		23		16.8	
T-2/HT-2 toxin	155		66		42.6	
Toxin Co-occurrence with OTA	**Sample Numbers, *n***				**Incidence, %**	
DON + HT-2 toxin + ZEA	1				1.0	
DON + 3-ADON + FB_1 + ZEA	1				1.0	

Table 5. *Cont.*

Number of Toxins Simultaneously Present	2	3	4	5	6	7
Samples, *n* (Incidence, %)	141/279 [a] (50.54)	81/279 (29.0)	36/279 (12.9)	17/279 (6.1)	1/279 (0.4)	3/279 (1.1)
Toxin/Metabolite	Sample Numbers with the toxin present, *n*	Co-occurrence, *n*		Incidence, %		
T-2 toxin + FB_1 + ZEA	1			1.0		
DON + FB1 + FB2 + ZEA	1			1.0		
3-ADON	1			1.0		
DON + 3-ADON + T-2 toxin + FB_1	1			1.0		
DON + HT-2 toxin + FB_1 + ZEA	2			2.0		
T-2 toxin + HT-2 toxin + FB_1 + ZEA	2			2.0		
DON + 3-ADON + T-2 toxin + HT-2 T-2 toxin + FB_1 + FB_2 + ZEA	2			2.0		
FB1 + ZEA	2			2.0		
T-2/HT-2 toxin + ZEA	3			2.9		
T-2 toxin + FB_1	3			2.9		
DON + T-2 toxin + HT-2 toxin	4			3.9		
DON + ZEA	4			3.9		
DON + T-2 + FB_1 + ZEA	6			5.9		
DON	7			6.9		
HT-2 toxin	8			7.8		
T-2 toxin	10			9.8		
FB_1/FB_2	12			11.8		
DON + FB_1	14			13.7		
ZEA	17			16.7		

[a] Corresponds to the total number of samples in which ≥ 2 simultaneous toxins occurred.

2.5. OTA Prevalence in Animal Feeds

Referring to OTA, the total prevalence from 2012 to 2017 was 40.6% (n = 146/360), ranging from 16.3% (n = 8/49) in 2013 to 76.6% (n = 49/64) in 2015. The maximum OTA reported level was 1810 μg kg^{-1}, in 2016 (Table 1). Only one sample exceeded the maximal advisory level for ochratoxin; this sample corresponded to poultry feed where the recommended concentration is 100 μg kg^{-1}. The overall OTA prevalence in non-traditional ingredients, poultry, and fish feed was of 56.3%, 44.4%, and 66.7%, respectively (Tables 2 and 3). Furthermore, in May and September, the highest global concentrations of OTA were presented, corresponding to the rainy season releasing an evident difference compared with the findings of the dry season (Table 4). As the presence of OTA involves other toxin-producing fungi (other than *Fusarium*), co-occurrence with other metabolites is a possibility. The most prevalent *Fusarium* toxins present in feed (different from OTA), in decreasing order of incidence, were ZEA, DON + FB_1, FB_1, and T-2 toxin with (n = 17/102) 16.7%, (n = 14/102) 13.7%, and (n = 12/102) 11.8% of incidence, respectively (Table 5). As expected, OTA incidence had a completely different geographical/spatial (Figure 1H) and thermo/temporal (Figure 2H) distribution, when compared with the other toxins.

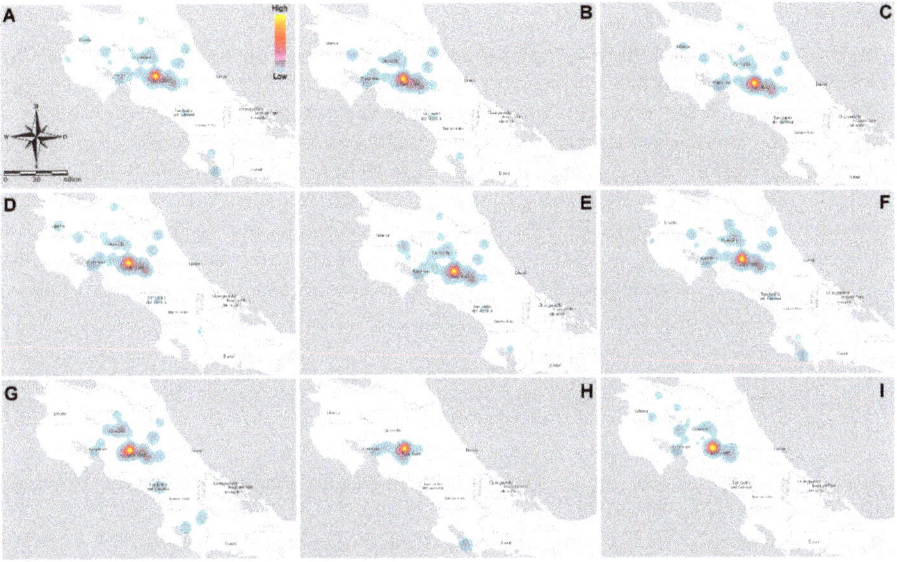

Figure 1. Heat map representing the geographical origin of samples and the mycotoxin concentration: (**A**) DON; (**B**) 3-ADON; (**C**) T-2 toxin; (**D**) HT-2 toxin; (**E**) ZEA; (**F**) FB_1; (**G**) FB_2; (**H**) OTA; and (**I**) AFM_1.

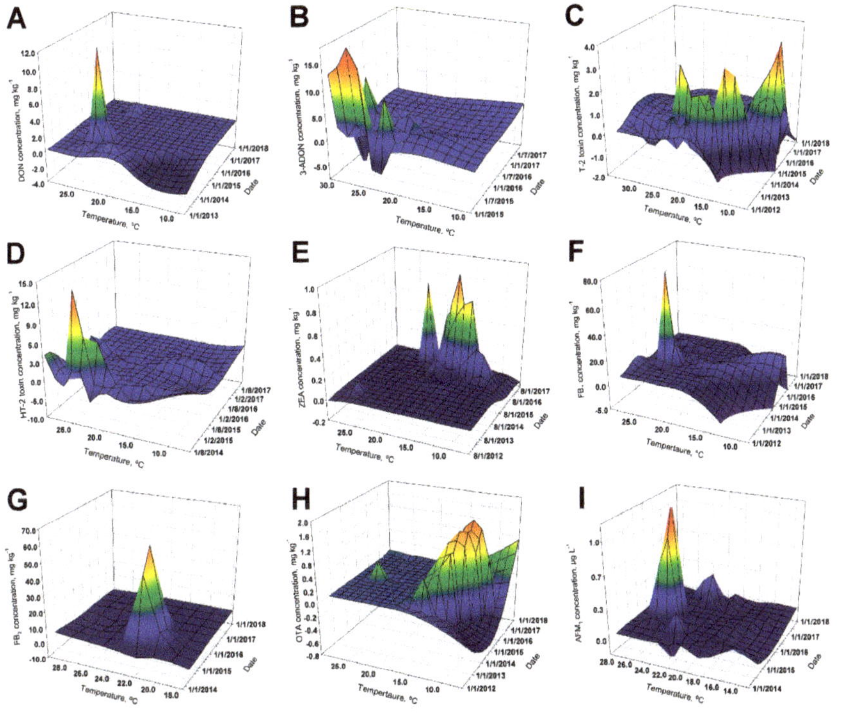

Figure 2. 3D mesh graphs representing the relationship among mycotoxin concentration, mean temperature, and sample date: (**A**) DON; (**B**) 3-ADON; (**C**) T-2 toxin; (**D**) HT-2 toxin; (**E**) ZEA; (**F**) FB_1; (**G**) FB_2; (**H**) OTA; and (**I**) AFM_1.

2.6. Aflatoxin M_1 in Liquid Milk

Water buffalo milk and butter samples were also analyzed for the presence of Aflatoxin M_1. Water buffalo (*Bubalus bubalis*) milk samples (n = 2) were reported below the limit of quantification (i.e., 0.014 µg kg^{-1}) and butter (n = 3) ranged from 0.021 to 0.024 µg kg^{-1}. Even though 2016 was the year with the lowest number of analyzed samples, it was also the year when fewer samples surpassed the 0.05 µg kg^{-1} threshold (Table 6). An increase in AFM_1 prevalence with 71.1% and 63.2%, respectively (Table 6), was observed during 2014 and 2017. Excluding three samples from 2015, there were no other samples surpassing the US FDA threshold of 0.5 µg kg^{-1}, thus representing a very small overall percentage for the four years of the study (i.e., n = 3/175, 1.7%). It was studied/monitored that, consistently, higher concentrations of AFM_1 were obtained during March, August, and September (Table 6 and Figure 2I).

Table 6. Prevalence and epidemiological data regarding AFM_1 in fresh bovine milk for four years.

				Concentration [b], ng mL^{-1}			
Year	**Positive Samples, n (Prevalence, %) [a]**	**Samples > 0.05 µg kg^{-1}, n (%)**	**Samples > 0.5 µg kg^{-1}, n (%)**	**Average ± SD**	**Median**	**Maximum**	**Minimum**
2017	24/38 (63.2)	16 (42.1)	0	0.083 ± 0.076	0.061	0.334	0.013
2016	8/27 (29.6)	2 (7.4)	0	0.042 ± 0.030	0.032	0.109	0.014
2015	34/73 (46.6)	16 (21.9)	3 (4.1)	0.154 ± 0.236	0.057	0.989	0.017
2014	32/45 (71.1)	11 (24.4)	0	0.042 ± 0.038	0.030	0.164	0.005
Overall	98/183 (53.5)	45 (45.9)	3 (3.1)	0.091 ± 0.155	0.049	0.989	0.005
Dry season [c]	28/45 (62.2)	14 (50.0)	0	0.075 ± 0.105	0.050	0.485	0.005
Rainy season [c]	69/138 (50.0)	34 (49.3)	3 (4.3)	0.098 ± 0.172	0.049	0.989	0.005
Overall months with higher levels and prevalence				March, August, and September			

[a] Prevalence understood as the number of samples > Limit of quantificaction of 0.014 µg kg^{-1}. [b] Values obtained using only positive samples, i.e., > limit of detection. [c] Dry season and rainy season defined as per mean precipitation, the former defined by the months between December and April where $x < 80$ mm rain.

3. Discussion

3.1. Mycotoxin Prevalence between 2013 and 2017 in Animal Feed

Most of the studied toxins (except for 3-ADON, FB_1, and HT-2) had prevalences higher than 40% during the five years. The average concentrations found in the different toxins in animal feed did not vary between one year and another, except for ZEA and T-2. The drastic increase of ZEA concentrations during 2017 was observed in corn meal and sorghum silo. There is a prior documented avidity of *Fusarium* spp. to produce ZEA when using moderately alkaline cereals (e.g., maize) as substrates [43]. A general drop in annual temperature may have provoked this upsurge in ZEA contamination. For example, *Fusarium graminearum* has demonstrated that conditions of pH 9 and incubation temperature of 15.05 °C are required to favor ZEA production [44]. Interestingly, the most toxicologically relevant levels for ZEA were encountered at relatively low temperatures (i.e., near 15 °C). Despite a relatively high prevalence for mycotoxins (i.e., between 46% and 99%, except for FB_1 + FB_2 and DON), the positive samples possessed comparatively low concentrations (Table 1) based on guidance values for mycotoxins in animal feeds within the European Union (see Appendix A Tables A1 and A2) [37,38]. This relatively low toxicological burden could be associated with the control of mycotoxin in animal feed and raw materials that were established in the country since 2007. This control policy covers the majority of the toxins analyzed in this study added to the control of imported raw materials, before its distribution. In coherence to what has been stated, since 2013, proficient manufacturing practices have been evaluated and audited by regulation in animal feed plants. These proficient practices involve the management of raw materials and storage measures, among others, contributing to the reduction of mycotoxin contamination [45].

However, some of the samples were observed with concentrations above the established guidelines with potentially adverse effects on animal health and productivity. It is worth of mentioning the fact that human health could be affected through the consumption of foods of animal origin contaminated with mycotoxins or their metabolites [24,27,28].

3.2. Mycotoxin Prevalence in Compound Feed and Feed Ingredients

3.2.1. Prevalence in Feed Ingredients

Vegetable ingredients may represent from 80% to 100% of the feed (e.g., in ruminants, animal origin ingredients are prohibited) [14,46,47]. For these vegetable-based formulations, corn and soybean meal may represent up to 60% of the input [14,15]. Costa Rican soybean meal and corn, as well as other relevant ingredients, are imported [18]. Quality grain assessment is a degree-based classification. Usually, grade 2 or 3 corn is purchased for feed production [18]. At least 97.9% of the samples contain around 3% of cracked material, and 36.2% of the samples exhibited higher moisture content (i.e., 17%); both factors promote the proliferation of fungi [48]. Toxin-wise, AFB_1, and DON were assayed and are regulated according to FDA criteria. Only 1.9% samples exceeded levels for AFB_1 but none for DON [49]. The data reveal coherence with the obtained results (Table 2). Notwithstanding, a high prevalence for DON was detected and reported by other researchers both for corn and wheat [49]. Conversely, a relatively lower incidence was found in OTA, different from what was conveyed elsewhere [50].

3.2.2. Prevalence in Cattle Feeds

In both dairy and meat cattle, forage, hay, and silage input must not be underplayed, especially in countries where extensive feeding systems based on grazing cattle predominate. Considering Costa Rica a particular case, 85% and 95.9% of the dairy and beef cattle are based on grazing farming, respectively [51]. Relatively favorable toxin profiles were still found in the tested samples. Thereby, surveillance efforts have been focused on compound feed. Generally speaking, ruminants are relatively less sensitive toward the effects of mycotoxins as rumen bacteria play a detoxification role [35,38]. For example, for DON (prevalence of 70.0% and 55.1% in beef cattle feed and dairy cattle feed, respectively), Charmley and collaborators determined that concentrations of 6000 $\mu g\ kg^{-1}$ neither affect feed intake nor are biotransferred to the milk [36,52].

3.2.3. Prevalence in Compound Feed destined for Poultry and Swine

Mycotoxin effects over monogastric animals are varied, depending on the species and physiological and productive stage [53]. For example, in pigs, fumonisin feed contamination is related to pulmonary, hepatic and cardiovascular lesions [54] while DON has been associated with a reduction of productive parameters and feed efficiency [54]. Besides, pigs are especially sensitive to ZEA, as it is directly related to reproductive disorders and low fertility rates [55]. Mycotoxin findings in poultry feed are also worrisome as birds are noticeably susceptible to molecules such as DON. For example, in broilers, trichothecene exposure (e.g., DON), through feed, increases mortality, reduces immune function, and impairs weight gain [56].

3.2.4. Prevalence in Pet Food

Mycotoxins in pet foods have already been reported by other countries, including industrialized ones (e.g., Portugal, USA, England, and Brazil) [57]. Mainly, *Fusarium* and *Penicillium* toxins have been described [51]. An elevated prevalence was described for DON and FB_1 (50.0% and 93.3%, respectively) [58]. Mycotoxicosis in pets is associated with chronic disease, liver and kidney damage, and cancer [58]. Finding mycotoxins in thermally treated foods is not uncommon as mycotoxins molecules can withstand relatively elevated temperature; low toxin reduction will occur during extrusion. Fungi colonization of pet extruded food is expected to be low as it possesses relatively low values of moisture and water activity [58,59]. Mycotoxin in pet foods may represent an additional burden to humans due to the pet closeness with their owners.

3.2.5. Prevalence in Fish Feed

Presence of mycotoxins in fish feed is another proof of an industry which has progressively substituted animal protein sources for vegetable ones [60,61]. In this regard, DON, OTA, and ZEA have been said to be responsible for weight loss, exacerbated feed conversion, and increased susceptibility to infection and disease in fish [61,62]. In line with the data reported herein, a recent report revealed that commercial fish feed samples were frequently contaminated with DON (i.e., over 80% of the samples) with mean concentrations of 289 μg kg^{-1} [49]. Levels as low as 4.5 mg DON kg^{-1} feed have already confirmed adverse effects in productive parameters and increased mortality in some fish. even in a relatively short period [62].

3.3. *Geographical Distribution and Climate Influence for Fusarium Toxins Present in Animal Feed*

A different spatial distribution profile was observed for AFM_1 and OTA, which are not produced by *Fusarium* species. *Fusarium* species have the potential of simultaneously producing the remainder of the toxins assayed [63,64]. OTA is a toxin produced by several fungal species including *Aspergillus ochraceus*, *A. carbonarius*, *A. niger* and *Penicillium verrucosum* [65]. On the other hand, AFM_1 is not only produced by *Aspergillus* species but it is also a product of metabolism [66]. Our data not only demonstrate that most sampling weight is centered on the Costa Rican Central Valley plateau, but the largest concentrations also occur therein (geographical zones with a high average relative humidity of 82%). The data also demonstrate that the intricate climate in tropical countries (such as Costa Rica) predicts the behavior of mycotoxin contamination as more challenging.

3.4. *Aflatoxin M_1 in Liquid Milk*

Milk is not only a staple commodity by itself, but it can accompany other potentially contaminated products (e.g., coffee, tea, or chocolate). Additionally, although AFM_1 is the most studied toxin in milk, other toxins have been described as well [67]. Other dairy products are derived from this raw material (e.g., cheese). Although processing is involved, these other dairy products can carry by themselves aflatoxin metabolites as well (see, for example, [68]). During 2017 alone, milk consumption was calculated to be 212 kg per capita [18]. Assuming the worst-case scenario (a sample with the highest concentration of 0.989 μg kg^{-1}), a Costa Rican citizen could be exposed up to 210 μg AFM_1 per year. Similarly, a Jersey calf weighing 25–30 kg at birth would be fed with 10% of its live weight with contaminated milk (from 2.5 to 3 kg of milk per day) [69]. Reiteratively, this means a daily exposure of 2.5–3 μg AFM_1 per day. Milk weaning can occur at ten weeks old [70]. Milk consumption level exposure is estimated to be 0.023 ng AFM_1 per kg body weight per day when a maximum level of 0.5 μg kg^{-1} is used.

Much higher average concentrations of AFM_1 have been documented in other Latin-American countries [71]. Interestingly, AFB_1 (the parent compound of AFM_1) has been reported to be present in milk samples [71]). Besides the toxic burden that AFB_1 and AFM_1 have in the liver, recent evidence suggests that kidney toxicity is a certainty [66]. On the other hand, considerably low (i.e., 0.037 μg kg^{-1}) AFM_1 levels in milk have been recently reported, although prevalence rates are also relatively high (i.e., 38.8%), [71]. Other Latin-American countries have reported similar percentages [72–75], and recent prevalence studies have been published in industrialized countries [76–79]. Epidemiological studies [1] and risk assessment [80–82] are paramount to reduce mycotoxin exposure to both humans and animals.

Aflatoxin-contaminated feed must also be monitored to avoid feeding dairy cows with contaminated batches [83]. For instance, the association among most aflatoxin-contaminated feed ingredients and prevalence has been detailed [36,73]. Although the samples reported herein come from a highly industrialized sector, similar prevalence has been reported in fresh milk from small farms [84]. Consistent with our results, the seasonal distribution does not seem to affect AFM_1 prevalence [71], probably because Costa Rica has a tropical climate. In general, Costa Rica has relatively high temperatures (19–30°C), humidity (60–91%) and abundant rainfall (1400–4500 mm per year) during a great part of the year (i.e., two distinct seasons), in opposition to an Iranian study exhibited a lower prevalence of AFM_1 in bovine milk during spring [85]. Seasonal variations (i.e., during rainy season) were also described for milk from other species (i.e., sheep, goat, and camel) [81]. Other researchers have not documented a clear tendency regarding AFM_1 occurrence during seasons [73]. It has been suggested, however, that climate change can bear an impact on human exposure to aflatoxins and health [85]. Finally, the burden of AFM_1 exposure for a human can be twice as much as breast milk contamination, as has also been well documented [86]. Although some methods for reducing AFM_1 contamination are available [87], pre- and post-harvest strategies are still the most effective strategies [88].

4. Conclusions

Toxicologically relevant concentrations were found during the five-year survey as some sample concentrations exceeded the regulatory guidelines. Fumonisin and deoxynivalenol feed contamination is worrisome since these toxins have the capacity of being found in significant levels in these matrices, and, in our case, higher levels of toxins are found in the Central Valley of the country. Therefore, surveillance programs should be expanded to the outermost productive regions of the country to suppress sampling bias, if existing any. Thermopluvial conditions do not seem to have a considerable effect on toxin levels, although some metabolites actually seem to behave concurrently. *Fusarium* metabolites must be stridently monitored as it is clear that contamination in feed and feed ingredients is unfortunately common; this is especially true for fumonisins and T-2. Feed manufacturers, farmers (both in the field and storage facilities) and pet owners alike should be educated as to the proper conditions for food storage to avoid mycotoxin-producing fungal colonization. Toxin metabolite analysis and co-occurrence are paramount for complete surveillance of toxin feeds, and efficiently execute systems for the control and reduction of mycotoxins, as well as their metabolites in feeds. In addition, a strict control of AFM_1 in milk is necessary, because the prevalence of AFM_1 in milk is considerable and several samples exceeded the regulatory thresholds. It must be remembered that milk is the raw material for a wide variety of dairy products (butter, cheese, and yogurt, among others), therefore, the exposure of the population to this mycotoxin is increased.

5. Materials and Methods

5.1. Reagents

An analytical standard with certified concentrations, dissolved in acetonitrile, for DON, 3-ADON, T-2 (TSL-314), HT-2 (TSL-333), ZEA (TSL-401), FB_1, FB_2 (TSL-202), and OTA (TSL-504) was purchased from Trilogy® Analytical Laboratory Inc (Washington, MO, USA). All standards have an initial concentration of 100 mg L^{-1}, except for FB_2 that was at 30 mg L^{-1}. Additionally, a naturally contaminated reference material (TRMT100, cornmeal) was used as a quality control sample (TS-108, Washington, MO, USA). Acetonitrile (ACN) and methanol (MeOH), both chromatographic grade, were purchased from J.T. Baker (Avantor Materials, Center Valley, PA, USA). Ultrapure water (type I, 0.055 µS cm^{-1} at 25°C, 5 µg L^{-1} TOC) was obtained using an A10 Milli-Q Advantage system and an Elix 35 system (Merck KGaA, Darmstadt, Germany).

5.2. Sampling

A total of n = 487 different feedstuffs of ca. 5 kg were collected during 2013–2017 by government inspectors from n = 107 Costa Rican feed manufacturers, as part of a countrywide surveillance program. Sample collection was composed of compound feed and feed ingredients, as follows: dairy cattle feed

28.9% (n = 141), cornmeal 9.9% (n = 48), citrus pulp 5.5% (n = 27), cattle feed 5.5% (n = 27), pig feed 5.3% (n = 26), calf feed 4.3% (n = 21), palm kernel meal 4.1% (n = 20), fish feed (Tilapia) 3.7% (n = 18), poultry feed 3.5% (n = 17), distillers dried grains 3.5% (n = 17), hay 3.3% (n = 16), dog food 3.3% (n = 16), wheat middlings 2.9% (n = 14), soybean meal 2.7% (n = 13), layer hen feed 2.0% (n = 10), horse feed 1.8% (n = 9), forage 1.8% (n = 7), pineapple byproducts 1.2% (n = 6), cassava meal 1.2% (n = 6), sorghum meal 0.6% (n = 3), rodent feed 0.6% (n = 3), ground roasted coffee 0.6% (n = 3), banana peel 0.6% (n = 3), rice bran 0.4% (n = 2), chamomile flowers 0.4% (n = 2), soybean hulls 0.2% (n = 1), shrimp feed 0.2% (n = 1), rice meal 0.2% (n = 1), rabbit feed 0.2% (n = 1), hydrolyzed feather meal 0.2% (n = 1), fish feed (snapper, n = 1), fish feed (salmon and trout, n = 1), corn silage (n = 1), and corn gluten (n = 1). Selection of feed and feed ingredients to be tested, number of samples, sampling sites, and specific toxins to assay (per matrix) were chosen by feed control officials. The selection considered the most common feedstuffs used in Costa Rica, import and export regulations, contamination risk factors, the productivity of the feed industry, and the risk for human and animal health associated with each feed or feed ingredient. Sampling was performed following the Association of American Feed Control Officials (AAFCO) recommendations for mycotoxin test object collection [89], and samples were taken from silos and storage reservoirs from feed manufacturing plants. All samples were quartered and sieved (1 mm particle size) [89]. Additionally, n = 180 dairy samples (mostly liquid bovine milk) from n = 13 different Costa Rican dairy farms were assayed; 50 mL subsamples were processed from 500 mL samples.

5.3. *Reference Methods for Toxin Determination*

Mycotoxins were assayed using the following methods: DON/3-ADON [90], T-2 and HT-2 toxins [91], ZEA AOAC 976.22, fumonisins AOAC 995.15, and OTA AOAC 991.44. AFM_1 was assayed according to the methods in [36,92] for milk and butter, respectively.

5.4. *Chromatographic System and Conditions*

All analytes were assayed using HPLC. Equipment consisted of an Agilent 1260 Infinity series HPLC with a quaternary pump (G1311B), a column compartment (G1316A), a variable wavelength and fluorescence detector (G1314B and G1321B) and an autosampler system (G1329A) (Agilent Technologies, Santa Clara, CA, USA). Peak separation was accomplished using a 5 mm Agilent Zorbax Eclipse C_{18} column (3.0 × 150 mm, 5 µm) except for T-2/HT-2 toxin analyses for which a Luna® Phenyl-Hexyl column (4.6 × 150 mm, 5 µm) was used (Phenomenex, Torrance, CA, USA). All analytes, except AFM_1, were extracted using Immunoaffinity columns (R-biopharm Rhône Ltd, Darmstadt, Germany).

5.4.1. DON/3-ADON

DONPREP® (R-biopharm) columns were used for sample extraction. Briefly, 200 mL of purified H_2O was added to 25 g of test portion. The mixture was dispersed using an Ultra-Turrax® (T25, IKA Works GmbH & Co, Staufen, Germany) at 8000 rpm. The supernatant was filtered by gravity over an ashless filter paper (Grade 541, Whatman®, GE Healthcare Life Sciences, Marlborough, MA, USA). Subsequently, an exact 2 mL aliquot from the supernatant was transferred to the IAC column and passed at 1 mL min^{-1} using an SPE 12 port vacuum manifold (57044, Visiprep™, Supelco Inc., Bellefonte, PA, USA) at 15 mm Hg vacuum. After a washing step using 2× 10 mL water, the columns were left to dry and then four MeOH fractions of 500 µL were passed through the IAC. The total volume recovered was concentrated to dryness under vacuum at 60°C. The sample was reconstituted with MeOH to 300 µL and transferred to an analytical HPLC conical vial insert (5182-0549, Agilent Technologies, Santa Clara, CA, USA) before injection into the chromatograph.

Gradient mode starting at 80:20 H_2O, Solvent A/CH_3OH, Solvent B as per chromatographic conditions. The rest of the program was as follows: at 0.5 min 80% A, at 5.50 min 90% A, at 10 min 90% A, at 11 min 80% A, and at 15 min 80% A. DON and 3-ADON absorption at 220 nm was exploited for detection purposes. Linear calibration curves ranging from 1.25 to 10.00 μg mL^{-1} were prepared during quantification. The limit of quantification for DON/3-ADON was 10.00 and 40.00 μg kg^{-1}.

5.4.2. T-2 and HT-2 Toxin

The extraction was similarly performed as detailed for DON/3ADON using an EASI-EXTRACT® T-2 and HT-2 IAC (R-biopharm). Extraction solvent consisted in 125 mL of MeOH/H_2O (90:10) and 2.5 g of NaCl. An aliquot of 5 mL 10-fold diluted in PBS (1.37 mol L^{-1}) was passed through the column. Precolumn derivatization was performed after the evaporation step using 50 μL of 4-dimethylaminopyridine (107700, Sigma-Aldrich, St. Louis, Mo, USA) and 50 μL of 1-anthroyl cyanide (017-12101, FUJIFILM (Wako Pure Chemical Corporation, Osaka, Japan) both at 1 mg mL^{-1} in toluene (TX0737, Sigma-Aldrich). Gradient mode started at 70:30 CH_3CN, Solvent A/H_2O, Solvent B as per chromatographic conditions. The rest of the program was as follows: at 5 min 70% A, at 15 min 70% A, at 25 min 85% A, at 27 min 100% A, at 32 min 100% A, and at 35 min 70% A. Flow rate was set at 1 mL min^{-1}. Adduct fluorescence was measured at λ_{ex} = 381 and λ_{em} = 470 nm. Linear calibration curves ranging from 125.00 to 1000.00 μg L^{-1} were prepared during quantification. The limit of quantification for T-2 and HT-2, was 5.00 and 3.00 μg kg^{-1}, respectively.

5.4.3. ZEA

Extraction was performed using 100 mL of CH_3CN/H_2O 60:40 and an EASI-EXTRACT® ZEARALENONE IAC (R-biopharm). Isocratic mode using a 40:10:50 $CH_3CN/CH_3OH/H_2O$ mixture at a flow rate of 0.7 mL min^{-1} was used as per chromatographic conditions. ZEA natural fluorescence (at λ_{ex} = 236, λ_{em} = 464 nm) was exploited for detection purposes. Linear calibration curves ranging from 300.00 to 1200.00 μg L^{-1} were prepared during quantification. The limit of quantification was 0.072 μg kg^{-1}.

5.4.4. FB_1 and FB_2

Extraction was performed using 100 mL of CH_3CN/MeOH/H_2O (25:25:50) and FUMONIPREP® IAC (R-biopharm). Fumonisin derivatization was based on the reaction with *o*-phthalaldehyde (Millipore Sigma, P0657) and 2-mercaptoethanol (Millipore Sigma, 97622) as stated on the reference method. However, pre-column derivatization was performed in situ in the autosampler injector, according to Bartolomeo and Maisano (2006), but increasing the sample and OPA reagent volume 5-fold. Adduct fluorescence was measured at λ_{ex} = 335 and λ_{em} = 440 nm. Isocratic mode using MeOH/0.1 mol L^{-1} NaH_2PO_4 (77:23), adjusted to apparent pH 3.3 with H_3PO_4, was used at a 0.8 mL min^{-1} flow rate. The limit of quantification was 0.05 μg kg^{-1} for both FB_1 and FB_2.

5.4.5. OTA

Extraction was performed using 100 mL of CH_3CN/H_2O 60:40 and an OCRAPREP® IAC column. OTA elution from column and resuspension after evaporation was achieved using a 98:2 MeOH and acetic acid solution to ensure OTA protonation. Isocratic mode using a 50:50 H_2O/CH_3CN mixture using 0.2 mol L^{-1} trifluoroacetic acid, pH = 2.1 (74564 Millipore Sigma) at a flow rate of 0.7 mL min^{-1} was used as per chromatographic conditions. OTA natural fluorescence (at λ_{ex} = 247, λ_{em} = 480 nm) was exploited for detection purposes. Linear calibration curves ranging from 2.50 to 40 μg L^{-1} were prepared during quantification. The limit of quantification was 0.011 μg kg^{-1}.

5.4.6. AFM_1 in Milk and Butter

AflaStar® M_1 (Romer Labs Diagnostic GmbH, Tulln an der Donau, Austria) columns were used for sample extraction. An exact 50 mL of raw or processed milk, previously homogenized and filtered by gravity over an ashless filter paper, was transferred to the IAC column. After a washing step using 3 × 10 mL of water, the columns were left to dry and eluted using MeOH and concentrated as described above in 5.4.1. Isocratic mode using a 10:35:55 $CH_3CN/CH_3OH/H_2O$ mixture at a flow rate of 0.6 mL min^{-1} was used as per chromatographic conditions. AFM_1 natural fluorescence (at λ_{ex} = 365, λ_{em} = 455 nm) was exploited for detection purposes. Linear calibration curves ranging from 0.50 to 2.00 μg L^{-1} were prepared during quantification. The limit of quantification was 0.014 μg kg^{-1}.

In the case of the butter samples, the preparation was performed according to the method in [84]. Briefly, 25 mL of aqueous methanol (70 mL/100 mL) was added to 5 g of butter. Afterwards, the solution was extracted by mixing gently for 10 min at room temperature using sonication. The extract was filtered through a paper filter, and 15 mL of distilled water was added to 5 mL of filtered solution. After that, 0.25 mL of Tween 20 were added and dispersed for 2 min, followed by the entire amount of the sample solution (20 mL) passing over the IAC.

5.5. Data Analysis

For Tables 1–3, prevalence is expressed as the ratio between the total of assays above the limit of detection and the total of assays performed for each toxin. Descriptive statistics displayed in Table 1 are expressed without considering samples below the limit of detection. Heat maps used in Figure 1 were rendered using ArcGIS Pro v2.2 (Esri™, Redlands, CA, USA). For each contaminant, Spearman Rank Order tests were applied to assess the association among the toxin concentration and climatic variables (i.e., precipitation, rainy days and temperature). In this particular case, toxin levels below the limit of detection were considered zero for association purposes; this analysis was performed using SigmaPlot 14 (Systat Software Inc., San Jose, CA, USA). Sampling date was linked to mean monthly values and data were retrieved from the closest climatological station to the sampling region. Meteorological data were provided by the Costa Rican National Weather Service (https://www.imn.ac.cr/boletin-meteorologico).

Author Contributions: Conceptualization, F.G.-C., and M.A.-C.; methodology, A.L., G.C., and F.G.-C.; validation, F.G.-C.; formal analysis, F.G.-C. and A.L.; resources, M.A.-C., G.C., and F.G.-C.; data curation, A.M. and F.G.-C.; writing—original draft preparation, A.M., A.L. and F.G.-C.; writing—review and editing, F.G.-C.; visualization, F.G.-C. and A.L.; supervision, F.G.-C.; project administration, M.A.-C. and G.C.; and funding acquisition, A.M.

Funding: The University of Costa Rica funded this research through grants ED-427 and ED-428, and the APC was supported by the Office of the Vice Provost for Research of the University of Costa Rica.

Acknowledgments: Geovanna Méndez is acknowledged for tabulating the data that corresponds to the year 2017. Special thanks to Mauricio Redondo-Solano and María Sabrina Sánchez for their suggestions, revising the manuscript and for language editing.

Conflicts of Interest: The authors declare no conflict of interest.

Appendix A

Table A1. Indicative Levels for T-2 and HT-2 in Cereals and Cereal products according to UE [a].

Matrix	Indicative Levels for the Sum of T-2 and HT-2 (μg kg^{-1}) from Which Onwards/above Which Investigations Should be Performed, Certainly in Case of Repetitive Findings
Unprocessed Cereals	
Barley (including malting barley) and maize	200
Oats (with husk)	1000
Wheat, rye and other cereals	100
Cereal Products for Feed and Compound Feed	
Oat milling products (husks)	2000
Other cereal products	500
Compound feed with the exception of feed for cats	250

[a] Based on Reference [38] and according to 2013/165/EU. Please see notes contained in each recommendation.

Table A2. Relevant guidance values for each mycotoxin in products intended for animal feed according to UE [a].

Mycotoxin	Products Intended for Animal Feed	Guidance Value in mg kg^{-1} Relative to a Feedstuff with a Moisture Content of 12 g/100 g
Deoxynivalenol	Feed materials	
	Cereals and cereal products with the exception	8
	Cereals and cereal products with the exception	12
	Compound feed (exception of compound feed for pigs, calves (<4 months), lambs, kids and dogs)	5
	Compound feed for pigs	0.9
	Compound feed for calves (<4 months), lambs, kids and dogs	2
Zearalenone	Feed materials	
	Cereals and cereal products with the exception of maize byproducts	2
	Maize byproducts	3
	Compound feed for:	
	Piglets, gilts (young sows), puppies, kittens, dogs and cats for reproduction	0.1
	Adult dogs and cats other than for reproduction	0.2
	Sows and fattening pigs	0.25
	Calves, dairy cattle, sheep (including lamb) and goats (kids)	0.5
Ochratoxin A	Feed materials	
	Cereals and cereal products	0.25
	Compound feed for	
	Pigs	0.05
	Poultry	0.1
	Cats and dogs	0.01
Fumonisin FB_1 + FB_2	Feed materials	
	Maize and maize products	60
	Compound feed for	
	Pigs, horses (*Equidae*), rabbits and pet animals	5
	Fish	
	Poultry, calves (<4 months), lambs and kids	20
	Adult ruminants (> 4 months) and mink	50
T2 + HT-2	Compound Feed for Cats	0.05

[a] Based on Reference [37] and according to 2006/576/EC, 2016/1319, and definitions stated in 68/2013/EC. Please see notes contained in each recommendation.

References

1. Tola, M.; Kebede, B. Occurrence, Importance and Control of Mycotoxins: A Review. *Cogent Food Agric.* **2016**. [CrossRef]
2. Lee, H.J.; Ryu, D. Worldwide occurrence of mycotoxins in cereals and cereal derived food products: Public Health Perspectives of their Co-occurrence. *J. Agric. Food Chem.* **2017**, *65*, 7034–7051. [CrossRef] [PubMed]
3. Arcella, D.; Gergelova, P.; Innocenti, M.L.; Steinkellner, H. Human and animal dietary exposure to T-2 and HT-2. *EFSA J.* **2017**, *15*, 4972.
4. Chen, S.S.; Li, Y.-H.; Lin, M.-F. Chronic Exposure to the *Fusarium* Mycotoxin Deoxynivalenol: Impact on Performance, Immune Organ, and Intestinal Integrity of Slow-Growing Chickens. *Toxins* **2017**, *9*, 334. [CrossRef] [PubMed]
5. Zhang, Y.; Han, J.; Zhu, C.-C.; Tang, F.; Cui, X.-S.; Kim, N.-H. Exposure to HT-2 toxins causes oxidative stress-induced apoptosis/autophagy in porcine oocytes. *Sci. Rep.* **2016**, *6*, 33904. [CrossRef]
6. Ismail, Z.; Basha, E.A.; Al-Nabulsi, F. Mycotoxins in animal feed, hazardous to both animals and human health. *J. Vet. Med. Res.* **2018**, *5*, 1145.
7. Bertero, A.; Moretti, A.; Spicer, L.J.; Caloni, F. Fusarium Molds and Mycotoxins: Potential Species-Specific Effects. *Toxins* **2018**, *10*, 244. [CrossRef] [PubMed]

8. Kinoshita, A.; Keese, C.; Meyer, U.; Starke, A.; Wrenzycki, C.; Dänicke, S.; Rehage, J. Chronic Effects of Fusarium Mycotoxins in rations with or without Increased Concentrate Proportion on the Insulin Sensitivity in Lactating Dairy Cows. *Toxins* **2018**, *10*, 188. [CrossRef] [PubMed]
9. Ashiq, S. Natural Occurrence of Mycotoxins in Food and Feed: Pakistan Perspective. *Compr. Rev. Food Sci. Food Saf.* **2015**, *14*, 159–175. [CrossRef]
10. Antonissen, G.; Van Immerseel, F.; Pasmans, F.; Ducatelle, R.; Haesebrouck, F.; Timbermont, L.; Verlinden, M.; Janssens, G.P.J.; Eeckhaut, V.; Eekhpout, M.; et al. The mycotoxin deoxynivalenol predisposes for the development of Clostridium perfringens-induced necrotic enteritis in broiler chickens. *PLoS ONE* **2014**, *9*, e108775. [CrossRef] [PubMed]
11. Streit, E.; Schatzmayr, G.; Tassis, P.; Tzika, E.; Marin, D.; Taranu, I.; Tabuc, C.; Nicoau, A.; Aprodu, I.; Puel, O.; et al. Current Situation of Mycotoxin Contamination and Co-occurrence in Animal Feed-Focus on Europe. *Toxins* **2012**, *4*, 788–809. [CrossRef] [PubMed]
12. Greco, M.; Pardo, A.; Pose, G. Mycotoxigenic Fungi and Natural Co-Occurrence of Mycotoxins in Rainbow Trout (*Oncorhynchus mykiss*) Feeds. *Toxins* **2015**, *7*, 4595–4609. [CrossRef] [PubMed]
13. Ismaeil, A.A.; Papenbrock, J. Mycotoxins: Producing Fungi and Mechanisms of Phytotoxicity. *Agriculture* **2015**, *5*, 492–537. [CrossRef]
14. Rostagno, H.; Teixeira, L.; Hannas, M.; Lopes, J.; Kazue, N.; Perazzo, F.; Saraiva, A.; Teixeira de Abreu, M.; Borges, P.; Flávia De Oliveira, R.; et al. *Tablas Brasileñas Para aves y Cerdos*, 4th ed.; Universidad Federal de Viçosa, Departamento de Zootecnia: Viçosa, Brasil, 2017; pp. 28–256.
15. De Blass, C.; Mateos, G.G.; García-Rebollar, P. *Tablas FEDNA de Composición y Valor Nutritivo de Alimentos Para la Fabricación de Piensos Compuestos*, 3rd ed.; Fundación Española para el Desarrollo de la Nutrición Animal: Madrid, Spain, 2010; Available online: http://www.fundacionfedna.org/ingredientes-para-piensos (accessed on 4 February 2019).
16. SEPSA [Secretaría Ejecutiva de Planificación Agropecuaria]. Informe de Comercio Exterior del Sector Agropecuario 2016–2017. 2018. Available online: http://www.sepsa.go.cr/docs/2018-004-Informe_Comercio_Exterior_Sector_Agropecuario_2016-2017.pdf (accessed on 4 February 2019).
17. Chacón, M. Evolución del Cultivo de Maíz en Costa Rica. Oficina Nacional de Semillas, 2017. Available online: http://ofinase.go.cr/certificacion-de-semillas/certificacion-de-semillas-de-maiz/evolucion-cultivo-maiz/ (accessed on 4 February 2019).
18. CIAB [Cámara de Industriales de Alimentos Balanceados]. Situación Actual de Alimentos Balanceados—Informe Anual. 2018. Available online: https://www.ciabcr.com/charlas/Nutrici%C3%B3n%20Animal%202018/Charlas/Carl_Oroz.pdf (accessed on 4 February 2019).
19. Karlovsky, P.; Suman, M.; Berthiller, F.; De Meester, J.; Eisenbrand, G.; Perrin, I.; Oswald, I.P.; Speijers, G.; Chiodini, A.; Recker, T.; et al. Impact of food processing and detoxification treatments on mycotoxin contamination. *Mycotoxin Res.* **2016**, *32*, 179. [CrossRef] [PubMed]
20. Ma, R.; Zhang, L.; Su, Y.-T.; Xie, W.-M.; Zhang, N.-Y.; Dai, J.-F.; Wang, Y.; Rajput, S.A.; Qi, D.-S.; Karrow, N.A.; et al. Individual and Combined Occurrence of Mycotoxins in Feed Ingredients and Complete Feeds in China. *Toxins* **2018**, *10*, 113. [CrossRef] [PubMed]
21. Chagwa, R.; Abia, W.; Msagati, T.; Nyoni, H.; Ndleve, K.; Njobeh, P. Multi-Mycotoxin Occurrence in Dairy Cattle Feeds from the Gauteng Province of South Africa: A Pilot Study Using UHPLC-QTOF-MS/MS. *Toxins* **2018**, *10*, 294. [CrossRef] [PubMed]
22. Franco, L.T.; Petta, T.; Rottinghaus, G.E.; Bordin, K.; Gomes, G.A.; Oliveira, C.A.F. Co-occurrence of mycotoxins in maize food and maize-based feed from small-scale farms in Brazil: A pilot study. *Mycotoxin Res.* **2018**. [CrossRef]
23. Ul Hassan, Z.; Al Thani, R.; Atia, F.A.; Al Meer, S.; Migheli, Q.; Jaoua, S. Co-occurrence of mycotoxins in commercial formula milk and cereal-based baby food in Qatar. *Food Addit. Contam. Part B* **2018**, *11*, 191–197. [CrossRef] [PubMed]
24. Bozzo, G.; Bonerba, E.; Ceci, E.; Valeriana, C.; Tantillo, G. Determination of ochratoxin A in eggs and target tissues of experimentally drugged hens using HPLC–FLD. *Food Chem.* **2011**, *126*, 1278–1282.
25. Payros, D.; Alassane-Kpembi, I.; Pierron, A.; Loiseau, N.; Pinton, P.; Oswald, I.P. Toxicology for deoxynivalenol and its acetylated and modified forms. *Arch. Toxicol.* **2016**, *90*, 2931–2957. [CrossRef]

26. Munkvold, G.P.; Arias, S.; Taschl, I.; Gruber-Dorninger, C. Chapter 9: Mycotoxin in Corn: Occurrence, Impacts and Management. In *Corn*; AACC International Press: St. Paul, MN, USA, 2019; pp. 235–287. [CrossRef]
27. Guerre, P. Fusariotoxins in Avian Species: Toxicokinetics, Metabolism, and Persistence in Tissues. *Toxins* **2015**, *7*, 2289–2305. [CrossRef] [PubMed]
28. Alshannaq, A.; Yu, J.H. Occurrence, Toxicity, and Analysis of Major Mycotoxins in Food. *Int. J. Envron. Res. Public Health* **2017**, *14*, 632. [CrossRef] [PubMed]
29. Krska, R.; Sulyok, M.; Berthiller, F.; Schuhmacher, R. Mycotoxin testing: From Multi toxin analysis to metabolomics. *JSM Mycotoxins* **2017**, *67*, 11–16. [CrossRef]
30. Van der Fels-Klerx, H.J.; Adamse, P.; Punt, A.; van Asselt, E.D. Data analyses and modeling for risk-based monitoring of mycotoxins in animal feed. *Toxins* **2018**, *10*, 54. [CrossRef] [PubMed]
31. Streit, E.; Naehrer, K.; Rodrigues, I.; Schatzmayr, G. Mycotoxin occurrence in feed and feed raw materials worldwide: Long-term analysis with special focus on Europe and Asia. *J. Sci. Food Agric.* **2013**, *93*, 2892–2899. [CrossRef]
32. Pinotti, L.; Ottoboni, M.; Giormini, C.; Dell'Orto, V.; Cheli, F. Mycotoxin Contamination in the EU Feed Supply Chain: A Focus on Cereal Byproducts. *Toxins* **2016**, *8*, 45. [CrossRef]
33. Rodrigues, I.; Naehrer, K. A Thre-Year Survey on the Worldwide Occurrence of mycotoxins in feedstuff and feed. *Toxins* **2012**, *4*, 663–675. [CrossRef]
34. Selvaraj, J.N.; Wang, Y.; Zhou, L.; Zhao, Y.; Xing, F.; Dai, X.; Liu, Y. Recent mycotoxin survey data and advanced mycotoxin detection techniques reported from China: A review. *Food Addit. Contam. Part A* **2015**, *32*, 440–452. [CrossRef]
35. Granados-Chinchilla, F.; Molina, A.; Chavarría, G.; Alfaro-Cascante, M.; Bogantes, D.; Murillo-Williams, A. Aflatoxins occurrence through the food chain in Costa Rica: Applying the One Health approach to mycotoxin surveillance. *Food Control* **2017**, *82*, 217–226. [CrossRef]
36. Chavarría, G.; Granados-Chinchilla, F.; Alfaro-Cascante, M.; Molina, A. Detection of Aflatoxin Mn milk, cheese and sour cream samples from Costa Rica using enzyme-assisted extraction and HPLC. *Food Addit. Contam. Part B* **2015**, *8*, 128–135. [CrossRef]
37. EU Commission Recommendations (2006/576/EC) of 17 August 2006 on the presence of deoxynivalenol, zearalenone, ochratoxin A, T-2 and HT-2 and fumonisins in products intended for animal feeding. *Off. J. Eur. Union* **2016**, *229*, 7–9.
38. EU Commission Recommendations (2013/165/EU) of March 2013 on the presence of T-2 and HT-2 toxin in cereals and cereal products. *Off. J. Eur. Union* **2013**, *91*, 12–15.
39. FAO (Food and Agriculture Organization of the United Nations). Aquaculture Feed and Fertilizer Resources Information System. 2018. Available online: http://www.fao.org/fishery/affris/species-profiles/nile-tilapia/tables/en/ (accessed on 19 July 2018).
40. INRA. *Equine Nutrition*, 1st ed.; Wageningen Academic Publishers: Wageningen, The Netherlands, 2015; pp. 97–120.
41. FEDIAF. *Nutritional Guidelines for Complete and Complementary Pet Food for Cats and Dog*; FEDIAF: Brussels, Belgium, 2016; pp. 1–102.
42. Martínez Marín, A.L. Inclusion of feeds in pelleted concentrates intended for stall-fed leisure horses. *Arch. Zootec* **2008**, *57*, 115–122.
43. Milani, J.M. Ecological conditions affecting mycotoxin production in cereals: A review. *Vet. Med.* **2013**, *58*, 405–411. [CrossRef]
44. Wu, L.; Qiu, L.; Zhang, H.; Sun, J.; Hu, X.; Wang, B. Optimization for the Production of Deoxynivalenol and Zearalenone by *Fusarium graminearum* Using Response Surface Methodology. *Toxins* **2017**, *9*, 57. [CrossRef] [PubMed]
45. CODEX. *Code of Practice for the Prevention and Reduction of Mycotoxin Contamination in Cereals*; CAC/RCP 51-2003; CODEX: Rome, Italy, 2014.
46. Pettersson, H. Mycotoxin contamination of animal feed. In *Woodhead Publishing Series in Food Science, Technology and Nutrition, Animal Feed Contamination*; Fink-Gremmels, J., Ed.; Woodhead Publishing: Cambridge, UK, 2012; ISBN 9781845697259. [CrossRef]

47. Leiva, A.; Granados-Chinchilla, F.; Redondo-Solano, M.; Arrieta-González, M.; Pineda Salazar, E.; Molina, A. Characterization of the animal by-product meal industry in Costa Rica: Manufacturing practices through the production chain and food safety. *Poult. Sci.* **2018**, *97*, 2159–2169. [CrossRef] [PubMed]
48. U.S. Grains Council. 2017/2018 Corn Harvest Quality Report 2018. Available online: https://grains.org/corn_report/corn-harvest-quality-report-2017-2018/ (accessed on 4 February 2019).
49. Xie, S.; Zheng, L.; Wan, M.; Niu, J.; Liu, Y.; Tian, L. Effect of deoxynivalenol on growth performance, histological morphology, anti-oxidative ability and immune response of juvenile Pacific white shrimp, Litopenaeus vannamei. *Fish Shellfish Immunol.* **2018**, *82*, 442–452. [CrossRef]
50. Di Stefano, V. Occurrence & Risk of OTA Food and Feed in Food and Feed. *Ref. Modul. Food Sci.* **2018**. [CrossRef]
51. INEC (Instituto Nacional de Estadística y Censos). Encuesta Nacional Agropecuaria 2017: Resultados Generales de las Actividades Ganaderas Vacuna y Porcina. 2019. Available online: http://www.inec.go.cr/multimedia/encuesta-nacional-agropecuaria-2017-datos-de-la-ganaderia-vacuna-y-porcina (accessed on 4 February 2019).
52. Charmley, E.; Trenholm, H.L.; Thompson, B.K.; Vudathala, D.; Nicholson, J.W.G.; Prelusky, B.D.; Charmley, L.L. Influence of level of deoxynivalenol in the diet of dairy cows on feed intake, milk production, and its composition. *J. Dairy Sci.* **1993**, *76*, 3580–3587. [CrossRef]
53. CAST. *Mycotoxins: Risks in Plant, Animal, and Human Systems. Council for Agricultural Science and Technology*; CAST: Ames, IA, USA, 2003; pp. 1–217.
54. Focht Müller, L.K.; Paiano, D.; Gugel, J.; Lorenzetti, W.R.; Morais Santurio, J.; de Castro Tavernari, F.; Micotti da Gloria, E.; Baldissera, M.D.; Da Silva, A.S. Post-weaning piglets fed with different levels of fungal mycotoxins and spray-dried porcine plasma have improved weight gain, feed intake and reduced diarrhea incidence. *Microb. Pathog.* **2018**, *117*, 259–264. [CrossRef]
55. Dänicke, S.; Winkler, J. Invited review: Diagnosis of zearalenone (ZEN) exposure of farm animals and transfer of its residues into edible tissues (carry over). *Food Chem. Toxicol.* **2015**, *84*, 225–249. [CrossRef] [PubMed]
56. Wang, A.; Hogan, N.S. Performance effects of feed-borne Fusarium mycotoxins on broiler chickens: Influences of timing and duration of exposure. *Anim. Nutr.* **2018**, *5*, 32–40. [CrossRef] [PubMed]
57. Boermans, H.J.; Leung, M.C.K. Mycotoxins and the pet food industry: Toxicological evidence and risk assessment. *Int. J. Food Microbiol.* **2007**, *119*, 95–102. [CrossRef] [PubMed]
58. Gazzotti, T.; Biagi, G.; Pagliuca, G.; Pinna, C.; Scardilli, M.; Grandi, M.; Zaghini, G. Occurrence of mycotoxins in extrude commercial dog food. *Anim. Feed Sci. Technol.* **2015**, *202*, 81–89. [CrossRef]
59. Atungulu, G.G.; Mohammadi-Shad, Z.; Wilson, S. Chapter 2—Mycotoxin Issues in Pet. In *Food and Feed Safety Systems and Analysis*; Academic Press: Cambridge, MA, USA, 2018; pp. 25–44.
60. García-Herranz, V.; Valdehita, A.; Navvas, J.M.; Fernández-Cruz, M.L. Cytotoxicity against fish and mammalian cells lines and endocrine activity of the mycotoxins beauvericin, deoxynivalenol and ochratoxin-A. *Food Chem. Toxicol.* **2019**. [CrossRef]
61. Gonçalves, R.A.; Navarro-Guillén, C.; Gilannejad, N.; Días, J.; Schatzmayr, D.; Bichl, G.; Czabany, T.; Moyano, F.J.; Rema, P.; Yúfera, M.; et al. Impact of deoxynivalenol on rainbow trout: Growth performance, digestibility, key gene expression regulation and metabolism. *Aquaculture* **2018**, *490*, 362–372. [CrossRef]
62. Woźny, M.; Obremski, K.; Hliwa, P.; Gomulka, P.; Rożyński, R.; Wojtacha, P.; Florczyk, M.; Segner, H.; Brzuzan, P. Feed contamination with zearalenone promotes growth but affects the immune system of rainbow trout. *Fish Shellfish Immunol.* **2019**, *84*, 680–694.
63. Ferrigo, D.; Raiola, A.; Causin, R. Fusarium Toxins in Cereals: Occurrence, Legislation, Factors Promoting the Appearance and Their Management. *Molecules* **2016**, *21*, 627. [CrossRef]
64. Shi, W.; Tan, Y.; Wang, S.; Gardiner, D.M.; De Saeger, S.; Liao, Y.; Wang, C.; Fan, Y.; Wang, Z.; Wu, A. Mycotoxigenic Potentials of Fusarium Species in Various Culture Matrices Revealed by Mycotoxin Profiling. *Toxins* **2017**, *9*, 6. [CrossRef]
65. Malir, F.; Ostry, V.; Pfohl-Leszkowicz, A.; Malir, J.; Toman, J. Ochratoxin A: 50 Years of Research. *Toxins* **2016**, *8*, 191. [CrossRef]
66. Li, H.; Xing, L.; Zhang, M.; Wang, J.; Zheng, N. The Toxic Effects of Aflatoxin B1 and Aflatoxin M1 on Kidney through Regulating L-Proline and Downstream Apoptosis. *BioMed Res. Int.* **2018**, *2018*, 9074861. [CrossRef] [PubMed]

67. Becker-Algeri, T.A.; Castagnaro, D.; de Bartoli, K.; de Souza, C.; Drunkler, D.A.; Badiale-Furlong, E. Mycotoxins in Bovine Milk and Dairy Products: A Review. *J. Food Sci.* **2016**, *81*, R545–R552. [CrossRef] [PubMed]
68. Ramírez-Martínez, A.; Camarillo-Hernández, E.; Carvajal-Moreno, M.; Vargas-Ortiz, M.; Wesolek, N.; Del Carmen, G.; Jimenes, R.; García Alvarado, M.A.; Roudot, A.-C.; Salgado Cervantes, M.A.; et al. Assessment of Aflatoxin M1 and M2 exposure risk through Oaxaca cheese consumption in southeastern Mexico. *Int. J. Environ. Health Res.* **2018**, *28*, 202–213.
69. US Jersey. A Quality Heifer. Cornell University, 2008. Available online: https://www.usjersey.com/Portals/0/AJCA/2_Docs/QualityHeiferBrochure.pdf (accessed on 27 February 2019).
70. Franklin, S.T.; Amaral-Phillips, D.M.; Jackson, J.A.; Campbell, A.A. Health and performance of Holstein calves that suckled or were hand-fed colostrum and were fed one of three physical forms of starter. *J. Dairy Sci.* **2003**, *86*, 2145–2153. [CrossRef]
71. Scaglioni, P.T.; Becker-Algeri, T.; Drunkler, D.; Badiale-Furlong, E. Aflatoxin B1 and M1 in milk. *Anal. Chim. Acta* **2014**, *829*, 68–74. [CrossRef] [PubMed]
72. Michlig, N.; Signorini, M.; Gaggiotti, M.; Chiericatti, C.; Basílico, J.C.; Repetti, M.R.; Beldomenico, H.R. Risk factors associated with the presence of aflatoxin M1 in raw bulk milk from Argentina. *Food Control* **2016**, *64*, 151–156. [CrossRef]
73. Quevedo-Garza, P.A.; Amador-Espejo, G.G.; Cantú-Martínez, P.C.; Trujillo-Mesa, J.A. Aflatoxin M1 occurrence in fluid milk commercialized in Monterrey, Mexico. *J. Food Saf.* **2018**, *38*, e12507. [CrossRef]
74. Peña-Rodas, O.; Martinez-Lopez, R.; Hernandez-Rauda, R. Occurrence of Aflatoxin M1 in cow milk in El Salvador: Results from a two-year survey. *Toxicol. Rep.* **2018**, *5*, 671–678. [CrossRef]
75. Sibaja, K.V.; Gonçalves, K.D.M.; Garcia, S.D.O.; Feltrin, A.C.P.; Noguiera, W.V.; Badiale-Furlong, E.; Garda-Buffon, J. Aflatoxin M_1 and B_1 in Colombian milk powder and estimated risk exposure. *Food Addit. Contam. Part B* **2019**, *30*, 1–8. [CrossRef] [PubMed]
76. Iqbal, S.Z.; Jinap, S.; Pirouz, A.A.; Faizal, A.R.A. Aflatoxin M1 in milk and dairy products, occurrence and recent challenges: A review. *Trends Food Sci. Technol.* **2015**, *46*, 110–119. [CrossRef]
77. Yoon, B.R.; Hong, S.-Y.; Cho, S.M.; Lee, K.R.; Kim, M.; Chung, S.H. Aflatoxin M1 levels in dairy products from South Korea determined by high-performance liquid chromatography with fluorescence detection. *J. Food Nutr. Res.* **2016**, *55*, 171–180.
78. Assunçao, R.; Martins, C.; Viegas, S.; Viegas, C.; Jakobsen, L.S.; Pires, S.; Alvito, P. Climate change and the health impact of aflatoxins exposure in Portugal—An overview. *Food Addit. Contam. Part A* **2018**, *35*, 1610–1621. [CrossRef]
79. Bellio, A.; Bianchi, D.M.; Gramaglia, M.; Loria, A.; Nucera, D.; Gallina, S.; Gili, M.; Decastelli, L. Aflatoxin M1 in Cow's Milk: Method Validation for Milk Sampled in Northern Italy. *Toxins* **2016**, *8*, 57. [CrossRef] [PubMed]
80. Gong, Y.Y.; Watson, S.; Routledge, M.N. Aflatoxin Exposure and Associated Human Health Effects, a Review of Epidemiological Studies. *Food Saf.* **2016**, *4*, 14–27. [CrossRef]
81. Milićević, D.R.; Spirić, D.; Radičević, T.; Velebit, B.; Steganović, S.; Milojević, L.; Janković, S. A review of the current situation of aflatoxin M1 in cow's milk in Serbia: Risk assessment and regulatory aspects. *Food Addit. Contam. Part A* **2017**, *34*, 1617–1631. [CrossRef] [PubMed]
82. Ahlberg, S.; Grace, D.; Kiarie, G.; Kirino, Y.; Lindahl, J. A Risk Assessment of Aflatoxin M1 Exposure in Low Mid-Income Dairy Consumers in Kenya. *Toxins* **2018**, *10*, 348. [CrossRef] [PubMed]
83. Walte, H.-G.; Schwake-Anduschus, C.; Geisen, R.; Fritsche, J. Afaltoxin: Food chain transference from feed to food. *J. Verbr. Lebensm* **2016**, *11*, 295–297. [CrossRef]
84. Gonçalves, L.; Dalla Rosa, A.; Gonzales, S.L.; Feltes, M.M.C.; Badiale-Furlong, E.; Dors, G.C. Incidence of aflatoxin M1 in fresh milk from small farms. *Food Sci. Technol.* **2017**, *37*, 11–15.
85. Fallah, A.A.; Fazlollahi, R.; Emami, A. Seasonal study of aflatoxin M1 contamination in milk of four dairy species in Yazd, Iran. *Food Control* **2016**, *68*, 77–82. [CrossRef]
86. Cantú-Cornelio, F.; Aguilar-Toalá, J.E.; de León-Rodríguez, C.I.; Esparza-Romero, J.; Vallejo-Córdoba, A.F.; García, H.S.; Hernández-Mendoza, A. Occurrence and factors associated with the presence of aflatoxin M1 in breast milk samples of nursing mothers in central Mexico. *Food Control* **2016**, *62*, 16–22. [CrossRef]
87. Naeimipour, F.; Aghajani, J.; Kojuri, S.A.; Ayoubi, S. Useful Approaches for Reducing Aflatoxin M1 Content in Milk and Dairy Products. *Biomed. Biotechnol. Res. J.* **2018**, *2*, 94–99.

88. Udomkun, P.; Wiredu, A.N.; Nagle, M.; Müller, J.; Vanlauwe, B.; Bandyopadhyay, R. Innovative technologies to manage aflatoxins in foods and feeds and the profitability of application—A review. *Food Control* **2017**, *76*, 127–138. [CrossRef] [PubMed]
89. Association of American Feed Control Officials (AAFCO). *Feed Inspector's Manual*, 7th ed.; AAFCO Inspection and Sampling Committee: Atlanta, GA, USA, 2017.
90. Czerwiecki, L.; Wilczyńska, G. Determination of Deoxynivalenol in cereal by HPLC-UV. *Mycotoxin Res.* **2003**, *19*, 31–34. [CrossRef]
91. Visconti, A.; Lattanzio, V.M.T.; Pascale, M.; Haidukowski, M. Analysis of T-2 and HT-2 toxins in cereal grains by immunoaffinity clean-up and liquid chromatography with fluorescence detection. *J. Chromatogr. A* **2005**, *1075*, 151–158. [CrossRef] [PubMed]
92. Aydemir Atasever, M.; Atasever, M.; Özturan, K.; Urçar, S. Determination of Aflatoxin M_1 level in Butter Samples Consumed in Erzurum, Turkey. *Kafkas Univ. Vet. Fak. Derg.* **2010**, *16* (Suppl. A), S159–S162.

toxins

MDPI

Article

Occupational Exposure to Mycotoxins in Swine Production: Environmental and Biological Monitoring Approaches

Susana Viegas [1,2,*], Ricardo Assunção [3,4], Carla Martins [2,3,4,5], Carla Nunes [2,5], Bernd Osteresch [6], Magdalena Twarużek [7], Robert Kosicki [7], Jan Grajewski [7], Edna Ribeiro [1] and Carla Viegas [1,2]

1 H&TRC—Health & Technology Research Center, ESTeSL—Escola Superior de Tecnologia da Saúde, Instituto Politécnico de Lisboa, 1990-096 Lisbon, Portugal; edna.ribeiro@estesl.ipl.pt (E.R.); carla.viegas@estesl.ipl.pt (C.V.)

2 Centro de Investigação em Saúde Pública, Escola Nacional de Saúde Pública, Universidade NOVA de Lisboa, 1600-560 Lisbon, Portugal; carla.martins@insa.min-saude.pt (C.M.); CNunes@ensp.unl.pt (C.N.)

3 Food and Nutrition Department, National Institute of Health Doutor Ricardo Jorge, I.P. (INSA), Av. Padre Cruz, 1649-016 Lisbon, Portugal; ricardo.assuncao@insa.min-saude.pt

4 Centre for Environmental and Marine Studies (CESAM), University of Aveiro, Campus de Santiago, 3810-193 Aveiro, Portugal

5 Escola Nacional de Saúde Pública, Universidade NOVA de Lisboa, 1600-560 Lisbon, Portugal

6 Group of Prof. Humpf, Institute of Food Chemistry, Westfälische Wilhelms-Universität Münster Corrensstraße 45, 48149 Münster, Germany; osteresch@uni-muenster.de

7 Faculty of Natural Sciences, Institute of Experimental Biology, Department of Physiology and Toxicology, Kazimierz Wielki University, 85-064 Bydgoszcz, Poland; twarmag@ukw.edu.pl (M.T.); robkos@ukw.edu.pl (R.K.); jangra@ukw.edu.pl (J.G.)

* Correspondence: susana.viegas@estesl.ipl.pt

Received: 2 December 2018; Accepted: 18 January 2019; Published: 1 February 2019

Abstract: Swine production workers are exposed simultaneously to multiple contaminants. Occupational exposure to aflatoxin B_1 (AFB_1) in Portuguese swine production farms has already been reported. However, besides AFB_1, data regarding fungal contamination showed that exposure to other mycotoxins could be expected in this setting. The present study aimed to characterize the occupational exposure to multiple mycotoxins of swine production workers. To provide a broad view on the burden of contamination by mycotoxins and the workers' exposure, biological (urine) samples from workers (n = 25) and 38 environmental samples (air samples, n = 23; litter samples, n = 5; feed samples, n = 10) were collected. The mycotoxins biomarkers detected in the urine samples of the workers group were the deoxynivalenol-glucuronic acid conjugate (60%), aflatoxin M_1 (16%), enniatin B (4%), citrinin (8%), dihydrocitrinone (12%) and ochratoxin A (80%). Results of the control group followed the same pattern, but in general with a lower number of quantifiable results (<LOQ). Besides air samples, all the other environmental samples collected presented high and diverse contamination, and deoxynivalenol (DON), like in the biomonitoring results, was the most prominent mycotoxin. The results demonstrate that the occupational environment is adding and contributing to the workers' total exposure to mycotoxins, particularly in the case of DON. This was confirmed by the biomonitoring data and the high contamination found in feed and litter samples. Furthermore, he followed multi-biomarker approach allowed to conclude that workers and general population are exposed to several mycotoxins simultaneously. Moreover, occupational exposure is probably described as being intermittent and with very high concentrations for short durations. This should be reflected in the risk assessment process.

Keywords: mycotoxins; occupational exposure; swine production; biomonitoring; mycotoxins mixture

Key Contribution: This study allowed to conclude that the workplace environment adds significantly to the mycotoxins exposure resulting from ingestion of contaminated food, and to recognize that inhalation is an important exposure route. Moreover, the findings showed us that workers and controls are exposed to several mycotoxins simultaneously. All these findings were possible due to the environmental and biological monitoring approaches.

---

1. Introduction

The confinement buildings used for swine production are recognized for their high levels of contamination with fungi and their metabolites [1–6]. Previous studies performed in swine farms demonstrated that this environment could be considered an occupational setting with high levels of exposure to dust aerosolization [4,7–9], and consequently it results in the widespread presence of fungi and their metabolites, such as volatile organic compounds and mycotoxins [1,2,4,9–11]. Therefore, it is expected that swine production workers are exposed simultaneously to multiple contaminants, as demonstrated previously by some authors [5,8]. Besides, the swine feed contamination by mycotoxins is also a well-known and frequently reported issue in Portugal [12] and all over the world [13–16].

Occupational exposure to aflatoxin B_1 (AFB_1) in Portuguese swine production farms has been reported [17]. However, data regarding fungal contamination showed that exposure to other mycotoxins besides AFB_1 could be expected in this setting. Indeed, in addition to the *Aspergillus* section *Flavi*, other fungal species recognized as mycotoxin producers were found in this occupational environment [5,10]. The most prevalent found in air (20.9%) and surface (26.6%) samples was the *Aspergillus* section *Versicolores*. However, other *Aspergillus* sections were also found, namely *Nigri*, *Circumdati* and *Fumigati* [5,10], and all of them have recognized toxigenic potential [18], besides the clinical relevance of *Fumigati* section [19].

Occupational exposure to mycotoxins is considered a complex process since it is associated with co-exposure to several mycotoxins by different exposure routes. In this context, human biomonitoring is of particular importance, characterizing the workers exposure to multiple mycotoxins and taking advantage of already available analytical methods that cover the detection and quantification of several mycotoxins and metabolites simultaneously in different biological samples [20–23]. Therefore, biomonitoring has an important role in the determination of the real human exposure to mycotoxins [17,20,22,24–27]. Biomonitoring covers not only mycotoxin intake from all dietary sources, but also exposure by other routes, such as inhalation of mycotoxins at the workplace [28]. Nowadays, the use of biomarkers has become more common, and research to discover new and more specific biomarkers has been proposed since the use of biomarkers is proven to be a successful method to assess exposure to xenobiotics. However, some challenges have to be addressed, such as the deep knowledge about the toxicokinetics and the possible metabolites for all relevant mycotoxins [29]. Other challenges include the frequent discovery of new metabolites for a specific mycotoxin and the need for understanding their possible use for biomonitoring studies, considering the measuring feasibility and the representativeness of the information regarding exposure to that mycotoxin [30]. Few studies have been performed with the use of biomarkers to study occupational exposure to mycotoxins [23,27,28].

Whether workplace-related exposure could represent a significant exposure source to mycotoxins as compared to exposure through ingestion of contaminated food constitutes a critical issue. As suggested by Reference [28], the comparison of results from workers and from non-occupationally exposed individuals (controls) should shed light on this issue contributing to the clarification of the importance of some occupational settings to multiple mycotoxins exposure in humans. The control group includes workers from administrative companies from the same locality and where the workplace environment does not have conditions to promote exposure to mycotoxins. This enables us to take into account the exposure by food intake and to have a better understanding of the role of the working environment in the total burden of mycotoxin exposure [4,24].

The present study aims to characterize the occupational exposure to multiple mycotoxins, including aflatoxin M_1 (AFM_1), aflatoxin B_1 (AFB_1), aflatoxin B_2 (AFB_2), aflatoxin G_1 (AFG_1), aflatoxin G_2 (AFG_2), patulin (PAT), nivalenol (NIV), deoxynivalenol (DON), deoxynivalenol-3-glucoside (DON-3-G), 15-acetyldeoxynivalenol (15-AcDON), 3-acetyldeoxynivalenol (3-AcDON), deepoxy-deoxynivalenol (DOM-1), deoxynivalenol-glucuronide (DON-GlcA), fusarenon-X (FUS-X), α-zearalanol (α-ZAL), β-zearalanol (β-ZAL), α-zearalenol (α-ZEL), β-zearalenol (β-ZEL), zearalenone (ZAN), zearalenone (ZEN), toxin T-2 (T-2), toxin HT-2 (HT-2), toxin HT-2-4-glucuronide (HT-2-4-GlcA), T-2 tetraol, T-2 triol, neosolaniol (NEO), monoacetoxyscirpenol (MAS), diacetoxyscirpenol (DAS), fumonisin B_1 (FB_1), fumonisin B_2 (FB_2), fumonisin B_3 (FB_3), roquefortine C (ROQ-C), griseofulvin (GRIS), ochratoxin A (OTA), ochratoxin B (OTB), ochratoxin alpha (OTα), mycophenolic acid (MPA), mevinolin (MEV), sterigmatocystin (STER), citrinin (CIT), dihydrocitrinone (DH-CIT), Enniatin B (EnB), of workers of swine production, in addition to the previously documented exposure to AFB_1.

2. Results

2.1. Biomonitoring

2.1.1. Participant Characteristics

The workers group of this study was composed of employees of five swine production farms. The volunteers of the "control group" were working in offices without expected occupational exposure to mycotoxins. The mean ages in control participants (n = 19) were similar to those of the workers (n = 25). For the control group, the median age was 40 years with a range of 32–54 years. The swine workers had a median age of 38.6 years with a range of 21–62 years (Table 1).

Table 1. Participants age and years of activity.

Groups	Female	Male	Age (Median; IQR)	Years of Activity (Median; IQR)
Workers (n = 25)	13	12	38.6; 30.0–46.0	3.5 ± 10.1
Controls (n = 19)	7	12	40.0; 38.5–44.0	-

IQR = Interquartile range.

2.1.2. Mycotoxins and Their Metabolites in Urine Samples

A summary of the biomonitoring data is presented in Tables 2 and 3. Samples with mycotoxins biomarkers above the respective Limit of Detection (LOD) were considered positive. The mycotoxins biomarkers detected in the urine samples of workers group were DON-GlcA (60%), AFM_1 (16%), EnB (4%), CIT (8%), DH-CIT (12%), and OTA (80%). Results for participants of the control group followed the same pattern, but in general with a lower number of positive samples (>LOD).

Here, DON 3 Glc was used as a reference that was chromatographically not separated from DON 15 GlcA, because both analytes are co-eluting in the used instrument set up. Consequently, the signal was accepted as the sum of both analytes [21,22]. As already reported in Reference [30], it is possible to separate the DON-3-GlcA, and DON-15-GlcA. However, in the instrument set-up, this would extend the liquid chromatography run up to 17 min. By doing so, the peak shapes of later eluting peaks would be worse off. It was not the aim of this study to distinguish between them, but to incorporate an early eluting polar metabolite.

Considering the values higher than LOD, DON-GlcA and OTA were the most prevalent biomarkers in the analyzed urine of the workers group, being 60% and 80% respectively. Data presented in Tables 2 and 3 showed that glucuronidation is a metabolic pathway for DON excretion since it was detected in samples from both workers and control groups.

Table 2. Mycotoxins biomarkers detected in urine samples from workers and controls.

Groups	DON-GlcA	AFM_1	EnB	CIT	DH-CIT	OTA
LOD (μg/L)	1.24	0.11	0.006	0.61	0.115	0.011
LOQ (μg/L)	4.14	0.38	0.020	2.00	0.383	0.036
Workers (n = 25)						
>LOQ (n, %)	13, 52%	4, 16%	-	1, 4%	1, 4%	1, 4%
LOD–LOQ (n, %)	2, 8%	-	1, 4%	1, 4%	2, 8%	19, 76%
<LOD (n, %)	10, 40%	21, 84%	24, 96%	23, 92%	22, 88%	5, 20%
Controls (n = 19)						
>LOQ (n, %)	-	-	-	1, 5%	-	-
LOD–LOQ (n, %)	11, 58%	1, 5%	2, 11%	10, 53%	2, 11%	13, 68%
<LOD (n, %)	8, 42%	18, 95%	17, 89%	8, 42%	17, 89%	6, 32%

Limit of Detection (LOD); Limit of Quantification (LOQ); Deoxynivalenol-glucuronide (DON-GlcA); Aflatoxin M_1 (AFM_1); Enniatin B (EnB); Citrinine (CIT); Dihydrocitrinone (DH-CIT); Ochratoxin A (OTA).

Table 3. Mycotoxins biomarkers levels (>LOQ) in urine samples from workers and controls (μg/L).

Groups	DON-GlcA	AFM_1	CIT	DH-CIT	OTA
Workers					
Range	22.0–71.1	2.1–5.4	-	-	-
Median	32.8	4.9	-	-	-
IQR	27.2–44.5	4.5–8.1	-	-	-
Single value	-	-	5.3	0.8	0.1
Controls (μg/L)					
Single value			24.2		

Interquartile range (IQR); Deoxynivalenol-glucuronide (DON-GlcA); Aflatoxin M_1 (AFM_1); Enniatin B (EnB); Citrinine (CIT); Dihydrocitrinone (DH-CIT); Ochratoxin A (OTA).

Most of the other mycotoxin biomarkers detected in urine samples followed a similar pattern to DON, that is, a higher proportion of positive samples (>LOD) in the workers group than in the control group (Table 4). However, the differences were not as remarkable for DON-GlcA detection. CIT and DH-CIT were also both detected in these participants, meaning that this compound is a metabolite of CIT detoxification (Table 4).

Table 4. Differences in the proportion of exposures between the control group and workers group.

Mycotoxins	Groups	Total	Workers	Controls	p Value
DON-GlcA	Not exposed	18 (40.9%)	10 (40.0%)	8 (42.1%)	1 *
	Exposed	26 (59.1%)	15 (60.0%)	11 (57.9%)	
AFM_1	Not exposed	39 (88.6%)	21 (84.0%)	18 (94.7%)	0.370 **
	Exposed	5 (11.4%)	4 (16.0%)	1 (5.3%)	
CIT	Not exposed	31 (70.5%)	23 (92.0%)	8 (42.1%)	0.001 *
	Exposed	13 (29.5%)	2 (8.0%)	11 (57.9%)	
DH-CIT	Not exposed	39 (88.6%)	22 (88.0%)	17 (89.5%)	1 **
	Exposed	5 (11.4%)	3 (12.0%)	2 (10.5%)	
EnB	Not exposed	41 (93.2%)	24 (96.0%)	17 (89.5%)	0.57 **
	Exposed	3 (6.8%)	1 (4.0%)	2 (10.5%)	
OTA	Not exposed	11 (25.0%)	5 (20.0%)	6 (31.6%)	0.598 *
	Exposed	33 (75%)	20 (80.0%)	13 (68.4%)	

* Chi-Square Test of Independence; ** Fisher Exact Test.

Regarding co-exposure to several mycotoxins, there are three workers that presented exposure to three mycotoxins/metabolites simultaneously: 2 workers with the combination of DON-GlcA, AFM_1, and OTA, and 1 worker with the combination of AFM_1, CIT, and OTA. However, the most common situation was the presence of the DON metabolite and OTA (8 workers). Regarding controls, most of the individuals showed exposure to two mycotoxins (42%) which was also the most common situation observed—the co-exposure to DON (through DON-GlcA measurement) and OTA (3 individuals). There were also 3 (21%) individuals with exposure to a mixture of 4 mycotoxins and another 3 individuals (21%) with simultaneous exposure to 3 mycotoxins.

In total, 18 (75%) workers and 15 (78%) individuals from the control group showed exposure to more than 1 mycotoxin.

2.2. Environmental Samples

All the collected environmental samples (air, liter, and feed) were analyzed for the presence of thirty-six mycotoxins and their metabolites (Tables 5 and 6).

Table 5. Mycotoxins present in environmental samples.

Farms	Environmental Samples	Mycotoxins *	Number of Mycotoxins		
			(>LOD)	LOD–LOQ	> LOQ
Farm A	Feed—Sample 1	NIV, DON-3-G, DON, ZEN, NEO, 15-AcDON, 3-Ac-DON, MAS, DAS, FB_1, FB_2, FB_3, GRI, T-2, HT-2, MPA, STER	17	2	15
	Feed—Sample 2	DON, ZEN, 15-AcDON, 3-AcDON, FB_1, FB_2, FB_3, T-2, HT-2, MPA, MEV	11	0	11
	Air				
	Litter	DON, ZEN, FB_1, STER	4	0	4
Farm B	Feed—Sample 1	DON-3-G, DON, ZEN, 15-AcDON, FB_1, FB_2, FB_3, T-2, HT-2, OTA, MPA, MEV	12	1	11
	Feed - Sample 2	DON-3-G, DON, ZEN, 15-AcDON, 3-AcDON, MAS, FB_1, FB_2, FB_3, T-2, HT-2, MPA	12	3	9
	Air				
	Litter	DON, ZEN, GRI, STER	4	0	4
Farm C	Feed—Sample 1	DON, ZEN, NEO, 15-AcDON, FB_1, FB_2, FB_3, GRI, T-2, HT-2, MPA	11	0	11
	Feed—Sample 2	DON-3-G, DON, ZEN, 15-AcDON, FB_1, FB_2, FB_3, T-2,HT-2, MPA, MEV	11	3	8
	Air				
	Litter	DON, ZEN, DOM-1, STER	4	0	4
Farm D	Feed—Sample 1	DON-3-G, DON, ZEN, 15-AcDON, FB_1, FB_2, FB_3, T-2, HT-2, MPA, MEV	11	1	10
	Feed—Sample 2	DON, ZEN, 15-AcDON, FB_1, FB_2, FB_3, T-2, HT-2, MPA	9	1	8
	Air				
	Litter	DON, ZEN, FB_1, GRI, STER	5	0	5
Farm E	Feed—Sample 1	DON-3-G, DON, ZEN, NEO, 15-AcDON, FB_1, FB_2, FB_3, T-2, HT-2, MPA	11	1	10
	Feed—Sample 2	DON, ZEN, 15-AcDON, FB_1, FB_2, T-2, HT-2, MPA, STER	9	1	8
	Air				
	Litter	DON, GRI, STER, MPA	4	0	4

* Mycotoxins with values >LOD; nivalenol (NIV), deoxynivalenol (DON), deoxynivalenol-3-glucoside (DON-3-G), fusarenon-X (FUS-X), α-zearalanol (α-ZAL), β-zearalanol (β-ZAL), β-zearalenol (β-ZEL), α-zearalanol (α-ZEL), zearalenone (ZAN), zearalenone (ZEN), Toxin T2 (T-2), Toxin HT2 (HT-2), deepoxy-deoxynivalenol (DOM-1), neosolaniol (NEO), 15-acetyldeoxynivalenol (15-AcDON), 3-acetyldeoxynivalenol (3-AcDON), monoacetoxyscirpenol (MAS), diacetoxyscirpenol (DAS), fumonisin B_1 (FB_1), fumonisin B_2 (FB_2), fumonisin B_3 (FB_3), roquefortine C (ROQ-C), griseofulvin (GRI), ochratoxin A (OTA), ochratoxin B (OTB), mycophenolic acid (MPA), mevinolin (MEV), sterigmatocystin (STER).

Table 6. The concentration of mycotoxins quantified in the feed (ng/g).

Mycotoxins	Range of Values/Mean
NIV	<LOQ
DON-3-G	<LOQ
DON	137–388/272
ZEN	6.83–32.35/14.4
NEO	0.96–12.4/4.84
15-AcDON	6.94–35.64/14.79
3-Ac-DON	4.48–10.9/7.66
MAS	<LOQ–0.70
DAS	1.18
FB_1	6.52–366/149
FB_2	2.06–97.6/48.3
FB_3	6.36–61.2/19.6
GRIS	1.59–1.88/1.74
T-2	<LOQ–24.6/3.81
HT-2	<LOQ–28.1/3.84
MPA	0.80–89.0/29.7
STER	<LOQ–0.72
MEV	0.43–0.62/0.55
OTA	0.30

Nivalenol (NIV), deoxynivalenol (DON), deoxynivalenol-3-glucoside (DON-3-G), fusarenon-X (FUS-X), α-zearalanol (α-ZAL), β-zearalanol (β-ZAL), β-zearalenol (β-ZEL), α-zearalanol (α-ZEL), zearalenone (ZAN), zearalenone (ZEN), Toxin T2 (T-2), Toxin HT2 (HT-2), deepoxy-deoxynivalenol (DOM-1), neosolaniol (NEO), 15-acetyldeoxynivalenol (15-AcDON), 3-acetyldeoxynivalenol (3-AcDON), monoacetoxyscirpenol (MAS), diacetoxyscirpenol (DAS), fumonisin B_1 (FB_1), fumonisin B_2 (FB2), fumonisin B_3 (FB_3), roquefortine C (ROQ-C), griseofulvin (GRIS), ochratoxin A (OTA), ochratoxin B (OTB), mycophenolic acid (MPA), mevinolin (MEV), sterigmatocystin (STER).

Regarding the air samples, only three samples from two different farms showed contamination by sterigmatocystin (STER) (<LOQ–1.42 ng/g). All the other air samples were found to be negative for the analyzed mycotoxins and metabolites. Regarding the litter samples, it was observed that the most prevalent mycotoxins were DON (<LOQ–76.4 ng/g) and STER (1.14–2.69 ng/g) which were detected in all litter samples and in considerably higher amounts than the other analyzed mycotoxins. Zearalenone was a mycotoxin that was also detected in 4 out of 5 farms, but in lower amounts (<LOQ–0.78 ng/g).

Concerning the feed samples, it is possible to observe that the common scenario is the co-occurrence of mycotoxins in the same sample (9–17 mycotoxins were detected in the same sample). The higher values were obtained for DON (values between 137–388 ng/g) and fumonisins, particularly FB1 (values between 6–366 ng/g). Others mycotoxins, such as ZEN, 3-AcDON, 15-AcDON, and DON-3-G, fumonisins (FB_1, FB_2 and FB_3), and type A trichothecenes such as T-2 and HT-2, were also detected in almost all the feed samples.

3. Discussion

This study is the result of previous work related to occupational exposure to mycotoxins and the need to identify the contribution of specific occupational settings to total mycotoxins exposure. At the same time, this study and previous ones [27,31] allow us to recognize mycotoxins as real and common occupational risk factors in specific occupational settings. Indeed, as in previous reports, results showed that the occupational environment and probably specific work tasks developed by the workers implicate exposure to mycotoxins by inhalation. Although no statistical significance was obtained in some tests, results demonstrated that only workers presented quantifiable levels of DON-GlcA (a biomarker of exposure to DON), AFM_1 (the hydroxylated metabolite of AFB_1, EnB (also a Fusarium toxin)), DH-CIT (the main metabolite of CIT) and OTA (the most-abundant food-contaminating mycotoxin). One possible reason for the absence of statistical significance in some tests could be due to the small sample size in both groups. Additionally, the type of urine samples used for this study (spot samples) might be responsible since 24 h urine (or first-morning void) are more concentrated with mycotoxins than one spot urine sample [32]. For instance, in the case of DON, previous studies showed that there is clear evidence that urinary DON excretion varies at different times of the day, and spot samples cannot describe these differences [33–35].

Consequently, the results were mainly discussed in the context of their values and not their statistical significance. However, and despite the small number, results indicate that even if workers are exposed through food consumption to some of these mycotoxins, occupational exposure is adding and contributing to the total exposure. This is not difficult to understand if we consider that, besides air samples, all the other environmental samples collected presented high and diverse levels of contamination, and DON was, like in the biomonitoring results, the most prominent mycotoxin. Additionally, the almost null results regarding air samples can be explained by the fact that mycotoxins are not volatile, and for the workers, exposure by inhalation occurs when exposure to organic dust happens in specific tasks since dust functions as a mycotoxins carrier and enters respiratory systems. A previous work developed by Reference [36] identified in swine farms the predictors for dust exposure being associated with tasks involving intense animal handling, such as castrating, ear tagging, and teeth cutting, as well as activities related to feeding, floor sweeping, and removal of dry manure. If we consider the results obtained in the current study concerning the high contamination found in the litter and feed samples, it is possible to estimate that feeding, floor sweeping, and removal/change of litter will be responsible for the workers' dust and mycotoxins exposure. Furthermore, dust particles containing mycotoxins can be deposited in the skin, leading to dermal absorption, or work surfaces contaminated with dust particles can also be touched, generating the opportunity for additional skin contact [4,37]. Consequently, this exposure route is also possible in this occupational setting since workers do not use gloves and most of the workers were using short leaves when performing their working tasks. Unfortunately, there is a lack of information on the adsorption rates from lungs and skin for mycotoxins in humans.

The results obtained regarding feed contamination (between 9–17 mycotoxins in the same sample) demonstrate that feed has a relevant role in workplace environment contamination with mycotoxins and the handling of feed is probably one of the tasks that implicates exposure. An important preventive action will be the choice of the raw materials used during feed formulation, avoiding the use of materials with high mycotoxin contaminations. Considering this aspect, it seems of interest to highlight the influence that the geographic origin of the raw material can have on the mycotoxin contamination of feed at different stages of production [38]. Previously, and similarly to our findings, DON has been reported as the more prevalent mycotoxin in the different types of raw materials used to produce feed, since it is common to find DON, for instance, in maize, wheat, soybean meal, and others [38]. This contamination has several consequences for pig health, such as increased susceptibility to infectious diseases, reactivation of chronic infection, and a decreased vaccine efficacy, with a huge economic impact on pig production [39]. Other mycotoxins present in all the feed samples analyzed, although in lower concentrations, such as ZEN, fumonisins (FB_1, FB_2, and FB_3), and type A trichothecenes (T-2 and HT-2) are also commonly reported as contaminants of feed and have several health consequences for the animals [38,39]. Therefore, preventive actions taken to avoid feed contamination will result in preventing/reducing workers exposure to mycotoxins and, at the same time, guarantee better production results.

Exposure to mycotoxins mixtures was also once more revealed in this biomonitoring study. Both group results in workers and controls showed that this is a common aspect. This is understandable since, besides the presence of multiple mycotoxins in the occupational environment, this is also a common feature of food commodities. Even the most frequent combination found in biological samples from workers and controls (DON and OTA) were already reported in several foods from European countries such as beer, pasta, cereals, and cereal-based foods [26,40].

A previous paper developed by Reference [41] assessed DON and OTA interactions using two different model systems appropriate for the evaluation of intestinal or liver toxicity and an experimental design that included realistic doses of each mycotoxin. The authors found that Caco-2 and HepG2 cells were more sensitive to DON alone than to OTA. Moreover, when combined, OTA-DON showed the most toxic combinations for Caco-2 and HepG2, respectively, having both synergistic effects at all inhibition levels [41]. The same trend was found for the combination AFB_1-DON, a mixture also observed in our study. Therefore, the results obtained in the present study, even if exposure route is mainly via inhalation, suggest that exposure to DON occurs in combination with other mycotoxins and this should be considered when performing risk assessment.

Regarding the high prevalence of OTA in the samples of both groups, previous studies developed in the Portuguese population found OTA in biologic fluids [40,42–44] relating to the consumption of some food commodities. Additionally, Reference [43] concluded that the estimated daily intake values in the Portuguese populations are higher than other European populations. Indeed, our results are probably explained once again by the fact that this mycotoxin is one of the most-abundant food-contaminating mycotoxins [44]. In Portugal, the bread is the major cereal-derived product consumed, and it is probably the main factor responsible for OTA exposure, also due to the contamination levels. Other products such as wine and pork also contribute to exposure but are more related to the high consumption rate of these products and not so much due to their contamination levels [44].

One aspect relevant to the analysis is the fact that in all environmental samples, including air samples, STER was detected, with a high frequency and concentration in the feed samples. STER synthesis is restricted to species in four sections in *Aspergillus* (*Ochraceorosei, Versicolores, Nidulantes,* and *Flavi*) [45]. However, most of the *Aspergillus* species from the section *Versicolores* are able to produce STER, and this was the most prevalent species on air and surface samples from the swine farms engaged in this study. Therefore, besides the feed contaminated with STER that has already been reported [45], it seems that the swine farm environment can promote this mycotoxin production by the *Versicolores* section. STER is extensively metabolized essentially by glucuronidation but the identification of the glucuronide forms in human biological samples has not been accomplished until now [29]. Further studies should be developed to determine the most suitable STER biomarkers for identifying exposure.

This study demonstrates once more the usefulness of biomonitoring tools. These tools not only allowed us to identify that the occupational environment is contributing to the swine workers' total exposure to mycotoxins but also it revealed that exposure occurs as a mixture of mycotoxins. Furthermore, and considering that some mycotoxin mixtures could lead to additive or synergistic effects, a significant threat to human and animal health could occur. However, most studies have been carried out over less than three days and at concentrations above the legal limits available in the context of food safety. There is therefore a lack of data about chronic exposure at sub-toxic mycotoxin concentrations, closer to real food and feed consumption habits [46]. This implies also the availability of enough sensitive analytical techniques for the quantification of biomarkers of multiple co-occurring mycotoxins [47]. Likewise, and concerning occupational exposure, probably we are dealing with intermittent exposures linked with very high concentrations within a short duration of time. This exposure is in addition to the exposure occurring via food intake (chronic exposure to low amounts). Subsequently, there is a gap in the knowledge concerning the approach which should be used to accomplish a suitable risk assessment methodology. Toxicokinetics and toxicodynamics data from exposure sources other than ingestion, as well as human biomonitoring guidance values, are needed in order to anticipate the associated risk. This implies that the involved stakeholders need to extend the dialogue across different chemical sectors (food safety vs. occupational health) in order to come to more overarching and harmonized approaches [48].

Moreover, the exposure scenario found in this occupational setting can suffer variations due to climate change that will affect cereals (used for feed), agricultural practices, and the ecological niches of mycotoxigenic fungi in a particular area. In the future, mycotoxin producers in temperate climates will be replaced by better-adapted species or mutants which may produce new secondary metabolites [49,50]. Therefore, monitoring programs considering biological and environmental samples should be developed continuously to allow for a better and more detailed exposure scenario. In addition to this, adequate health surveillance programs should be applied.

4. Conclusions

Despite the small numbers of individuals in both groups (workers and controls), this study allowed us to recognize that the occupational environment is adding and contributing to the workers' total exposure to mycotoxins. This was also confirmed by the high contamination found in feed and litter samples. Additionally, the multi-biomarker approach permitted us also to conclude that exposure to mycotoxins, in workers and in the general population, is characterized by being a mixture of mycotoxins, and this should be reflected in risk assessment processes.

5. Materials and Methods

5.1. Setting Characteristics

This study was conducted between June and July 2017 in five Portuguese swine locations in the Lisbon district and is part of an enlarged exploratory study aiming to characterize occupational exposure to microorganisms and mycotoxins in this setting (Instituto Politécnico de Lisboa: IPL/2016/BBIOR_ESTeSL, Date of approval: 7 December 2016). While being part of a larger study in which additional environmental characterization was carried out, this paper presents the results regarding environmental samples collected by active (air) and passive (feed and litter) methods in which mycotoxins assessment was performed. Additionally, biomonitoring was performed involving the workers who agreed to participate.

Five Portuguese swine farms were selected according to three specific criteria: Location within the Lisbon district, a high number of animals, and the number of workers. All the farms were divided into five pavilions dedicated to different phases of animal growth/age, namely pig gestation, maternity, stalls, pig fattening areas, and quarantine confinement. The five farms had been assessed in a previous study from our group [17], but no modifications in working activities or safety procedures were made until this new sampling campaign was performed in the scope of a new study. The floor in the swine maternities was covered with newspaper. Manure removal systems were present in all farm facilities, with complete removal from the building several times a day. The ventilation systems in the studied farm buildings consisted of mechanical ventilation by wall exhaust fans coupled with natural ventilation through the operation of a winch-curtain. Swine farm workers did not use respiratory protection devices during tasks performance.

Fungal burden found in the different environmental matrices from the assessed swine was already reported [5]. Besides the most prevalent (*Cladosporium* sp. and *Penicillium* sp.), other fungal species with recognized toxigenic potential were also identified, namely the *Fusarium graminearum* complex on air samples, *Fusarium culmorum* on feed samples, and *Aspergillus* section *Circumdati* on surfaces. *Aspergillus* section *Circumdati* was the most prevalent (55%) on MEA followed by *Aspergilli* (25%). Different *Aspergillus* sections were more prevalent on DG18, *Versicolores* being the most identified (50%), followed by *Usti* (20.8%).

5.2. Sampling

In order to provide a broad view on the burden of contamination by mycotoxins and the workers' exposure to these toxins, biological (human biomonitoring) samples from workers (n = 25) and environmental (air, litter, and feed) (n = 38 samples) samples were collected.

5.2.1. Human Biomonitoring Approach

Qualitative and quantitative determinations of mycotoxins with the objective of occupational exposure assessment at an individual level for each study participant were performed using a multi-analyte approach since it allows for a more precise and realistic exposure assessment over a broad range of different analytes [51,52]. Workers that developed tasks which implicate the handling of piglets, feed, or litter are normally inside the pavilions and were all invited to participate in this study. In the end, 25 workers (out of 26) were enrolled in this study.

A control group (not exposed) was also enrolled in the study (n = 19) in order to investigate mycotoxin background levels for the Portuguese population and to evaluate and easily detect putative possible differences regarding the exposure of the workers group. Therefore, the control group was composed of individuals who conducted administrative tasks in an educational institution without recognized activities known to involve or promote occupational exposure to mycotoxins [4]. Additionally, the building of the educational institution was well maintained, not showing signs of degradation that can implicate optimal conditions for fungal growth. In this study, it is assumed that both groups (workers and controls) have similar diets and consequently it was hypothesized that the main difference of exposure to mycotoxins was work activities. The same control group was used in another research project [27] since both projects were developed almost simultaneously and the workers groups are from companies located in the same region of Portugal.

This study was conducted in full accordance with the World Medical Association Declaration of Helsinki and European Commission recommendations [53,54]. Written consents from the participants involved in this study were obtained. All participants were informed about the scope and the aim of this study and signed a consent form. After data collection, all the personal data was anonymized to avoid identification of the participants. Moreover, all the data was pseudonymized in order to protect the privacy and minimize the risk in the event of unauthorized access to the participant's data.

Additionally, during a personal interview, participants answered a questionnaire to collect personal data such as age, detailed current and previous occupational history, and tasks performed in the two previous days prior urine collection, as well as activities outside the company, e.g., agriculture or animal production. However, it only collected data needed to meet the research objectives and to obtain contextual information to enable a better analysis of the biomonitoring data. In each unit, workers collected spot urine samples (more or less 25 mL) at the end of the morning (between 11 a.m. and 1 p.m.) in a dedicated room in each swine farm facility. This schedule was the one indicated by the companies as the most suitable for samples collection.

5.2.2. Environmental Sampling

Air, litter, and feed from the swine farms (identified as A, B, C, D, and E) were analyzed to assess mycotoxins contamination. The objective of considering these environmental samples was to recognize the most relevant contamination source of the occupational environment and to identify potential preventive measures that could be more adequate to reduce workers exposure to mycotoxins. In each area of the swine farms considered in the study (the pig gestation site, maternity site, stalls, the pig fattening area, and quarantine confinement) air samples were collected. In total, 23 air samples were collected. Air samples (600 L) were collected using the impinger Coriolis® μ air sampler (Bertin Technologies, Montigny-le-Bretonneux, France) with a flow rate of 300 L of air per minute. Samples were collected using 10 mL sterile phosphate-buffered saline (PBS) with 0.05% Triton^{tm} X-100 and were subsequently used for the mycotoxins assay.

Five litter samples (one from each unit) were collected into sterilized bags in the maternity area, the only area off the swine farm that had litter. Ten feed samples (two from each swine farm) from different areas of the swine farms were collected into sterilized bags.

5.3. *Analytical Methods for the Determination of Mycotoxins and Metabolites*

5.3.1. Urine Samples Analysis

Urine samples were stored at 4 °C after collection and during transportation to the laboratory. After aliquotation, 15 mL of these samples were kept frozen at −20 °C until analysis in the next two weeks. After the collection of all samples, dilute-and-shoot sample preparation was used that consists only of centrifugation as well as a dilution step of thawed samples in combination with a HPLC-MS/MS measurement.

In short, samples were centrifuged at 15,000× *g* for five minutes at 8 °C followed by dilution of 10 µL of the supernatant with 90 µL mobile phase at LC-starting conditions, namely a solvent mixture of acetonitrile, water, and formic acid (95+5+0.1, *v*/*v*/*v*), following the sample preparation from an earlier published approach [21]. Sample 30 µL of this solution was injected to an Infinity 1260 system (Agilent, Waldbronn, Germany) on a C18 Pyramid column (100 × 2 mm, 3 µm, Macherey-Nagel, Düren, Germany) connected to a pre-column filled with the same material (4 × 2 mm, 3 µm). Column oven temperature was set to 45 °C, and the flow rate was 600 µL/min. After chromatographic separation, the detection was carried out by a QTRAP 6500 triple quadrupole mass spectrometer (SCIEX, Santa Clara, CA, USA) run by Analyst 1.6.2 software (SCIEX, Santa Clara, CA, USA). Source parameters were as follows: Temperature was set to 500 °C, as well as curtain gas at 40, nebulizer gas at 45, and heater gas at 55 arbitrary units. Electrospray ionization was used in both polarities at −4500 V or +5500 V, respectively. Further parameters and characteristics, for example, the used gradient of the mobile phases or the Multiple Reaction Monitoring (MRM) transitions, can be found in the original publication of this method application [22]. Analytes of interest are presented in Table 3. Additionally, the presence of structurally-related compounds and important metabolites was investigated. Since spot urine samples were used to determine the workers' exposure to mycotoxins, it was necessary to perform an adjustment in order to correct for differences in inter-individual dilution and excretion rates [27]. The determination of urinary creatinine was chosen to perform this adjustment. Creatinine was determined with a spectrophotometric method based on Jaffe reaction in automatized equipment (Dimension RXL, Siemens®, Munich, Germany). Results for mycotoxins urinary concentrations were expressed as µg mycotoxin/g creatinine.

5.3.2. Analyses of the Environmental Samples

Aliquots from feed (0.50 g) and litter (0.25 g) were extracted with 2.0 mL of extraction solvent (acetonitrile (ACN): water (H_2O): acetic acid (AcOH) 79:20:1) on MultiReax shaker (Heidolph, Germany) for 60 min. Raw extracts after dilution with water (1:1) and centrifugation were injected into the LC-MS/MS system. Air samples (600 L) were diluted 1:7 (*v*/*v*) with extraction solvent and water mixture (1:1) (Table 7).

Table 7. Limits of Detection (LOD) and Limits of Quantitation (LOQ) for mycotoxins analyzed by LC-MS/MS in environmental samples.

Mycotoxins	LOD (µg/Kg)	LOQ (µg/Kg)	Calibration Range	Recovery (%) ± RSD (*n* = 3)
Aflatoxin M_1	0.06	0.20	0.1–8.1	79 ± 6
Aflatoxin B_1	0.06	0.20	0.3–32.1	80 ± 2
Aflatoxin B_2	0.06	0.20	0.1–8.0	101 ± 12
Aflatoxin G_1	0.10	0.10	0.3–32.4	81 ± 2
Aflatoxin G_2	0.12	0.40	0.1–8.0	74 ± 1
Deoxynivalenol	2.70	9.00	3.2–1060	90 ± 2
Deoxynivalenol-3-glucoside	5.41	18.00	5.5–548	85 ± 7
15-Acetyldeoxynivalenol	0.81	2.70	3.3–1100	88 ± 6
3-Acetyldeoxynivalenol	0.81	2.70	3.2–1070	90 ± 1
Deepoxydeoxynivalenol	0.36	1.20	1.7–558	92 ± 5
Nivalenol	4.50	15.00	10.7–1070	83 ± 4
Neosolaniol	0.09	0.30	2.2–740	92 ± 2
Zearalanone	0.45	1.50	3.2–107	85 ± 5
Zearalenone	0.18	0.60	0.5–151	87 ± 3
α-Zearalanol	1.98	6.60	2.0–47.4	83 ± 7
β-Zearalanol	0.93	3.10	1.0–47.2	85 ± 7
β-Zearalenol	1.44	4.80	2.0–47.2	81 ± 1
α-Zearalenol	1.02	3.40	1.0–48.6	89 ± 1

Table 7. *Cont.*

Mycotoxins	LOD (µg/Kg)	LOQ (µg/Kg)	Calibration Range	Recovery (%) ± RSD (n = 3)
Ochratoxin A	0.06	0.20	2.0–199	103 ± 1
Ochratoxin B	0.09	0.30	1.6–164	99 ± 1
Fumonisin B_1	0.51	1.70	8.1–811	64 ± 9
Fumonisin B_2	0.36	1.20	8.1–809	70 ± 9
Fumonisin B_3	0.45	1.50	2.4–235	66 ± 11
T2 toxin	0.12	0.40	3.2–319	104 ± 4
HT2 toxin	0.27	0.90	3.2–322	98 ± 1
T2 Tetraol	5.41	18.00	7.4–741	87 ± 5
T2 Triol	0.33	1.10	2.2–222	103 ± 6
Monoacetoxyscirpenol	0.12	0.40	1.9–634	93 ± 5
Diacetoxyscirpenol	0.30	1	3.2–322	97 ± 2
Roquefortine C	0.21	0.70	3.5–352	87 ± 4
Griseofulvin	0.09	0.30	2.4–239	94 ± 3
Patulin	1.05	3.50	4.1–405	93 ± 7
Fusarenon-X	4.80	16.00	6.4–319	81 ± 8
Mycophenolic acid	0.21	0.70	2.4–815	101 ± 2
Mevinolin	0.09	0.30	2.4–239	98 ± 1
Sterigmatocystin	0.20	0.60	1.0–101	100 ± 3

Mycotoxins were detected using high-performance liquid chromatography (HPLC) Nexera (Shimadzu, Tokyo, Japan) with a mass detector API 4000 (Sciex, Foster City, CA, USA). Separation of mycotoxins was carried out on a chromatographic column Gemini NXC18 (150 × 4.6 mm, 3 µm) (Phenomenex, Torrance, CA, USA); eluent A was composed of water/acetic acid (99:1, v/v) and eluent B of methanol /acetic acid (99:1, v/v), both contained 5mM ammonium acetate; eluent flow rate: 0.75 mL/min, injection volume: 7 µL. The concentrations of mycotoxins were calculated using external calibration. The Limits of Detection (LOD) and Limits of Quantitation (LOQ) obtained for each mycotoxin with the analytical method are presented in Table 7. The LOD (signal-to-noise ratio of 3) and LOQ (signal-to-noise ratio of 10), respectively, were estimated (using the Analyst® 1.6.2 software (Sciex, Foster City, CA, USA), by spiking blank feed extract before extraction at low concentrations.

5.4. Statistical Analysis

Statistical analysis was performed using IBM® SPSS Statistics 20 software (IBM, Armonk, NY, USA). Descriptive statistics are presented as medians (IQR) and range (minimum and maximum). Assuming the research (alternative) hypothesis "there is a difference in the distribution of responses to the outcome variable among the comparison groups" (i.e., that the distribution of responses "depends" on the group), differences in the proportion of exposures between the control group and workers were evaluated through the Chi-Square Test of Independence (with continuity correction or the Fisher Exact Test—in case the conditions of the applied Chi-Square Test of Independence were not satisfied). For this, the classification of "not exposed" were considered to be the values below the LOD, and "exposed" considers the values higher than the LOD. The level of $p \leq 0.05$ was considered statistically significant.

Author Contributions: Conceptualization, S.V., R.A. and C.V.; Methodology, S.V.; Validation, S.V., R.A., C.M., C.N., B.O., M.T., R.K., J.G., E.R. and C.V.; Formal Analysis, C.N.; Investigation, S.V., R.A., C.M., C.N., B.O., M.T., R.K., J.G., E.R. and C.V.; Resources, S.V., E.R.; Data Curation, S.V., R.A., C.M., C.N., B.O., M.T., R.K., J.G., E.R. and C.V.; Writing—Original Draft Preparation, S.V.; Writing—Review & Editing, S.V., R.A., C.N., C.M., E.R. and C.V.; Visualization, S.V., R.A., C.M., C.N., B.O., M.T., R.K., J.G., E.R. and C.V.; Supervision, S.V.; Project Administration, E.R.; Funding Acquisition, E.R., S.V. and C.V.

Funding: This research was funded by Instituto Politécnico de Lisboa, Lisbon, Portugal: Project "Bacterial Bioburden assessment in the context of occupational exposure and animal health of swine productions (IPL/2016/BBIOR_ESTeSL)" and also by FCT—Fundação para Ciência e Tecnologia: Project "EXPOsE – Establishing protocols to assess occupational exposure to microbiota in clinical settings (02/SAICT/2016 – Project nº 23222)".

Acknowledgments: The authors are grateful to the swine farms employers and workers that collaborate in this research project. R.A. and C.M. are grateful to INSA and to CESAM (UID/AMB/50017/2013) through national funds (FCT), and the co-funding by the Fundo Europeu de Desenvolvimento Regional (FEDER) (POCI-01-0145-FEDER-00763), within the PT2020 Partnership Agreement and Compete 2020.

Conflicts of Interest: The authors declare no conflict of interest.

References

1. Millner, P.D. Bioaerosols associated with animal production operations. *Bioresour. Technol.* **2009**, *100*, 5379–5385. [CrossRef] [PubMed]
2. Tsapko, V.; Chudnovets, A.; Sterenbogen, M.; Papach, V.; Dutkiewicz, J.; Skórska, C.; Krysinska-Traczyk, E.; Golec, M. Exposure to bioaerosols in the selected agricultural facilities of the Ukraine and Poland—A review. *Ann. Agric. Environ. Med.* **2011**, *18*, 19–27. [PubMed]
3. Mackiewicz, B.; Skórska, C.; Dutkiewicz, J. Relationship between concentrations of microbiological agents in the air of agricultural settings and occurrence of work-related symptoms in exposed persons. *Ann. Agric. Environ. Med.* **2015**, *3*, 473–477. [CrossRef] [PubMed]
4. Viegas, S.; Viegas, C.; Oppliger, A. Occupational Exposure to Mycotoxins: Current Knowledge and Prospects. *Ann. Work Expo. Health* **2018**, 1–19. [CrossRef] [PubMed]
5. Viegas, C.; Faria, T.; Monteiro, A.; Caetano, L.A.; Carolino, E.; Quintal Gomes, A.; Viegas, S. A novel multi-approach protocol for the characterization of occupational exposure to organic dust—Swine production case study. *Toxics* **2018**, *6*, 5. [CrossRef] [PubMed]
6. Viegas, S.; Mateus, V.; Almeida-Silva, M.; Carolino, E.; Viegas, C. Occupational Exposure to Particulate Matter and Respiratory Symptoms in Portuguese Swine Barn Workers. *J. Toxicol. Environ. Health Part A Curr. Issues* **2013**, *76*, 1007–1014. [CrossRef] [PubMed]
7. Jo, W.; Kang, J. Exposure levels of airborne bacteria and fungi in Korean swine and poultry sheds. *Arch. Environ. Occup. Health* **2005**, *60*, 140–146. [CrossRef]
8. Kim, K.Y.; Ko, H.J.; Kim, H.T.; Kim, Y.S.; Roh, Y.M.; Lee, C.M.; Kim, C.N. Influence of Extreme Seasons on Airborne Pollutant Levels in a Pig-Confinement Building. *Arch. Environ. Occup. Health* **2007**, *62*, 27–32. [CrossRef]
9. Viegas, C.; Gomes, A.Q.; Abegão, J.; Sabino, R.; Graça, T.; Viegas, S. Assessment of fungal contamination in waste sorting and incineration—Case study in Portugal. *J. Toxicol. Environ. Heal. Part A* **2014**, *77*, 57–68. [CrossRef]
10. Sabino, R.; Faísca, V.M.; Carolino, E.; Veríssimo, C.; Viegas, C. Occupational Exposure to Aspergillus by Swine and Poultry Farm Workers in Portugal. *J. Toxicol. Environ. Health A* **2012**, *75*, 1381–1391. [CrossRef]
11. D'Ovidio, D.; Grable, S.L.; Ferrara, M.; Santoro, D. Prevalence of dermatophytes and other superficial fungal organisms in asymptomatic guinea pigs in Southern Italy. *J. Small Anim. Pract.* **2014**, *55*, 355–358. [CrossRef] [PubMed]
12. Abrunhosa, L.; Morales, H.; Soares, C.; Calado, T.; Vila-Chã, A.S.; Pereira, M.; Venâncio, A. Review of Mycotoxins in Food and Feed Products in Portugal and Estimation of Probable Daily Intakes. *Crit. Rev. Food Sci. Nutr.* **2016**, *56*, 249–265. [CrossRef] [PubMed]
13. Streit, E.; Schatzmayr, G.; Tassis, P.; Tzika, E.; Marin, D.; Taranu, I.; Tabuc, C.; Nicolau, A.; Aprodu, I.; Puel, O.; et al. Current situation of mycotoxin contamination and co-occurrence in animal feed focus on Europe. *Toxins* **2012**, *4*, 788–809. [CrossRef] [PubMed]
14. Kovalsky, P.; Kos, G.; Nährer, K.; Schwab, C.; Jenkins, T.; Schatzmayr, G.; Sulyok, M.; Krska, R. Co-occurrence of regulated, masked and emerging mycotoxins and secondary metabolites in finished feed and maize—An extensive survey. *Toxins* **2016**, *8*, 363. [CrossRef] [PubMed]
15. Abdallah, M.F.; Girgin, G.; Baydar, T.; Krska, R.; Sulyok, M. Occurrence of multiple mycotoxins and other fungal metabolites in animal feed and maize samples from Egypt using LC-MS/MS. *J. Sci. Food Agric.* **2017**, *97*, 4419–4428. [CrossRef] [PubMed]
16. Viegas, S.; Caetano, L.A.; Korkalainen, M.; Faria, T.; Pacífico, C.; Carolino, E.; Quintal Gomes, A.; Viegas, C. Cytotoxic and Inflammatory Potential of Air Samples from Occupational Settings with Exposure to Organic Dust. *Toxics* **2017**, *5*, 8. [CrossRef] [PubMed]
17. Viegas, S.; Veiga, L.; Verissimo, C.; Sabino, R.; Figueiredo, P.; Almeida, A.; Carolino, E.; Viegas, C. Occupational Exposure to Aflatoxin B1 in Swine Production and Possible Contamination Sources. *J. Toxicol. Environ. Health Part A Curr. Issues* **2013**, *76*, 944–951. [CrossRef]
18. Varga, J.; Baranyi, N.; Chandrasekaran, M.; Vágvölgyi, C.; Kocsubé, S. Mycotoxin producers in the Aspergillus genus: An update. *Acta Biol. Szeged.* **2015**, *59*, 151–167.

19. Spikes, S.; Xu, R.; Nguyen, K.; Chamilos, G.; Kontoyiannis, D.; Jacobson, R.; Ejzykowicz, D.; Chiang, L.; Filler, S.; May, G. Gliotoxin Production in Aspergillus fumigatus Contributes to Host-Specific Differences in Virulence. *J. Infect. Dis.* **2008**, *197*, 479–486. [CrossRef]
20. Warth, B.; Sulyok, M.; Fruhmann, P.; Mikula, H.; Berthiller, F.; Schuhmacher, R.; Hametner, C.; Abia, W.A.; Adam, G.; Frohlich, J.; et al. Development and validation of a rapid multi-biomarker liquid chromatography/tandem mass spectrometry method to assess human exposure to mycotoxins. *Rapid Commun. Mass Spectrom.* **2012**, *26*, 1533–1540. [CrossRef]
21. Warth, B.; Sulyok, M.; Krska, R. LC-MS/MS-based multi-biomarker approaches for the assessment of Human exposure to mycotoxins. *Anal. Bioanal. Chem.* **2013**, *405*, 5687–5695. [CrossRef] [PubMed]
22. Gerding, J.; Cramer, B.; Humpf, H.U. Determination of mycotoxin exposure in Germany using an LC-MS/MS multibiomarker approach. *Mol. Nutr. Food Res.* **2014**, *58*, 2358–2368. [CrossRef] [PubMed]
23. Osteresch, B.; Viegas, S.; Cramer, B.; Humpf, H.-U. Multi-mycotoxin analysis using dried blood spots and dried serum spots. *Anal. Bioanal. Chem.* **2017**, *409*, 3369–3382. [CrossRef] [PubMed]
24. Degen, G. Tools for investigating workplace-related risks from mycotoxin exposure. *World Mycotoxin J.* **2011**, *4*, 315–327. [CrossRef]
25. Viegas, S.; Veiga, L.; Malta-Vacas, J.; Sabino, R.; Figueredo, P.; Almeida, A.; Viegas, C.; Carolino, E. Occupational exposure to aflatoxin (AFB1) in poultry production. *J. Toxicol. Environ. Health Part A* **2012**, *75*, 1330–1340. [CrossRef] [PubMed]
26. Assunção, R.; Silva, M.J.; Alvito, P. Challenges in risk assessment of multiple mycotoxins in food. *World Mycotoxin* **2016**, *9*, 791–811. [CrossRef]
27. Viegas, S.; Assunção, R.; Nunes, C.; Osteresch, B.; Twaruzek, M.; Kosicki, R.; Grajewski, J.; Martins, C.; Alvito, P.; Almeida, A.; et al. Exposure Assessment to Mycotoxins in a Portuguese Fresh Bread Dough Company by Using a Multi-Biomarker Approach. *Toxins* **2018**, *10*, 342. [CrossRef] [PubMed]
28. Föllmann, W.; Ali, N.; Blaszkewicz, M.; Degen, G.H. Biomonitoring of Mycotoxins in Urine: Pilot Study in Mill Workers. *J. Toxicol. Environ. Heal. Part A* **2016**, *79*, 1015–1025. [CrossRef]
29. Vidal, A.; Mengelers, M.; Yang, S.; De Saeger, S.; De Boevre, M. Mycotoxin Biomarkers of Exposure: A Comprehensive Review. *Compr. Rev. Food Sci. Food Saf.* **2018**, *17*, 1127–1155. [CrossRef]
30. Schwartz-Zimmermann, H.E.; Hametner, C.; Nagl, V.; Fiby, I.; Macheiner, L.; Winkler, J.; Dänicke, S.; Clark, E.; Pestka, J.J.; Berthiller, F. Glucuronidation of deoxynivalenol (DON) by different animal species: Identification of iso-DON glucuronides and iso-deepoxy-DON glucuronides as novel DON metabolites in pigs, rats, mice, and cows. *Arch. Toxicol.* **2017**, *91*, 3857. [CrossRef]
31. Viegas, S.; Osteresch, B.; Almeida, A.; Cramer, B.; Humpf, H.-U.; Viegas, C. Enniatin B and ochratoxin A in the blood serum of workers from the waste management setting. *Mycotoxin Res.* **2017**. [CrossRef] [PubMed]
32. Papageorgiou, M.; Wells, L.; Williams, C.; White, K.; De Santis, B.; Liu, Y.; Debegnach, F.; Miano, B.; Moretti, G.; Greetham, S.; et al. Assessment of Urinary Deoxynivalenol Biomarkers in UK Children and Adolescents. *Toxins* **2018**, *10*, 50. [CrossRef] [PubMed]
33. Turner, P.C.; White, K.L.M.; Burley, V.J.; Hopton, R.P.; Rajendram, A.; Fisher, J.; Cade, J.E.; Wild, C.P. A comparison of deoxynivalenol intake and urinary deoxynivalenol in UK adults. *Biomarkers* **2010**. [CrossRef] [PubMed]
34. Turner, P.C.; Hopton, R.P.; White, K.L.M.; Fisher, J.; Cade, J.L.; Wild, C.P. Assessment of deoxynivalenol metabolite profiles in UK adults. *Food Chem. Toxicol.* **2010**, *49*, 132–135. [CrossRef] [PubMed]
35. EFSA. Scientific opinion on the risk to human and animal health related to the presence of deoxynivalenol and its acetylated and modified forms in food and feed. *EFSA J.* **2017**, *15*, 345.
36. Basinas, I.; Sigsgaard, T.; Kromhout, H.; Heederik, D.; Wouters, I.M.; Schlünssen, V. A comprehensive review of levels and determinants of personal exposure to dust and endotoxin in livestock farming. *J. Expo. Sci. Environ. Epidemiol.* **2015**, *25*, 123. [CrossRef] [PubMed]
37. Boonen, J.; Malysheva, S.V.; Taevernier, L.; Diana Di Mavungu, J.; De Saeger, S.; De Spiegeleer, B. Human skin penetration of selected model mycotoxins. *Toxicology* **2012**, *301*, 21–32. [CrossRef] [PubMed]
38. Guerre, P. Worldwide Mycotoxins Exposure in Pig and Poultry Feed Formulations. *Toxins* **2016**, *8*, 350. [CrossRef]
39. Pierron, A.; Alassane-Kpembi, I.; Oswald, I.P. Impact of mycotoxin on immune response and consequences for pig health. *Anim. Nutr.* **2016**, *2*, 63–68. [CrossRef]

40. Šegvić Klarić, M.; Rašić, D.; Peraica, M. Deleterious Effects of Mycotoxin Combinations Involving Ochratoxin A. *Toxins* **2013**, *5*, 1965–1987. [CrossRef]
41. Sobral, M.M.C.; Faria, M.A.; Cunha, S.C.; Ferreira, I.M. Toxicological interactions between mycotoxins from ubiquitous fungi: Impact on hepatic and intestinal human epithelial cells. *Chemosphere* **2018**, *202*, 538–548. [CrossRef] [PubMed]
42. Pena, A.; Seifrtová, M.; Lino, C.; Silveira, I.; Solich, P. Estimation of ochratoxin A in portuguese population: New data on the occurrence in human urine by high performance liquid chromatography with fluorescence detection. *Food Chem. Toxicol.* **2006**, *44*, 1449–1454. [CrossRef] [PubMed]
43. Lino, C.M.; Baeta, M.L.; Henri, M.; Dinis, A.M.P.; Pena, A.S.; Silveira, M.I.N. Levels of ochratoxin A in serum from urban and rural Portuguese populations and estimation of exposure degree. *Food Chem. Toxicol.* **2008**, *46*, 879–885. [CrossRef] [PubMed]
44. Duarte, S.; Bento, J.; Pena, A.; Lino, C.M.; Delerue-Matos, C.; Oliva-Teles, T.; Morais, S.; Correia, M.; Oliveira, M.B.P.P.; Alves, M.R.; et al. Monitoring of ochratoxin A exposure of the Portuguese population through a nationwide urine survey—Winter 2007. *Sci. Total Environ.* **2010**, *408*, 1195–1198. [CrossRef]
45. Viegas, C.; J Nurme, J.; Piecková, E.; Viegas, S. Sterigmatocystin in foodstuffs and feed: Aspects to consider. *Mycology* **2018**. [CrossRef]
46. Smith, M.C.; Madec, S.; Coton, E.; Hymery, N. Natural Co-Occurrence of Mycotoxins in Foods and Feeds and Their in vitro Combined Toxicological Effects. *Toxins* **2016**, *8*, 94. [CrossRef]
47. Sarkanj, B.; Ezekiel, C.N.; Turner, P.C.; Abia, W.A.; Rychlik, M.; Krska, R.; Sulyok, M.; Warth, B. Ultra-sensitive, stable isotope assisted quantification of multiple urinary mycotoxin exposure biomarkers. *Anal. Chim. Acta* **2018**, *1019*, 84–92. [CrossRef]
48. Bopp, S.K.; Barouki, R.; Brack, W.; Costa, S.D.; Dorne, J.C.M.; Drakvik, P.E.; Faust, M.; Karjalainen, T.K.; Kephalopoulos, S.; van Klaveren, J.; et al. Current EU research activities on combined exposure to multiple chemicals. *Environ. Int.* **2018**, *120*, 544–562. [CrossRef]
49. Assunção, R.; Martins, C.; Viegas, S.; Viegas, C.; Jakobsen, L.S.; Pires, S.; Alvito, P. Climate change and the health impact of aflatoxins exposure in Portugal—An overview. *Food Addit. Contam. Part A* **2018**, *35*, 1610–1621. [CrossRef]
50. Battilani, P.; Toscano, P.; Van der Fels-Klerx, H.J.; Moretti, A.; Camardo Leggieri, M.; Brera, C.; Rortais, A.; Goumperis, T.; Robinson, T. Aflatoxin B1 contamination in maize in Europe increases due to climate change. *Sci. Rep.* **2016**, *6*, 24328. [CrossRef]
51. WHO (World Health Organization). *Biological Monitoring of Chemical Exposure in the Workplace*; World Health Organization: Geneva, Switzerland, 1996; Volume 1.
52. Choi, J.; Mørck, T.A.; Polcher, A.; Knudsen, L.E.; Joas, A. Review of the state of the art of human biomonitoring for chemical substances and its application to human exposure assessment for food safety. *EFSA Support. Publ.* **2015**, *12*, 724E. [CrossRef]
53. World Medical Association. Declaration of Helsinki Ethical Principles for Medical Research Involving Human Subjects. *JAMA* **2013**, *310*, 2191–2194. [CrossRef] [PubMed]
54. European Commission. *Ethics and Data Protection*; European Commission: Brussels, Belgium; Luxembourg, November 2018.

toxins

MDPI

Article

Porcine Hepatic Response to Fumonisin B_1 in a Short Exposure Period: Fatty Acid Profile and Clinical Investigations

Omeralfaroug Ali [1,*], Judit Szabó-Fodor [2], Hedvig Fébel [3], Miklós Mézes [4], Krisztián Balogh [4], Róbert Glávits [5], Melinda Kovács [1,2], Arianna Zantomasi [6] and András Szabó [1,2]

1 Faculty of Agricultural and Environmental Sciences, Kaposvár University, 7400 Kaposvár, Hungary; kovacs.melinda@ke.hu (M.K.); szan1125@freemail.hu (A.S.)
2 "MTA-KE Mycotoxins in the Food Chain" Research Group, Hungarian Academy of Sciences, Kaposvár University, 7400 Kaposvár, Hungary; szabo.fodor.judit@gmail.com
3 Research Institute for Animal Breeding, Nutrition and Meat Science, National Agricultural Research Center, 2053 Herceghalom, Hungary; febel.hedvig@atk.naik.hu
4 Department of Nutrition, Faculty of Agricultural and Environmental Sciences, Szent István University, 2103 Gödöllő, Hungary; mezes.miklos@mkk.szie.hu (M.M.); balogh.krisztian@mkk.szie.hu (K.B.)
5 Autopsy Ltd., Telepes u. 42, 1147 Budapest, Hungary; glavits.robert.dr@gmail.com
6 Department of Animal Science, University of Padova, Agripolis, Viale dell'Università 16, 35020 Legnaro, Padova, Italy; mania9123@gmail.com
* Correspondence: omeralfaroug.ali@gmail.com; Tel.: +36-304-642-369

Received: 2 October 2019; Accepted: 8 November 2019; Published: 10 November 2019

Abstract: Scarce studies have investigated the impact of fumonisin B_1 (FB_1) on the hepatic tissue fatty acid (FA) profile, and no study is available on piglets. A 10-day in vivo experiment was performed on seven piglets/group: control and FB_1-fed animals (diet was contaminated with fungal culture: 20 mg FB_1/kg diet). Independent sample *t*-test was carried out at $p < 0.05$ as the significance level. Neither growth, nor feed efficiency, was affected. The hepatic phospholipid (PL) fatty acids (FAs) were more susceptible for FB_1, while triglyceride (TG) was less responsive. The impact of FB_1 on hepatic PL polyunsaturated fatty acids (PUFAs) was more pronounced than on saturated fatty acids. Among all PUFAs, predominant ones in response were docosapentaenoicacid (DPA) (↓), docosahexaenoic DHA (↓) and arachidonic acids (↑). This led to a higher omega-6:omega-3 ratio, whereas a similar finding was noted in TGs. Neither total saturation (SFA) nor total monousaturation (MUFA) were affected by the FB_1 administration. The liver showed an increase in malondialdehyde, as well as antioxidant capacity (reduced glutathione and glutathione peroxidase). The plasma enzymatic assessment revealed an increase in alkaline phosphatase (ALP), while alanine transaminase (ALT), aspartate transaminase (AST), lactate dehydrogenase (LDH), and gamma-glutamyltransferase (GGT) were not influenced. The microscopic sections provided evidence of vacuolar degeneration of the hepatocytes' cytoplasm, but it was not severe. Furthermore, the lung edema was developed, while the kidney was not affected. In conclusion, regarding FB_1-mediated hepatotoxicity in piglets, the potential effect of slight hepatotoxicity did not compromise growth performance, at least at the dose and exposure period applied.

Keywords: fumonisin B_1; piglet; liver; lipids; blood serum; oxidation; clinical chemistry; histopathology; phospholipids

Key Contribution: Fumonisin B_1 for piglets at 20 mg/kg dietary dose was found not to compromise growth and production traits, but was found to negatively influence histology, cellular enzyme leakage, and hepatocellular membrane lipid fatty acid profile in a comprehensive manner, after an exposure time of 10 days.

1. Introduction

Fumonisin B1 (FB_1) can be regarded as one of the most important mycotoxins, due to its toxicity and carcinogenic mode of action [1,2]. FB_1 can induce hepatotoxicity (proven in vitro and in vivo) and kidney cancer in mammals [3–7]. FB_1 has a structure similar to the ceramide precursor sphinganine and therefore it inhibits the de novo ceramide synthesis (CerS); it catalyzes the acylation of sphinganine (Sa) and recycling of sphingosine (So) and interferes with the sphingolipid metabolism. This results in a higher concentration of intracellular Sa and other sphingoid bases in cells and tissues [8], which are proapoptotic, cytotoxic, and growth inhibitors [9]. The Sa:So ratio has been reported to increase in the plasma by FB_1 exposure from a 3.7 mg FB_1 + FB_2/kg diet [10]. Also, it was found to increase from a 5 mg FB_1/kg diet in several organs of the piglet, including the liver [11].

Pigs have been considered as the most relevant and sensitive animal model with a digestive system highly similar to the human [12,13]. Basically, the kidney and liver are very important organs in mycotoxicity experiments, since both are involved in FB_1 (and metabolized forms) elimination and detoxification [14]. In swine, specifically, FB_1 was found to exert development of pulmonary edema and hepatotoxicity [4], moreover, it has been suggested as the key player behind pulmonary fibrosis [15]. With regard to the liver, several studies reported the ability of FB_1 in inducing histomorphological alterations with dose range of 3.7–190 mg/kg diet and exposure time range of 5–83 days, using different exposure methods: contaminated diet, orally gavaged, and intravenously [10,16–21]. Also, it induced clinical signs, such as respiratory distress [11]. On the other hand, assessment of the liver function relies on the serum biochemical levels, including the enzymatic matrix of alanine transaminase (ALT), aspartate transaminase (AST), alkaline phosphatase (ALP), lactate dehydrogenase (LDH), and gamma-glutamyltransferase (GGT). Moreover, sometimes the alteration in serum enzymatic matrix occurred coupled with higher total cholesterol level [18,22]. The negative effects of FB_1 decrease after the regulation establishment, in which numerous regulations are available. Regulations are locally different, varying in the maximum recommended level of FB_1 in the food/feed. The U.S. Food and Drug Administration (FDA) has published guidance level (20 mg/kg) as the maximum level for total fumonisins (FBs: FB_1 + FB_2 + FB_3) in corn or its byproducts intended for swine nutrition [23]. In addition, the FDA states the contaminated corn should not exceed 50% of swine diet. Therefore, the total FBs in a complete diet should not exceed 10 mg/kg. On the other hand, in Europe, the European Commission (EC) has recommended maximally 5 mg FB_1 + FB_2 kg feed in all complementary and complete feedstuffs for swine [24].

The cellular fatty acid profile is acknowledged as a useful biomarker to monitor disease status. To date, it is well known that the disruption for the membrane lipid profile is FB_1 toxicity mechanism, as numerous in vivo and in vitro; relevant literatures are available and well documented on rodents, such as those by Gelderblom et al. [25–27], Riedel et al. [5,6], Burger et al. [7,28], Szabó et al. [29–31], and to a lesser extent on rabbits [32,33]. However, in many cases, in vivo studies of FB_1 altered the lipid metabolism in the rat which displayed different patterns than in in vitro studies. FB_1 was found to interfere with the metabolism of sphingolipids and ceramides-subjective lipid regulatory enzymes and was found to induce lipid peroxidation [6,27]. Lipid peroxidation influences the lipid/FA composition of cellular membranes, as it highly depends on the degree of FA unsaturation in membranes. In addition, FB_1 was suggested not only to modulate lipid profile integrity of the hepatocellular membranes by changing the FA composition and enzyme activities, but also through modifying its membrane microdomains [7]. Systematically, such changes in the intracellular and extracellular levels of lipid mediators alter the expression and activity of signaling and regulatory pathways that control physiological processes critical for cell growth, differentiation, and normal cell function [34]. In this regard, FB_1 has been suggested to induce cancer development through modulating the membrane integrity and lipid raft of cells [5,7].

Despite a recent study illustrating that 12.2 mg FBs/kg diet developed hepatotoxicity in piglets after 28 days of exposure [10], it is interesting to study the sub-acute effect of FB_1 on the liver. From this point of view, earlier reports which applied 20 mg FB_1/kg diet [18,21] on piglets did not provide alteration in the membrane profile of the liver, in connection with its hepatotoxicity. Monitoring alterations in lipids may assist for better understanding of FB_1 toxicity mechanism of action. The pathophysiology mechanism of FB_1 in the piglets' liver is not yet well understood. The pig was our animal model in this study, with a primary focus on the liver. Thus, this study aimed to investigate the effect of orally administrated FB_1 on the FA profile of membrane phospholipids (PLs) and that of tissue triglycerides (TGs) from the hepatic tissue of weaned piglets exposed to a diet contaminated with fungal culture (20 mg FB_1/kg diet) for 10 days. Furthermore, the study seeks to illustrate the hepatotoxicity status at the shorter exposure period through investigating the clinical chemistry and histomorphological changes.

2. Results

2.1. Body, Organ Weight, Feed Intake, and Its Utilization Efficiency

It is worth highlighting that during the study period no mortality case was found. Regarding the results in Table 1, for the liver weights no significant difference was detected among the study groups (control and FB_1-fed group), even when expressed as relative weight of the total body weight. Similarly, the body weight, absolute weight of other organs (kidney, spleen, lung, and heart), and feeding parameters were not significantly affected by FB_1.

Table 1. The somatic and feeding parameters of the control and fumonisin B_1 (FB_1)-fed piglets.

Somatic Traits	Control			FB_1		
	Mean	±	SD	Mean	±	SD
BW initial (kg)	13.3	±	1.90	13.1	±	1.60
BW final (kg)	15.9	±	2.40	15.8	±	1.80
DBWG (g)	266	±	66.3	269	±	33.3
FC (kg/10 days)	4458	±	1022	4650	±	443
FCR (g diet/g BWG)	1.69	±	0.13	1.74	±	0.20
Liver (g)	359	±	78.9	358	±	56.2
Kidney (g)	85.2	±	9.99	81.3	±	11.4
Spleen (g)	38.3	±	4.29	36.1	±	5.16
Lung (g)	198	±	34.4	189	±	37.7
Heart (g)	99.2	±	14.9	106	±	12.5

BW, body weight; DBWG, daily body weight gain; FC, feed consumption; FCR, feed conversion ratio.

2.2. Fatty Acid Profile of the Hepatic Phospholipids

When evaluating the hepatic PL FA (Table 2) composition, among all saturated FAs (SFAs), only lignoceric acid (C24:0) decreased to FB_1 exposure ($p < 0.01$). Unsaturated FAs (UFAs) were more responsive, as compared to SFAs. Proportions of the C18:3n-6 (γ-linolenic acid, $p < 0.05$) and C20:4n-6 (arachidonic acid, $p < 0.05$) were significantly higher in FB_1-fed piglets, while both of the C22:5n-3 (docosapentaenoic acid, DPA; $p < 0.001$) and C22:6n-3 (docosahexaenoic acid, DHA; $p < 0.01$) proportions were lower. Consequences of DPA and DHA proportional reduction are reductions in total polyunsaturation (PUFA; $p < 0.05$) and omega-3 FAs ($p < 0.001$). In contrast, significant increases were detected in total omega-6 FAs ($p < 0.05$) and n-6:n-3 ratio ($p < 0.001$). Total monounsaturation (MUFA) and total saturation (SFA) were not altered by FB_1 feeding. From the calculated indices, unsaturation index (UI) and average fatty acyl chain length (ACL) decreased in the FB_1-treated group ($p < 0.05$).

Table 2. Fatty acid profiles of the total phospholipid (PL) and triglycerides (TGs) from the hepatic tissue for control and FB_1-fed piglets.

Fatty Acids	Hepatic Total PL (%)							Hepatic Total TG (%)						
	Control			FB_1				Control			FB_1			
	Mean	±	SD	Mean	±	SD	Sig.	Mean	±	SD	Mean	±	SD	Sig.
C12:0	-	±	-	-	±	-	-	0.04	±	0.01	0.03	±	0.01	NS
C14:0	0.13	±	0.03	0.16	±	0.03	NS	0.35	±	0.14	0.26	±	0.09	NS
C15:0	0.13	±	0.07	0.17	±	0.11	NS	0.10	±	0.04	0.12	±	0.06	NS
C16:0	15.5	±	0.60	15.2	±	0.95	NS	12.3	±	2.25	11.1	±	0.70	NS
C16:1n-7	0.30	±	0.07	0.38	±	0.16	NS	0.56	±	0.30	0.38	±	0.14	NS
C17:0	0.72	±	0.23	1.09	±	0.65	NS	0.63	±	0.22	0.88	±	0.61	NS
C18:0	29.0	±	0.93	29.6	±	1.62	NS	26.6	±	1.88	28.6	±	1.11	*
C18:1n-9c	5.75	±	0.54	6.48	±	1.17	NS	8.17	±	2.83	6.62	±	0.92	NS
C18:2n-6c	20.6	±	1.04	20.7	±	0.75	NS	18.4	±	1.77	18.0	±	0.74	NS
C18:3n-6	0.14	±	0.03	0.18	±	0.05	NS	0.14	±	0.08	0.19	±	0.05	NS
C18:3n-3	0.21	±	0.05	0.17	±	0.03	NS	0.56	±	0.28	0.40	±	0.13	NS
C20:0	0.07	±	0.01	0.08	±	0.02	NS	0.13	±	0.06	0.11	±	0.01	NS
C20:1n-9	0.12	±	0.02	0.12	±	0.02	NS	0.15	±	0.11	0.20	±	0.08	NS
C20:2n-7	0.66	±	0.08	0.63	±	0.06	NS	0.70	±	0.10	0.64	±	0.05	NS
C20:3n-6	1.34	±	0.35	1.29	±	0.25	NS	1.29	±	0.38	1.33	±	0.25	NS
C20:4n-6	12.1	±	1.36	13.4	±	0.41	*	15.5	±	1.66	17.9	±	1.12	**
C20:3n-3	0.14	±	0.04	0.12	±	0.02	NS	0.21	±	0.06	0.20	±	0.04	NS
C20:5n-3	1.35	±	0.55	1.37	±	0.32	NS	1.44	±	0.57	1.54	±	0.26	NS
C22:0	0.03	±	0.00	0.04	±	0.01	NS	0.10	±	0.09	0.05	±	0.02	NS
C22:5n-3	3.04	±	0.14	2.38	±	0.29	***	3.13	±	0.34	2.89	±	0.25	NS
C22:6n-3	8.34	±	0.79	6.28	±	1.11	*	9.03	±	1.41	8.14	±	0.82	NS
C24:0	0.34	±	0.03	0.26	±	0.04	**	0.38	±	0.07	0.33	±	0.04	NS
SFA	46.0	±	0.75	46.6	±	0.77	NS	40.7	±	2.73	41.6	±	0.99	NS
UFA	54.0	±	0.75	53.4	±	0.77	NS	59.3	±	2.73	58.4	±	0.99	NS
MUFA	6.17	±	0.59	6.89	±	1.33	NS	8.88	±	3.21	7.19	±	1.10	NS
PUFA	47.8	±	1.07	46.5	±	1.39	*	50.4	±	4.92	51.2	±	1.32	NS
Omega-6	34.1	±	0.81	35.5	±	0.53	*	35.4	±	3.03	37.4	±	0.85	NS
Omega-3	13.0	±	0.91	10.3	±	1.35	***	14.4	±	2.09	13.2	±	1.05	NS
n-6:n-3	2.62	±	0.21	3.49	±	0.44	***	2.49	±	0.23	2.86	±	0.26	*
Odd Chain	0.85	±	0.29	1.26	±	0.76	NS	0.73	±	0.26	1.00	±	0.66	NS
UI	174.3	±	5.43	164.8	±	6.50	*	192.8	±	16.4	193.3	±	5.36	NS
ACL	18.5	±	0.05	18.4	±	0.08	*	18.6	±	0.15	18.6	±	0.06	NS

* $p < 0.05$; ** $p < 0.01$; *** $p < 0.001$; NS, not significant, $p > 0.05$; SFA, saturated fatty acids; UFA, unsaturated fatty acids; MUFA, monounsaturated fatty acids; PUFA, polyunsaturated fatty acids; n-6:n-3, omega-6:omega-3; UI, unsaturation index; ACL, average chain length.

2.3. Fatty Acid Profile of the Triglycerides from Hepatic Tissue

In the hepatic TG FA profile (Table 2), C18:0 (stearic acid) proportion increased significantly ($p < 0.05$) in the FB_1-fed group, as well as that in C20:4n-6 (arachidonic acid, AA; $p < 0.01$). The omega-6:omega-3 FA ratio increased significantly ($p < 0.05$) in piglets exposed to FB_1. This increase was combined with a higher proportion of arachidonic acid, being the only responder FA (higher proportion) among all UFAs. No alterations were detected in the other calculated indices.

2.4. Lipid Peroxidation and Antioxidant Parameters

Based on the results of the oxidative stress assessment parameters obtained from the liver, significant alterations were noticed (Figure 1). The tissue concentration of malondialdehyde (MDA) increased significantly ($p < 0.05$) due to FB_1 administration. In a similar manner, the activity of glutathione peroxidase (GPx) increased ($p < 0.001$), as well as the level of the reduced glutathione (GSH, $p < 0.05$).

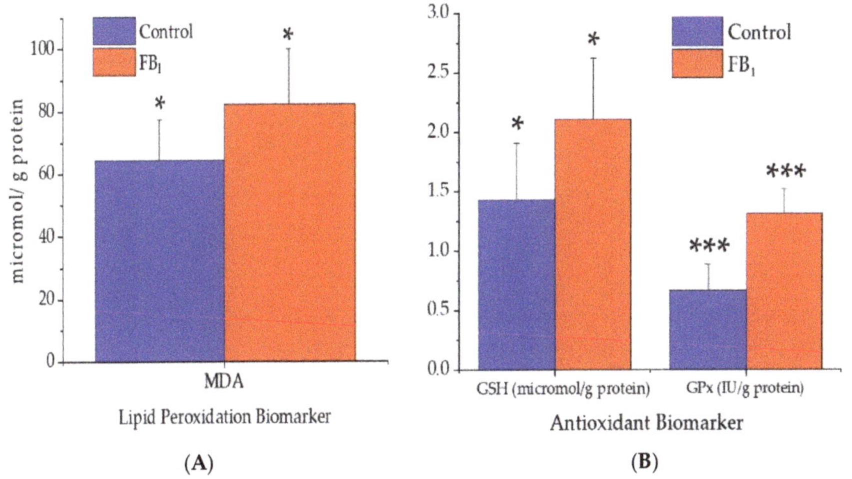

Figure 1. (**A**) Lipid peroxidation and (**B**) antioxidant biomarkers of the hepatic tissue of control and FB_1-fed animals (data represent mean ± SD, $n = 7$ per group). * $p < 0.05$; *** $p < 0.001$; MDA, malondialdehyde; GSH, reduced glutathione; GPx, glutathione peroxidase.

2.5. Serum Biochemical Parameters

The blood serum biochemical parameters ALT, AST, ALP, LDH, and GGT can be seen in Figure 2.

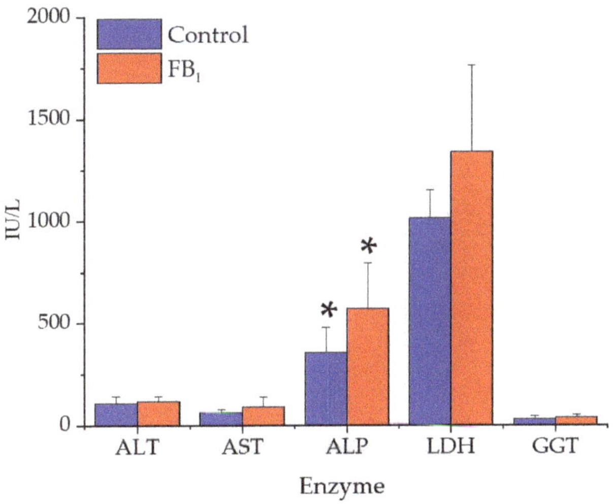

Figure 2. Alteration in serum enzymes for control and FB_1-fed groups (20 mg FB_1/kg feed) during the 10-day feeding period (data represent mean ± SD, $n = 7$ per group). * $p < 0.05$; ALT, alanine transaminase; AST, aspartate transaminase; ALP, alkaline phosphatase; LDH, lactate dehydrogenase; GGT, gamma-glutamyltransferase.

Only alkaline phosphatase (ALP) showed a significant activity increase after 10 days of toxin administration, while activity differences of the ALT, AST, LDH, and GGT in the blood serum were insignificant. Similarly, to the latter enzymes, concentrations of total protein, albumin, cholesterol, and bilirubin were not different (Table 3).

Table 3. The liver associated serum biochemical parameters for control and FB_1-fed piglets (20 mg FB_1/kg feed).

Parameter	Control			FB_1		
	Mean	±	SD	Mean	±	SD
Total protein (g/L)	55.4	±	3.64	52.6	±	3.41
Albumin (g/L)	34.0	±	1.82	32.7	±	3.15
Total cholesterol (mmol/L)	1.98	±	0.21	2.10	±	0.18
Total bilirubin (μmol/L)	2.44	±	1.50	1.10	±	0.83

2.6. Histopathological Results

The histopathological assessment of the hepatic and lung tissues (see Table 4) has revealed changes in FB_1-fed animals. In regard to the renal and spleen tissues, no lesion was found in any of the animals.

Table 4. The histopathological alteration in the hepatic and lung tissues for control and FB_1-fed animals individually (20 mg FB_1/kg feed) after a 10-day feeding period.

Organ	Parameters	Control							FB_1						
		Animal Number													
		1	2	3	4	5	6	7	1	2	3	4	5	6	7
Liver	Vacuolar degeneration	-	-	-	-	-	-	-	1	1	-	1	1	2	-
Lung	Alveolar edema	-	-	-	-	-	-	-	2	-	1	-	1	-	-
	Interstitial edema	-	-	-	-	-	-	-	-	-	-	1	1	-	-

(-) = no alteration; 1 = slight/small scale/few; 2 = medium degree/medium scale/medium number.

In some FB_1-fed animals (5 piglets), slightly different degrees of vacuolar degeneration of the hepatocytes' cytoplasm were observed (Figure 3). Those lesions were considered to be mild in severity (not substantially affecting the organ function) and were prone to recovery (healing).

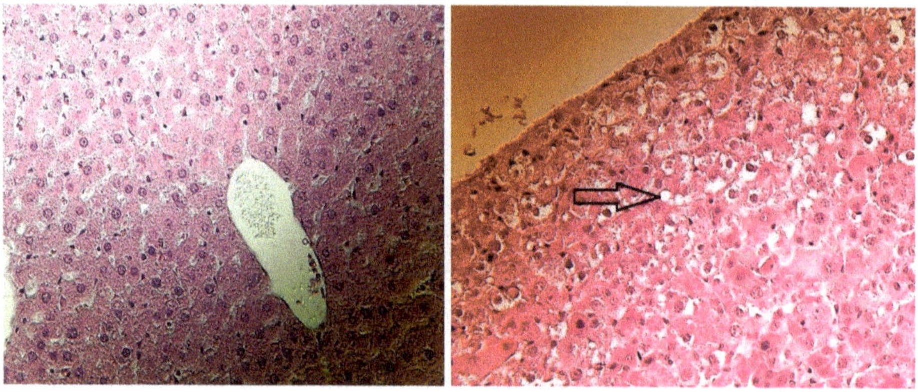

(**A**) (**B**)

Figure 3. (**A**) Healthy (no lesion detected) liver of the control and (**B**) vacuolar degeneration of the hepatocytes (arrow) of weaned piglets after 20 mg FB_1/kg diet exposure for 10 days (hematoxylin-eosin, 400×).

In the lung, some animals fed FB_1 have shown histopathological alterations. Most findings were mild edema in the lung interstitium (3 animals) and cavity of some alveolar groups (3 animals), which was associated with the effect of the FB_1 toxin fed.

3. Discussion

The research area of FB_1-induced modulation of tissue FA profile is receiving attention. Numerous studies reported the interfering ability of FB_1 with FAs, PLs, and sphingolipids, but their exact role and extent is still unknown, especially in piglets.

3.1. Growth, Feed Intake, and Organ Weights

The administration of 20 mg FB_1/kg diet for 10 days resulted in no mortality case. Mortality caused by FB_1 is highly associated with high doses (FB_1 >100 mg/kg diet) and/or a longer exposure period (>8 weeks and above) [35]. Furthermore, it associates with acute porcine pulmonary edema [36]. In addition, the growth, feed intake, and efficiency were not different between groups. The body weight highly relied on the feed intake, which was influenced by feed palatability. The authors suggest that the artificial FB_1 contamination in our setting did not alter the feed palatability. Regarding the body weight gain and feed consumption, similar results to our findings were observed in weaned piglets fed 10, 20, and 40 mg/kg FB_1 for four weeks [15]. Furthermore, 9 mg FB_1/piglet/day for four weeks did not induce alteration in the production performance: growth, organ weights, and feed intake [10,37]. FB_1 at 10–15 mg/kg diet is able to delay the piglet sexual maturity during longer exposure period at 24 weeks [38]. In animals, FBs (mostly FB_1) typically damage the liver and kidneys (in a species-dependent manner), decrease body weight gain, and increase mortality rates [39]. In our setting, FB_1 did not affect the kidney weight, which is interesting since its elimination happens via renal filtration [14], and partly through feces. Our results are in full agreement with the study of Souto et al. [37] and partially with results of Andretta et al. [40], in which FBs did not affect the weight of the kidney, spleen, and heart, but increased the relative weight of the liver and lung. The probable weight alteration of the liver was based on the hypothesis that FB_1 provides slight hepatotoxicity in swine and rats [12,25]. The onset of hepatotoxicity was proven (mild and not severe), thereby no alteration was noticed in body weight, feed efficiency, and liver weight. With regards to the lung, FB_1 has a rather strong effect on pig lung [4], thereby edema development has been hypothesized. A very slight pulmonary edema was proven in this study (Table 4, Figure 4), but since this has been reported earlier by Haschek et al. [4], we avoided discussing this in detail. However, our findings provide support to the statement of Haschek et al. [4] that lung and liver of swine are sensitive organs to FB_1.

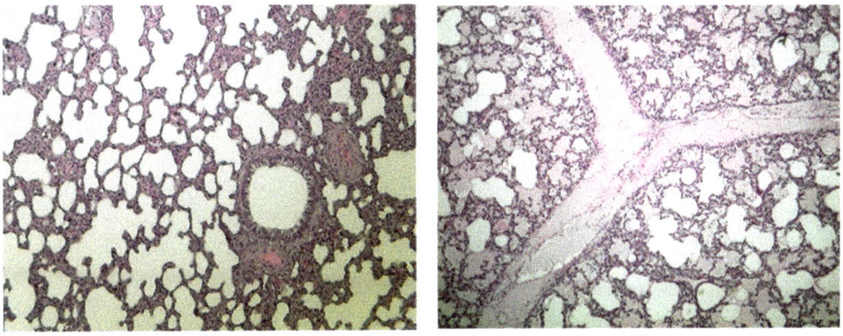

(**A**) (**B**)

Figure 4. (**A**) Healthy (no lesion detected) lung of the control, and (**B**) alveolar and interstitial edema of the lung of weaned piglets after 20 mg FB_1/kg diet exposure for 10 days (hematoxylin-eosin, 100×).

3.2. Fatty Acid Profile of the Hepatic Phospholipid FA Profile

A few in vivo and in vitro studies have investigated the effects of FB_1 on lipid metabolism in hepatic tissue, mainly in rodents. A novelty of this study is adding value to the piglet-relevant literature available. Results have shown numerous alterations in the hepatic PL FA profile, although they were not intense/severe. Only a minor modification was detected in SFAs, where the lignoceric acid proportion decreased. Lignoceric acid is a member of the long chain SFA group; an important component of sphingomyelins (SPH). The biosynthesis of SPH is relying on ceramides production, a key intermediate of sphingolipid metabolism and major precursor of long chain FA and complex sphingolipids [41,42]. Therefore, such a proportional reduction of lignoceric acid in the PLs is indirectly referring to the inhibition in the production of ceramide and sphingomyelin, a characteristic of the FB_1 mode of action.

FB_1 seems to attack hepatic PLs more intensely, as compared to TGs (Table 2). Essential FAs are commonly esterified to the *sn*-1 position and occasionally to the *sn*-2 position of the PLs. Within omega-3 FAs, except for DPA and DHA (decreases), none of their ALA long chain derivatives were modified. DPA and DHA cumulative effects were more visible in the total n-3 FA proportion, decreasing significantly. In rats exposed to 50 mg/kg feed FB_1 for five days, omega-3 FAs were found to decrease in the hepatic total PLs [28]. A similar reduction was reported by Szabó et al. [33] in the hepatic mitochondrial membrane of rabbits exposed to 10 mg/kg feed dose of FB_1. Equal ALA proportion between groups is related to resemble feed consumption, since its only source is the diet. Accordingly, alteration in ALA derivatives (namely the DPA and DHA) must be with high probability a toxin effect. Moreover, reactive oxygen species attack FAs according to their degree of polyunsaturation [43], in which omega-3 FAs are more prone.

The omega-6 FAs in the membrane have different roles from the omega-3 ones, although they may have common indications. C18:2n-6 (linoleic acid or LA, essential FA) equality among all groups in PLs and TGs may indirectly represent the identical diet uptake, similar to the ALA finding. FB_1 exposure has increased the proportions of γ-linolenic and arachidonic acids (C20:4n-6). There are contradicting literatures [25,26] from the prolonged FB_1 feeding studies on rats. Several studies reported the increase of arachidonic acid, such as Burger et al. [28], in rats treated for 21 days with 250 mg FB_1/kg feed dosage. Authors supposed a shift towards prostanoid synthesis of the E2 series and added that alterations in the phosphatidyl-ethanolamine FA composition and arachidonic acid proportion in the plasma membrane could alter growth regulatory factors and cell receptors in lipid rafts. Furthermore, some adverse effects (i.e., cancer development, tumor angiogenesis, cell adhesion, and an increase in DNA synthesis) have been correlated with high proportions of arachidonic derived eicosanoids [44]. Therefore, the proportional increase of arachidonic acid in the piglet liver may be likewise a targeted accretion of the root fatty acid component for eicosanoid synthesis.

The higher γ-linolenic and arachidonic acids' proportions have thus increased the proportion of total omega-6 FAs, alongside with the increase of omega-6:omega-3 ratio. This ratio is a biological marker for disruption of enzymes that regulate lipid metabolism. In the study of Burger et al. [28] on rats, the omega-6:omega-3 ratio increased with toxin administration, which is similar to ours in piglets. Most probably, the lipid peroxidation process is the key player behind this result through oxidative stress propagation, an indirect toxin effect. For this reason, our study revealed that the porcine liver is a sensitive organ to FB_1, and its toxicity can be linked with its membrane profile.

Regarding FA indices, a reduction was noted for the UI as a result of depletion in total PUFA proportions of FB_1-fed piglets. As a consequence, ACL decreased, highly influenced by the reduction of DPA and DHA. The reduction in PUFA and UI may refer to a more rigid cell membrane, as a protective way against FB_1, likely by manipulating membrane receptors and enzymes activities that are involved in the biosynthesis of proteins, lipids, and sterols. However, the MUFA level was also not responsive for the treatment applied. These insignificant results were unexpected, since relevant studies illustrated the increase in total saturation and monounsaturation is a way to increase the membrane rigidity, a resistance mechanism against oxidative stress [6].

3.3. *Fatty Acid Profile of the Hepatic Triglycerides*

Only a few modifications were observed in the hepatic TGs. Compositional changes of TGs are seldom reported and are generally referring to energy metabolism. TG stores have fewer other functions than energy supply and are thus mostly reflecting the need for specific FAs at an extra-hepatic site. Once we only registered minor changes, our TG dataset may be handled as secondary data. Similar to PL results, the omega-6:omega-3 ratio increased, as well as that in arachidonic acid. Despite TGs major role to provide energy, their compositional modifications were linked to alterations in the physical properties of cellular membranes [45]. The main reason behind this is that they are incorporated into the lipid bilayer and assist the maintenance of cell membranes.

3.4. *Lipid Peroxidation and Antioxidant Parameters*

Oxidative stress is a condition produced by free radical accumulation that is not entirely eliminated by antioxidants. Studies demonstrate the ability of FB_1 in the oxidation stress induction via generation of reactive oxygen species (ROS). ROS over-production by mitochondrial indicates damage on its membrane, associated with the transient activation of cytosolic phospholipases A2 ($cPLA_2$) [46]. Activity of cPLA2 is influenced by SPH concentration [47], in which FB_1 mechanism of action involves SPH disruption. Within a specific time-frame, ROS attack within the cell will contribute to its depletion and deterioration of its biomolecules and favor cell death conditions through stimulating certain stress-sensitive signaling pathways (e.g., nuclear factor κB, p38MAPK, and c-Jun N-terminal kinase) [48,49]. Lipid peroxidation (lipid attacked by ROS) is a consequence of FB_1 toxicity mode of action, whereas MDA level is acknowledged as a reliable biomarker for FA peroxidation and cell membrane damage [50]. MDA is cytotoxic and results from the terminal phase of FA peroxidation, majority three double bond containing FAs and with a considerable amount less than three double bond FAs [51,52]. In this study MDA level was significantly modified, indicating that the liver was undergoing oxidative stress. Consequently, alterations in its membrane lipid profile are possibly linked with oxidative stress.

When the MDA level was increasing, the free radical scavenger (GSH) and activities of GPx enzymes were stimulated as well. The increase of GSH and GPx in the hepatic tissue were unfamiliar since they were decreasing in rabbits, rats, and pigs exposed to FB_1. In the study of Szabó et al. [33] on weaned rabbits exposed for four weeks to 10 mg FB_1/kg dietary, reduction in the GSH and GPx of the plasma was present. Similar reductions in the GSH level were reported in the rat hepatic tissue [29], blood, and hemolyzed red blood cells (RBCs) of piglets [14]. In our study, no reduction was observed in levels of GSH and GPx, we suggest that oxidative stress and its derived byproduct production were less pronounced to compromise (decrease) compounds involved in the antioxidant defense mechanism.

The steady state level of cellular GSH builds on the equilibrium between production and consumption, extrusion and reduction in the cell, and oxidation and bond forming [53]. It is well known that GSH biological roles are not exclusive on the antioxidant defense mechanism. However, the GSH reinforced in hepatic tissue was achieved by increasing the activity of GPx enzymes, and thus eliminating the mitochondrial free radicals and byproducts of lipid peroxidation.

3.5. *Serum Clinical Chemistry*

In mammals, albumin represents most protein of the blood plasma [54], almost 60% of the total. Albumin levels were not different between groups. This refers to the non-compromised hepatic protein synthesis. It means no alteration at the glomerular permeability as well. This probably means the kidney was functioning well without nephrotoxicity. However, it is interesting to note that the concentration of albumin was in correlation with histopathological assessment, although its concentration was not statistically different between groups. Probably, the duration of exposure was the key player behind such a finding, since the mild hepatotoxicity was confirmed.

FB_1 administration has not altered the serum lipid total cholesterol concentration. This is unfamiliar with what was observed in piglets gavaged 1.5 mg FB_1/kg BW (equal to 25–30 mg FB_1/kg diet) for nine days [22], and also in piglets fed 12.2 mg FBs for 28 days [10]. In addition, this was observed in rats [55], due to the negative regulation of liver X receptors, the nuclear receptor family regulates the expression of genes involved in cholesterol and lipid homeostasis [56]. The reason behind this insignificant result in our study might be that the response is species-specific, thereby piglets had a different reaction than rats. In addition, the consumed FB_1 (93 mg/piglet) during the exposure period was lesser than that exposed in the study of Loiseau et al. [22]. Furthermore, Loiseau et al. [22] used oral gavage of a single FB_1 dose on a daily basis, and total daily dose was received at a specified moment. This is not similar to the case when the animal is exposed to FB_1 through diet, as animals receive a similar dose amount at a longer period, depending on the feeding system. Moreover, the longer exposure period (almost 300% as compared to ours) in a study of Terciolo et al. [10] was able to alter the serum cholesterol, which was not similar to our findings due to the shorter exposure period.

Hepatotoxicity is generally characterized by alterations in organ weight and serum enzyme activities [22]. The serum bilirubin was not responsive for FB_1, referring to normal physio-activities of the liver and pancreas. However, further investigations are needed to confirm this hypothesis. The ALT, AST, GGT, and LDH were not statistically altered by toxin exposure. In a study on piglets [21] at the same FB_1 level, but longer exposure period (two weeks), neither ALT, nor AST differed from the control. In pigs, ALP is a strongly responsive enzyme to FB_1 toxicity [57]. Such an increase was toxin-impact, as this has been proven in pigs [16,18,19,58], and male and female Sprague Dawley rats [59]. Once measured enzymes were not responsive for the treatment, except ALP, it is a likely indicator for the commencement hepatotoxicity phase and/or generalized bone dysfunction.

When rats were exposed to 90 mg FB_1/kg body weight for 21 days, hepatotoxicity was found to be sufficient to trigger the mineral balance leading into alterations in bone metabolism and its mechanical endurance, although bone mass was not affected [60]. The role of ALP in bone development has been well acknowledged [61], therefore, we suggest that alteration in ALP activity, as induced by FB_1 has a role in the impairment of mineral homeostasis. However, authors assumed that the dysfunction in mineral metabolism was absent (serum ions were unchanged, data not shown), under the present slight/initial hepatotoxicity. Accordingly, possible mild hepatotoxicity action was the key factor behind ALP induction and no other enzymes. Another possible scenario is FB_1 has altered the intestinal structure [62] of the enterocytes (not tested here).

3.6. Histopathological Investigation

Hepatotoxicity induced by FB_1 is well documented in the relevant literature, mostly tested in rats while scarcely on swine, horses, and rabbits. From the literature in swine, FB_1 induces pulmonary edema and provides slight hepatotoxicity [4,10,12]. Pigs are highly susceptible to FB_1-induced hepatotoxicity, regardless of the administration method, orally or intravenously [16]. In the present investigation, the most striking modifications seen in the liver of piglets exposed to 20 mg FB_1/kg diet are the vacuolar degeneration of hepatocyte cytoplasm. This finding was markedly categorized as a mild to moderate effect, in agreement with the findings of Dilkin et al. [20] and Kovács et al. [21]. The vacuolar degeneration of hepatic cell cytoplasm is highly associated with disturbance of cellular water or lipid metabolism, indicative of an exertion of the cell's metabolic and/or detoxification activity. However, no other change was detected in the liver, which is not similar to earlier reports [16,18]. Such variance might be mainly attributed to the relatively low dose applied in our study.

Cholestasis is a condition involving interruption of the bile production and/or secretion [63], whereas it is associated with vacuolar degeneration. Analyzing Table 3, the unchanged serum bilirubin level is indirectly indicating the absence of hepatocellular-cholestasis, and therefore our microscopic findings do not refer to cholestasis. It has been reported that FB_1 can modify protein biosynthesis [64], which may imply degenerative alterations in the tissue. This finding was not observed here, since albumin concentrations were equal among the experimental groups, meaning no protein synthesis fallback. We suggest that oxidative stress modulation in lipid metabolism was the indirect player/factor behind FB_1 which induced start-up hepatotoxicity and developed vacuolar degeneration, a result of stress and not inflammation since the liver weight was unchanged, although it is not a precise biochemical indicator. In this regard the Sa:So biomarker (not tested) may assist in clarifying the histopathological lesion observed, and also other measured parameters. In summary, the histopathological assessment indicated mild status, which in general provides evidence for the onset necrotic process, in which it is reversible (healing).

Interestingly, histopathological assessment of the renal tissue has revealed no intergroup difference, referring to absent nephrotoxicity. Such a result means the renal tissue is less sensitive to FB_1 than the liver in piglets. This result is not consistent with the recent published data, even at a lower FB_1 level 12 mg FBs/kg diet [10]. Most probably the longer exposure period (as compared to ours) played an important role in the development of kidney lesions. A similar finding to our result was reported by Gumprecht et al. [20], when 20 mg FB_1/kg diet for four days did not develop a microscopic lesion in the kidney, only in the lung and liver. This is rather different from the sensitivity of rats, where the kidney is the most relevant organ for FB_1 toxicity [30,65].

4. Conclusions

From the study point of view, the orally administrated 20 mg FB_1/kg diet induced the commencement of hepatotoxicity in piglets. Therefore, this study suggests that the applied dose (20 mg FB_1/kg diet) is not safe for weaned piglets two months age and with a body weight below 16 kg, even under a short exposure period (10 days), although the production performance was not compromised. This study illustrates the sub-acute negative effects of FB_1 in a shorter period on the liver, as compared to earlier reports. Alterations of membrane lipid profile could be due to the destruction of UFAs and/or disturbance of FA desaturase enzymes. In addition, alterations of PLs can be due to the destruction of the PL domain and/or disruption of CerS. Apparently, further investigation on Sa:So ratio would be important for finer clarification, since they are efficient biomarkers for assessing CerS disruption and even toxicity status of the liver, induced by FB_1.

In general, our results may facilitate to better perceive the modulation in lipid sites associated with cellular damage, induced by FB_1. However, this is the first in vivo study reporting the lipid profile alterations as a result of FB_1 impact on the hepatic tissue of weaned piglets. The study has handled total PL and TG, whereas investigating PL subclasses is more worthy. Furthermore, a clear visualization requires a bigger population size (i.e., more piglets). Therefore, further investigations are necessary to determine FA involvement in hepatocellular damage of pigs, which can be performed by handling the different phospholipid subclasses, applying multiple doses, and exposure periods.

5. Material and Methods

5.1. Ethical Allowance

The experiment was carried out according to the Hungarian Animal Protection Act, in compliance with the relevant EU rules. The experimental protocol has been authorized by the Food Chain Safety and Animal Health Directorate of the Somogy County Agricultural Office, under permission number XV-I-31/1509-5/2012 (approved on 27 November 2012).

5.2. Experimental Design and Nutrition

Fourteen weaned barrows of the same genotype (Landrace X Yorkshire), weighing 13–14 kg (50 days of age) were used in the experiment. The piglets were weighed and then divided into two groups: an experimental group (FB_1-fed) and a control (n = 7/group). Animals were kept individually during the trial. Feed was given twice a day, in two equal portions, and the amount of feed not consumed by the animals was measured back; drinking water was available ad libitum via automatic drinkers.

Animals were kept for 7 days as an adaptation period, while the duration of the feeding trial was 10 days. Experimental animals were fed a basic ration of a nutrient composition corresponding to their age, containing feed of identical proximate component (Table 5). After this period, a *Fusarium verticillioides* fungal culture (strain MRC 826, for production details see: [66]) was added to the diet and homogenized. This contaminated diet was fed to the FB_1-fed group, so as to provide a daily FB_1 intake of approximately 10 mg FB_1/animal/day (equivalent to 0.5 kg feed consumption/animal/day).

Table 5. The proximate and fatty acide (FA) composition of the basal feed.

Component	Diet
DM (%)	90.8
Metabolizable energy (MJ/kg)	14.8
Digestible energy (MJ/kg)	14.2
Crude protein (% of DM)	19.7
Ether extract (% of DM)	5.8
Crude fiber (% of DM)	3.2
Ash (% of DM)	5.1
FA weight % of total FA methyl esters	
C10:0	0.02
C12:0	0.03
C14:0	0.4
C15:0	0.05
C16:0	15.2
C16:1n-7	0.44
C17:0	0.15
C17:1n-7	0.07
C18:0	4.85
C18:1n-9	26.7
C18:1n11t	0.09
C18:2n-6c	49
C18:3n-3	0.23
C20:0	0.36
C20:1n-9	2.13
C20:2 n-6	0.1
C22:0	0.11

DM, dry matter; FA, fatty acid.

The fungal culture typically contained 3.4 mg FB_1/g, and small quantities of less toxic compounds FB_2 and FB_3, 0.6 and 1 mg/g, respectively. The mycotoxin concentration of the control and the experimental feed was determined with LC-MS (Shimadzu, Kyoto, Japan) with 3 μg/kg limit of detection (LOD) for FB_1. The diet fed to the control group did not contain detectable amounts of FB_1 (below the LOD), while deoxinivalenol, zearalenone, and T-2 toxin were well-controlled and absence was confirmed.

Animals were kept with only drinking water available (without feed) 12 h before the scarification. At the end of the trial, the piglets were euthanized and exsanguinated after sedation (euthanyl-pentobarbital sodium, 240 mg/mL) and liver and blood were sampled for analysis.

5.3. *Lipid Analysis of the Hepatic Tissue*

The liver sample (after storage at −20 °C) and the feed were homogenized (IKA T25 Digital Ultra Turrax, Staufen, Germany) in 20-fold volume of chloroform-methanol (2:1, *v:v*) and total lipid content was extracted according to Folch et al. [67]. Solvents were ultrapure-grade (Merck Sigma-Aldrich, Schnelldorf, Germany) and 0.01 % *w:v* butylated hydroxytoluene was added to prevent fatty acid oxidation.

For the separation of lipid fractions (TG and PL), extracted total lipids were transferred to glass chromatographic columns, containing 300 mg silica gel (230–400 mesh) for 10 mg of total lipids [68]. Neutral lipids were eluted with 10 mL chloroform for the above fat amount, then 15 mL acetone: methanol (9:1, *v/v*) was added, while 10 mL pure methanol eluted the total phospholipids. This latter fraction was evaporated under a nitrogen stream and was trans-methylated with a base-catalyzed $NaOCH_3$ method [69].

Fatty acid methyl esters were extracted into 300 μL ultrapure n-hexane for gas chromatography, which was performed on a GCMS-QP2010 Plus equipment (AOC 20i automatic injector), equipped with a Phenomenex Zebron ZB-WAX Capillary GC column (30 m × 0.25 mm ID, 0.25 micrometer film, Phenomenex Inc., Torrance, CA, USA). Characteristic operating conditions were as follows: injector temperature: 270 °C; helium flow: 28 cm/sec. The oven temperature was graded from 80 to 205 °C: 2.5 °C/min, 5 min at 205 °C and from 205 to 250 °C: 10 °C/min, 5 min at 210 °C. The makeup gas was nitrogen. To identify the individual FAs, an authentic external FA standard (37 Component FAME Mix, Merck Sigma-Aldrich, Cat. No.: CRM47885) was used. Fatty acid results were expressed as weight % of total fatty acid methyl esters.

Unsaturation index was defined as the number of double bonds in 100 fatty acyl chains. From the FA results, UI was calculated as: UI = ((1 × Σ monoenoic FA) + (2 × Σ dienoic FA) + (3 × Σ trienoic FA) + (4 × Σ tetraenoic FA) + (5 × Σ pentaenoic FA) + (6 × Σ hexaenoic FA)) [70]. The average fatty acyl chain length was calculated from the multiplication of the chain length values and the respective proportion of each FA.

5.4. Determination of Lipid Peroxidation and Antioxidant Capacity

Samples of hepatic tissue were stored at −82 °C before analysis. Lipid peroxidation was assessed with the determination of MDA levels with 2-thiobarbituric acid method [71] in the 10-fold volume of tissue homogenate in physiological saline. The amount of GSH and GPx activity was measured in the 10,000 g supernatant fraction of tissue homogenate. The quantification of the GSH was measured as non-protein thiols by Ellmann's reagent [72], while the activity of GPx was according to Lawrence and Burk [73]. GSH concentration and GPx activity were calculated to protein content of the 10,000 g supernatant which was measured by the Folin-phenol reagent [74]. In all instances the color was measure with UV–Vis spectrophotometry in 10 mm pathway optical glass cuvettes.

5.5. Serum Clinical Chemistry Analysis

The different clinical parameters of serum-total protein, albumin, creatinine, glucose, urea, and the total cholesterol concentrations and the activity of aspartate aminotransferase (AST) and alanine aminotransferase (ALT) were determined in a veterinary laboratory (Vet-Med Laboratory, Budapest, Hungary), using Roche Hitachi 917 Chemistry Analyzer (Hitachi, Tokyo, Japan) with commercial diagnostic kits (Diagnosticum LTD., Budapest, Hungary).

5.6. Histopathological Analysis

Immediately after piglets were sacrificed, the liver and lung samples were collected and stored in 10% neutrally buffered formalin and embedded in paraffin for the histopathologic investigation, under light microscope. Regarding the microscope analysis, the microtome slides of 5 micron (μ) were prepared and stained with hematoxylin-eosin.

The main pathological alterations were described and scored, according to their extent and severity as follows: (-) = no alteration; 1 = slight/small scale/few; 2 = medium degree/medium scale/medium number.

The histopathological analysis was carried out according to the Act #2011 (03.30) of the Hungarian Ministry of Agriculture and Rural Development and was in accordance with the ethical guidelines of the Organization for Economic Cooperation and Development (OECD) Good Laboratory Practice for Chemicals (1997).

5.7. Statistical Evaluation

All data were tested for normality (Shapiro–Wilk test); after this, control and FB_1-fed groups' means were compared with an independent sample *t*-test, using IBM SPSS for Windows version 20 (2009). However, for group differences, the calculating probability (*p*-value < 0.05) used as the significance level.

Author Contributions: O.A., J.S.-F., A.S. and M.K. conceived the study design, collected and analyzed data. O.A. and A.S. wrote the manuscript. H.F. analyzed lipids; antioxidants were analyzed by M.M. and K.B., R.G. performed and interpreted histopathological analysis. A.Z. was working with the animals and samples.

Funding: The work was supported by the project GINOP-2.2.1.-15-2016-00046 and the EFOP-3.6.3.-Vekop-16-2017-00005 projects.

Conflicts of Interest: The authors declare no conflict of interest.

References

1. Anttila, A.; Bhat, R.V.; Bond, J.A.; Borghoff, S.J.; Bosch, F.X.; Carlson, G.P.; Castegnaro, M.; Cruzan, G.; Wentzel, C.A.; Hass, U.; et al. IARC Monographs on the evaluation of carcinogenic risks to humans: some traditional herbal medicines, some mycotoxins, naphthalene and styrene. *IARC Monogr. Eval. Carcinog. Risks Hum.* **2002**, *82*, 301–366.
2. Voss, K.A.; Riley, R.T. Fumonisin Toxicity and Mechanism of Action: Overview and Current Perspectives. *Food Saf.* **2013**, *1*, 2013006. [CrossRef]
3. Gelderblom, W.C.; Kriek, N.P.; Marasas, W.F.; Thiel, P.G. Toxicity and carcinogenicity of the *Fusarium moniliforme* metabolite, fumonisin B1, in rats. *Carcinogenesis* **1991**, *12*, 1247–1251. [CrossRef] [PubMed]
4. Haschek, W.M.; Gunnprecht, L.A.; Snnith, G.; Tumbleson, M.E.; Constable, P.D. Fumonisin Toxicosis in Swine: An Overview of Porcine Pulmonary Edema and Current Perspectives. *Environ. Health Perspect.* **2001**, *109*, 251–257.
5. Riedel, S.; Abel, S.; Swanevelder, S.; Gelderblom, W.C.A. Induction of an altered lipid phenotype by two cancer promoting treatments in rat liver. *Food Chem. Toxicol.* **2015**, *78*, 96–104. [CrossRef]
6. Riedel, S.; Abel, S.; Burger, H.M.; van der Westhuizen, L.; Swanevelder, S.; Gelderblom, W.C.A. Differential modulation of the lipid metabolism as a model for cellular resistance to fumonisin B_1—Induced cytotoxic effects in vitro. *Prostaglandins Leukot. Essent. Fat. Acids* **2016**, *109*, 39–51. [CrossRef]
7. Burger, H.M.; Abel, S.; Gelderblom, W.C.A. Modulation of key lipid raft constituents in primary rat hepatocytes by fumonisin B_1—Implications for cancer promotion in the liver. *Food Chem. Toxicol.* **2018**, *115*, 34–41. [CrossRef]
8. Riley, R.T.; Voss, K.A.; Yoo, H.-S.; Gelderblom, W.C.A.; Merrill, A.H. Mechanism of Fumonisin Toxicity and Carcinogenesis. *J. Food Prot.* **1994**, *57*, 638–644. [CrossRef]
9. Voss, K.A.; Smith, G.W.; Haschek, W.M. Fumonisins: Toxicokinetics, mechanism of action and toxicity. *Anim. Feed Sci. Technol.* **2007**, *137*, 299–325. [CrossRef]
10. Terciolo, C.; Bracarense, A.P.; Souto, P.C.; Cossalter, A.-M.; Dopavogui, L.; Loiseau, N.; Oliveira, C.A.F.; Pinton, P.; Oswald, I.P. Fumonisins at Doses below EU Regulatory Limits Induce Histological Alterations in Piglets. *Toxins* **2019**, *11*, 548. [CrossRef]
11. Riley, R.T.; An, N.H.; Showker, J.L.; Yoo, H.S.; Norred, W.P.; Chamberlain, W.J.; Wang, E.; Merrill, A.H.L.; Motelin, G.; Beasley, V.R.; et al. Alteration of tissue and serum sphinganine to sphingosine ratio: An early biomarker of exposure to Fumonisin-containing feeds in pig. *Toxicol. Appl. Pharmacol.* **1993**, *118*, 105–112. [CrossRef] [PubMed]
12. EFSA (European Food Safety Authority). Opinion of the Scientific Panel on contaminants in the food chain [CONTAM] related to fumonisins as undesirable substances in animal feed. *EFSA J.* **2005**, *235*, 1–32. Available online: https://efsa.onlinelibrary.wiley.com/doi/epdf/10.2903/j.efsa.2005.235 (accessed on 6 September 2019).
13. Guilloteau, P.; Zabielski, R.; Hammon, H.M.; Metges, C.C. Nutritional programming of gastrointestinal tract development. Is the pig a good model for man? *Nutr. Res. Rev.* **2010**, *23*, 4–22. [CrossRef] [PubMed]
14. Fodor, J.; Balogh, K.; Weber, M.; Mézes, M.; Kametler, L.; Pósa, R.; Mamet, R.; Bauer, J.; Horn, P.; Kovács, F.; et al. Absorption, distribution and elimination of fumonisin B_1 metabolites in weaned piglets. *Food Addit. Contam. Part A* **2008**, *25*, 88–96. [CrossRef] [PubMed]
15. Zomborszkyné-Kovács, M.; Vetés, I.F.; Kovács, F.; Bata, Á.; Repa, I.; Horn, P. A fusarium moniliforme fumonizin-B_1 toxinjának tolerálható határértékére és perinatalis toxikózist eloîdézo hatására vonatkozó vizsgálatok sertésben (Investigations on the tolerable limit values and the perinatal toxic effect of mycotoxins produced by Fus. *Magy. Allatorvosok Lapja* **2000**, *122*, 168–175.

16. Haschek, W.M.; Motelin, G.; Ness, D.K.; Harlin, K.S.; Hall, W.F.; Vesonder, R.F.; Peterson, R.E.; Beasley, V.R. Characterization of fumonisin toxicity in orally and intravenously dosed swine. *Mycopathologia* **1992**, *117*, 83–96. [CrossRef]
17. Casteel, S.W.; Turk, J.R.; Cowart, R.P.; Rottinghaus, G.E. Chronic toxicity of fumonisin in weanling pigs. *J. Vet. Diagn. Investig.* **1993**, *5*, 413–417. [CrossRef]
18. Gumprecht, L.A.; Beasley, V.R.; Weigel, R.M.; Parker, H.M.; Tumbleson, M.E.; Bacon, C.W.; Meredith, F.I.; Haschek, W.M. Development of fumonisin-induced hepatotoxicity and pulmonary edema in orally dosed swine: Morphological and biochemical alterations. *Toxicol. Pathol.* **1998**, *26*, 777–788. [CrossRef]
19. Harvey, R.B.; Edrington, T.S.; Kubena, L.F.; Rottinghaus, G.E.; Turk, J.R.; Genovese, K.J.; Ziprin, R.L.; Nisbet, D.J. Toxicity of fumonisin from *Fusarium verticillioides* culture material and moniliformin from Fusarium fujikuroi culture material when fed singly and in combination to growing barrows. *J. Food Prot.* **2002**, *65*, 373–377. [CrossRef]
20. Dilkin, P.; Zorzete, P.; Mallmann, C.A.; Gomes, J.D.F.; Utiyama, C.E.; Oetting, L.L.; Corrêa, B. Toxicological effects of chronic low doses of aflatoxin B_1 and fumonisin B_1-containing Fusarium moniliforme culture material in weaned piglets. *Food Chem. Toxicol.* **2003**, *41*, 1345–1353. [CrossRef]
21. Kovács, M.; Pósa, R.; Tuboly, T.; Donkó, T.; Repa, I.; Tossenberger, J.; Szabó-Fodor, J.; Stoev, S.; Magyar, T. Feed exposure to FB1 can aggravate pneumonic damages in pigs provoked by P. multocida. *Res. Vet. Sci.* **2016**, *108*, 38–46. [CrossRef] [PubMed]
22. Loiseau, N.; Polizzi, A.; Dupuy, A.; Therville, N.; Rakotonirainy, M.; Loy, J.; Viadere, J.L.; Cossalter, A.M.; Bailly, J.D.; Puel, O.; et al. New insights into the organ-specific adverse effects of fumonisin B_1: Comparison between lung and liver. *Arch. Toxicol.* **2015**, *89*, 1619–1629. [CrossRef] [PubMed]
23. US-Food and Drug Administration (FDA). *Guidance for Industry: Fumonisin Levels in Human Foods and Animal Feeds*; Washington, DC, USA, November 2001. Available online: https://www.fda.gov/regulatory-information/search-fda-guidance-documents/guidance-industry-fumonisin-levels-human-foods-and-animal-feeds (accessed on 24 September 2019).
24. European Union. Commission Recommendation of 17 August 2006 on the presence of deoxynivalenol, zearalenone, ochratoxin A, T-2 and HT-2 and fumonisins in products intended for animal feeding. *Off. J. Eur. Union* **2006**, *229*, 7–9.
25. Gelderblom, W.C.A.; Smuts, C.M.; Abel, S.; Snyman, S.D.; Van Der Westhuizen, L.; Huber, W.W.; Swanevelder, S. Effect of fumonisin B_1 on the levels and fatty acid composition of selected lipids in rat liver in vivo. *Food Chem. Toxicol.* **1997**, *35*, 647–656. [CrossRef]
26. Gelderblom, W.C.A.; Lebepe-Mazur, S.; Snijman, P.W.; Abel, S.; Swanevelder, S.; Kriek, N.P.J.; Marasas, W.F.O. Toxicological effects in rats chronically fed low dietary levels of fumonisin B_1. *Toxicology* **2001**, *161*, 39–51. [CrossRef]
27. Gelderblom, W.C.A.; Moritz, W.; Swanevelder, S.; Smuts, C.M.; Abel, S. Lipids and Δ6-desaturase activity alterations in rat liver microsomal membranes induced by fumonisin B_1. *Lipids* **2002**, *37*, 869–877. [CrossRef] [PubMed]
28. Burger, H.M.; Abel, S.; Snijman, P.W.; Swanevelder, S.; Gelderblom, W.C.A. Altered lipid parameters in hepatic subcellular membrane fractions induced by fumonisin B_1. *Lipids* **2007**, *42*, 249–261. [CrossRef]
29. Szabó, A.; Szabó-Fodor, J.; Fébel, H.; Mézes, M.; Repa, I.; Kovács, M. Acute hepatic effects of low-dose fumonisin B_1 in rats. *Acta Vet. Hung.* **2016**, *64*, 436–448.
30. Szabó, A.; Szabó-Fodor, J.; Fébel, H.; Mézes, M.; Balogh, K.; Bázár, G.; Kocsó, D.; Ali, O.; Kovács, M. Individual and combined effects of fumonisin B_1, deoxynivalenol and zearalenone on the hepatic and renal membrane lipid integrity of rats. *Toxins* **2018**, *10*, 4.
31. Szabó, A.; Fébel, H.; Ali, O.; Mézes, M.; Balogh, K.; Kovács, M. Fumonisin B_1 induced compositional modifications of the renal and hepatic membrane lipids in rats—Dose and exposure time dependence. *Food Addit. Contam. Part A* **2019**, *36*, 1722–1739.
32. Szabó, A.; Szabó-Fodor, J.; Fébel, H.; Romvári, R.; Kovács, M. Individual and combined haematotoxic effects of fumonisin B_1 and T-2 mycotoxins in rabbits. *Food Chem. Toxicol.* **2014**, *72*, 257–264.
33. Szabó, A.; Szabó-Fodor, J.; Fébel, H.; Mézes, M.; Bajzik, G.; Kovács, M. Oral administration of fumonisin B_1 and T-2 individually and in combination affects hepatic total and mitochondrial membrane lipid profile of rabbits. *Physiol. Int.* **2016**, *103*, 321–333.

34. FAO/WHO. Safety evaluation of certain mycotoxins in food. Fifty-sixth report of the Joint FAO/WHO Expert Committee on Food Additives. *Int. Program. Chem. Saf. World Health Organ.* **2001**, *47*, 420–555.
35. Knutsen, H.K.; Alexander, J.; Barregård, L.; Bignami, M.; Brüschweiler, B.; Ceccatelli, S.; Cottrill, B.; Dinovi, M.; Edler, L.; Grasl-Kraupp, B.; et al. Risks for animal health related to the presence of fumonisins, their modified forms and hidden forms in feed. *EFSA J.* **2018**, *16*, e05242.
36. Marasas, W.F.O. Discovery and occurrence of the fumonisins: A historical perspective. *Environ. Health Perspect.* **2001**, *109*, 239–243.
37. Souto, P.C.M.C.; Ramalho, L.N.Z.; Ramalho, F.S.; Gregorio, M.C.; Bordin, K.; Cossalter, A.M.; Oswald, I.P.; Oliveira, C.A.F. Ganho de peso, consumo de ração e histologia de órgãos de leitões alimentados com rações contendo baixos níveis de fumonisina B1. *Pesqui. Vet. Bras.* **2015**, *35*, 451–455. [CrossRef]
38. Gbore, F.A. Reproductive organ weights and semen quality of pubertal boars fed dietary fumonisin B_1. *Animal* **2009**, *3*, 1133–1137. [CrossRef]
39. Akande, K.E.; Abubakar, M.M.; Adegbola, T.A.; Bogoro, S.E. Nutritional and Health Implications of Mycotoxins in Animal Feeds: A Review. *Pakistan J. Nutr.* **2006**, *5*, 398–403.
40. Andretta, I.; Kipper, M.; Lehnen, C.R.; Hauschild, L.; Vale, M.M.; Lovatto, P.A. Meta-analytical study of productive and nutritional interactions of mycotoxins in broilers. *Poult. Sci.* **2011**, *90*, 1934–1940. [CrossRef]
41. Dobrzyń, A.; Górski, J. Ceramides and sphingomyelins in skeletal muscles of the rat: Content and composition. Effect of prolonged exercise. *Am. J. Physiol. Metab.* **2015**, *282*, E277–E285. [CrossRef]
42. Müller, S.; Dekant, W.; Mally, A. Fumonisin B_1 and the kidney: Modes of action for renal tumor formation by fumonisin B_1 in rodents. *Food Chem. Toxicol.* **2012**, *50*, 3833–3846.
43. Hulbert, A.J. On the importance of fatty acid composition of membranes for aging. *J. Theor. Biol.* **2005**, *234*, 277–288. [CrossRef] [PubMed]
44. Larsson, S.C.; Kumlin, M.; Ingelman-Sundberg, M.; Wolk, A. Dietary long-chain n−3 fatty acids for the prevention of cancer: A review of potential mechanisms. *Am. J. Clin. Nutr.* **2004**, *79*, 935–945. [CrossRef] [PubMed]
45. Pakkanen, K.I.; Duelund, L.; Qvortrup, K.; Pedersen, J.S.; Ipsen, J.H. Mechanics and dynamics of triglyceride-phospholipid model membranes: Implications for cellular properties and function. *Biochim. Biophys. Acta Biomembr.* **2011**, *1808*, 1947–1956. [CrossRef] [PubMed]
46. Lee, J.C.M.; Simonyi, A.; Sun, A.Y.; Sun, G.Y. Phospholipases A_2 and neural membrane dynamics: Implications for Alzheimer's disease. *J. Neurochem.* **2011**, *116*, 813–819. [CrossRef] [PubMed]
47. Klapisz, E.; Masliah, J.; Béréziat, G.L.; Wolf, C.; Koumanov, K.S. Sphingolipids and cholesterol modulate membrane susceptibility to cytosolic phospholipase A_2. *J. Lipid. Res.* **2000**, *41*, 1680–1688. [PubMed]
48. Piccirella, S.; Czegle, I.; Lizák, B.; Margittai, É.; Senesi, S.; Papp, E.; Csala, M.; Fulceri, R.; Csermely, P.; Mandl, J.; et al. Uncoupled redox systems in the lumen of the endoplasmic reticulum: Pyridine nucleotides stay reduced in an oxidative environment. *J. Biol. Chem.* **2006**, *281*, 4671–4677. [CrossRef]
49. Bánhegyi, G.; Margittai, I.; Szarka, A.; Mandl, J.; Csala, M. Crosstalk and barriers between the electron carriers of the endoplasmic reticulum. *Antioxid. Redox Signal.* **2012**, *16*, 772–780. [CrossRef]
50. Esterbauer, H.; Schaur, R.J.; Zollner, H. Chemistry and biochemistry of 4-hydroxynonenal, malonaldehyde and related aldehydes. *Free Radic. Biol. Med.* **1991**, *11*, 81–128. [CrossRef]
51. Grotto, D.; Santa Maria, L.; Valentini, J.; Paniz, C.; Schmitt, G.; Garcia, S.C.; Pomblum, V.J.; Rocha, J.B.T.; Farina, M. Importance of the lipid peroxidation biomarkers and methodological aspects for malondialdehyde quantification. *Quim. Nova* **2009**, *32*, 169–174. [CrossRef]
52. Cheng, J.; Wang, F.; Yu, D.F.; Wu, P.F.; Chen, J.G. The cytotoxic mechanism of malondialdehyde and protective effect of carnosine via protein cross-linking/mitochondrial dysfunction/reactive oxygen species/MAPK pathway in neurons. *Eur. J. Pharmacol.* **2011**, *650*, 184–194. [CrossRef] [PubMed]
53. Lushchak, V.I. Glutathione Homeostasis and Functions: Potential Targets for Medical Interventions. *J. Amino Acids* **2012**, *2012*, 736837. [CrossRef] [PubMed]
54. Majorek, K.A.; Porebski, P.J.; Dayal, A.; Zimmerman, M.D.; Jablonska, K.; Stewart, A.J.; Chruszcz, M.; Minor, W. Structural and immunologic characterization of bovine, horse, and rabbit serum albumins. *Mol. Immunol.* **2012**, *52*, 174–182. [CrossRef] [PubMed]
55. Kouadio, J.; Moukha, S.; Brou, K.; Gnakri, D. Lipid metabolism disorders, lymphocytes cells death, and renal toxicity induced by very low levels of deoxynivalenol and fumonisin B_1 alone or in combination following 7 days oral administration to mice. *Toxicol. Int.* **2013**, *20*, 218. [CrossRef] [PubMed]

56. Régnier, M.; Polizzi, A.; Lukowicz, C.; Smati, S.; Lasserre, F.; Lippi, Y.; Naylies, C.; Latte, J.; Bétoulières, C.; Montagner, A.; et al. The protective role of liver X receptor (LXR) during fumonisin B_1-induced hepatotoxicity. *Arch. Toxicol.* **2019**, *93*, 505–517.
57. Oswald, I.P.; Desautels, C.; Laffitte, J.; Fournout, S.; Peres, S.Y.; Odin, M.; Le Bars, P.; Le Bars, J.; Fairbrother, J.M. Mycotoxin Fumonisin B_1 Increases Intestinal Colonization by Pathogenic Escherichia coli in Pigs. *Appl. Environ. Microbiol.* **2003**, *69*, 5870–5874. [CrossRef] [PubMed]
58. Smith, G.W.; Constable, P.D.; Smith, A.R.; Bacon, C.W.; Meredith, F.I.; Wollenberg, G.K.; Haschek, W.M. Effects of fumonisin-containing culture material on pulmonary clearance in swine. *Am. J. Vet. Res.* **1996**, *57*, 1233–1248.
59. Voss, K.A.; Chamberlain, W.J.; Bacon, C.W.; Norred, W.P. A preliminary investigation on renal and hepatic toxicity in rats fed purified fumonisin B_1. *Nat. Toxins* **1993**, *1*, 222–228. [CrossRef]
60. Rudyk, H.; Tomaszewska, E.; Kotsyumbas, I.; Muszyński, S.; Tomczyk-Warunek, A.; Szymańczyk, S.; Dobrowolski, P.; Wiącek, D.; Kamiński, D.; Brezvyn, O. Bone homeostasis in experimental fumonisins intoxication of rats. *Ann. Anim. Sci.* **2019**, *19*, 403–419. [CrossRef]
61. Sharma, U.; Pal, D.; Prasad, R. Alkaline phosphatase: An overview. *Indian J. Clin. Biochem.* **2014**, *29*, 269–278. [CrossRef]
62. Pierron, A.; Alassane-Kpembi, I.; Oswald, I.P. Impact of two mycotoxins deoxynivalenol and fumonisin on pig intestinal health. *Porc. Health Manag.* **2016**, *2*, 1–8. [CrossRef] [PubMed]
63. Li, M.K.; Crawford, J.M. The Pathology of Cholestasis. *Semin. Liver Dis.* **2004**, *24*, 21–42. [PubMed]
64. Abado-Becognee, K.; Mobio, T.A.; Ennamany, R.; Fleurat-Lessard, F.; Shier, W.T.; Badria, F.; Creppy, E.E. Cytotoxicity of fumonisin B_1: Implication of lipid peroxidation and inhibition of protein and DNA syntheses. *Arch. Toxicol.* **1998**, *72*, 233–236. [CrossRef] [PubMed]
65. Bondy, G.; Barker, M.; Mueller, R.; Fernie, S.; Miller, J.D.; Armstrong, C.; Hierlihy, S.L.; Rowsell, P.; Suzuki, C. Fumonisin B_1 Toxicity in Male Sprague-Dawley Rats. In *Fumonisins in Food*; Springer: Boston, MA, USA, 1996; pp. 251–264.
66. Fodor, J.; Kametier, L.; Kovács, M. Practical aspects of fumonisin production under laboratory conditions. *Mycotoxin Res.* **2006**, *22*, 211–216. [CrossRef]
67. Folch, J.; Lees, M.; Sloane Stanley, G.H. A simple method for the isolation and purification of total lipides from animal tissues. *J. Biol. Chem.* **1957**, *226*, 497–509.
68. Leray, C.; Andriamampandry, M.; Gutbier, G.; Cavadenti, J.; Klein-Soyer, C.; Gachet, C.; Cazenave, J.P. Quantitative analysis of vitamin E, cholesterol and phospholipid fatty acids in a single aliquot of human platelets and cultured endothelial cells. *J. Chromatogr. B Biomed. Appl.* **1997**, *696*, 33–42. [CrossRef]
69. Christie, W.W. A simple procedure for rapid transmethylation of glycerolipids and cholesteryl esters. *J. Lipid Res.* **1982**, *23*, 1072–1075.
70. Buttemer, W.A.; Battam, H.; Hulbert, A.J. Fowl play and the price of petrel: Long-living Procellariiformes have peroxidation-resistant membrane composition compared with short-living Galliformes. *Biol. Lett.* **2008**, *4*, 351–354. [CrossRef]
71. Placer, Z.A.; Cushman, L.L.; Johnson, B.C. Estimation of product of lipid peroxidation (malonyl dialdehyde) in biochemical systems. *Anal. Biochem.* **1966**, *16*, 359–364. [CrossRef]
72. Sedlak, J.; Lindsay, R.H. Estimation of total, protein-bound, and nonprotein sulfhydryl groups in tissue with Ellman's reagent. *Anal. Biochem.* **1968**, *25*, 192–205. [CrossRef]
73. Lawrence, R.A.; Burk, R.F. Species, Tissue and Subcellular Distribution of Non Se-Dependent Glutathione Peroxidase Activity. *J. Nutr.* **1978**, *108*, 211–215. [CrossRef] [PubMed]
74. Lowry, O.H.; Rosebrough, N.J.; Farr, A.L.; Randall, R.J. Protein measurement with the Folin phenol reagent. *J. Biol. Chem.* **1951**, *193*, 265–275. [PubMed]

toxins

MDPI

Article

Differential Transcriptome Responses to Aflatoxin B_1 in the Cecal Tonsil of Susceptible and Resistant Turkeys

Kent M. Reed [1,*], Kristelle M. Mendoza [1] and Roger A. Coulombe Jr. [2]

[1] Department of Veterinary and Biomedical Sciences, College of Veterinary Medicine, University of Minnesota, Saint Paul, MN 55108, USA; mendo008@umn.edu

[2] Department of Animal, Dairy and Veterinary Sciences, College of Agriculture and Applied Sciences, Utah State University, Logan, UT 84322, USA; roger@usu.edu

* Correspondence: reedx054@umn.edu; Tel.: +1-612-624-1287

Received: 7 December 2018; Accepted: 14 January 2019; Published: 18 January 2019

Abstract: The nearly-ubiquitous food and feed-borne mycotoxin aflatoxin B_1 (AFB_1) is carcinogenic and mutagenic, posing a food safety threat to humans and animals. One of the most susceptible animal species known and thus a good model for characterizing toxicological pathways, is the domesticated turkey (DT), a condition likely due, at least in part, to deficient hepatic AFB_1-detoxifying alpha-class glutathione S-transferases (GSTAs). Conversely, wild turkeys (Eastern wild, EW) are relatively resistant to the hepatotoxic, hepatocarcinogenic and immunosuppressive effects of AFB_1 owing to functional gene expression and presence of functional hepatic GSTAs. This study was designed to compare the responses in gene expression in the gastrointestinal tract between DT (susceptible phenotype) and EW (resistant phenotype) following dietary AFB_1 challenge (320 ppb for 14 days); specifically in cecal tonsil which functions in both nutrient absorption and gut immunity. RNAseq and gene expression analysis revealed significant differential gene expression in AFB_1-treated animals compared to control-fed domestic and wild birds and in within-treatment comparisons between bird types. Significantly upregulated expression of the primary hepatic AFB_1-activating P450 (*CYP1A5*) as well as transcriptional changes in tight junction proteins were observed in AFB_1-treated birds. Numerous pro-inflammatory cytokines, *TGF-β* and *EGF* were significantly down regulated by AFB_1 treatment in DT birds and pathway analysis suggested suppression of enteroendocrine cells. Conversely, AFB_1 treatment modified significantly fewer unique genes in EW birds; among these were genes involved in lipid synthesis and metabolism and immune response. This is the first investigation of the effects of AFB_1 on the turkey gastro-intestinal tract. Results suggest that in addition to the hepatic transcriptome, animal resistance to this mycotoxin occurs in organ systems outside the liver, specifically as a refractory gastrointestinal tract.

Keywords: Poultry; Turkey; Transcriptome; Aflatoxin B_1; Cecal Tonsil; Cecum; RNAseq

Key Contribution: This study is the first to examine the transcriptome of the turkey cecal tonsil region of gastro-intestinal tract. Importantly it combines RNAseq and gene expression analysis and identifies key gene transcripts modulated in response to dietary AFB_1 treatment.

1. Introduction

Aflatoxin B_1 (AFB_1) is a hepatotoxic, hepatocarcinogenic and immunosuppressive mycotoxin commonly found in food and feed, especially corn [1]. Poultry are particularly sensitive to the toxic effects of AFB_1 and commercial domesticated turkeys are perhaps the most susceptible animal thus far studied [2,3]. Exposure to AFB_1 through contaminated feed is practically unavoidable and can result in reduced feed intake, weight gain and feed efficiency and increased mortality, hepatotoxicity and GI hemorrhaging (reviewed in Monson et al. [4]). As a potent immunotoxin, AFB_1 suppresses cell-mediated, humoral and phagocytic immunological functions, thereby increasing susceptibility to bacterial and viral diseases [5–7].

In contrast to their modern domesticated counterparts, wild turkeys are relatively resistant to aflatoxicosis [8]. Metabolism of AFB_1 requires bioactivation by hepatic cytochrome P450s (CYPs) to the electrophilic exo-AFB1-8,9-epoxide (AFBO), which is catalyzed primarily, at pharmacological concentrations by the high-efficiency CYP1A5 and to a minor extent by the lower-affinity CYP3A37 which predominates only at high, environmentally-irrelevant substrate concentrations [9]. In most animals, AFBO is detoxified primarily by hepatic glutathione S-transferases (GSTs) [3]. The most likely mechanism for the extreme susceptibility in domesticated turkeys is dysfunctional hepatic GSTs rendering them unable to detoxify AFB_1 [10–14]. In this regard, domesticated turkeys closely resemble humans in that they also lack hepatic alpha-class GSTs (GSTA) with high activity toward AFB_1 (seen in mice and rats) suggesting that turkeys may represent a better model to study aflatoxin toxicology than either of these rodent species [9]. Expression of GSTA in the intestine and the potential for extra-hepatic bioactivation and metabolism of AFB_1 in turkeys is unknown.

To better understand the response of the domestic turkey to AFB_1 exposure, we initiated transcriptomic analysis of AFB_1-challenged domestic birds [15], where genes and gene pathways in the liver were significantly dysregulated by dietary AFB_1 challenge, such as pathways associated with cancer, apoptosis, cell cycle and lipid regulation. These changes reflect the molecular mechanisms underlying DNA alkylation and mutation, inflammation, proliferation and liver damage in aflatoxicosis. Analysis of spleen tissues from the same birds examined in the Monson et al. [15] study found that short AFB_1 exposure suppressed innate immune transcripts, especially from antimicrobial genes associated with either increased cytotoxic potential or activation-induced cell death during aflatoxicosis [16].

The differential response of domestic and wild turkey to AFB_1 was examined in a controlled feeding trial [17]. Analysis by RNAseq of the hepatic transcriptome found genes dysregulated as a response to toxic insult with significant differences observed between these genetically distinct birds in the expression of Phase I and Phase II drug metabolism genes. Genes important in cellular regulation, modulation of apoptosis and inflammatory responses were also affected. Unique responses in wild birds were seen for genes that negatively regulate cellular processes, serve as components of the extracellular matrix or modulate coagulation factors. Wild turkey embryos also showed differential AFB_1 effects compared to their commercial counterparts presumably due to lower levels of AFBO [18]. When treated with AFB_1, embryos showed up-regulation in cell cycle regulators, Nrf2-mediated response genes and coagulation factors [18]. Results of these studies supported the hypothesis that the reduced susceptibility of wild turkeys is related to higher constitutive expression of *GSTA3*, coupled with an inherited (genetic) difference in functional gene expression in domesticated birds.

The molecular basis for the differences in AFB_1 detoxification observed between domesticated commercial and wild birds has been extensively studied in our laboratories. However, extra-hepatic effects, such as those occurring at the site of initial toxicant exposure, the intestine, are needed to fully understand the systemic effects of AFB_1 in this susceptible species. Unlike many mycotoxins, AFB_1 is efficiently absorbed (>80%) in the avian upper gastrointestinal tract (GIT) [19]. Recent studies of broiler chickens have found conflicting evidence for the potential impact of AFB_1 on gut permeability, from no effect [20] to increased permeability [21]. The avian small intestine is a primary site of nutrient absorption [22] but is often overlooked from an immunological perspective. The cecal tonsils are the largest aggregates of avian gut-associated lymphoid tissue, yet basic information on gene expression in the cecal tonsil is lacking in the turkey. This study focused on the effects of dietary AFB_1 on gene expression in the turkey GIT and specifically the region at the junction of the distal ileum and cecum (the cecal tonsil region) that functions in AFB_1 absorption and gut immunity. The purpose of this study was to examine the transcriptomic response of the cecal tonsil region of the turkey intestine to dietary AFB_1 treatment and contrast these in susceptible (domesticated) and resistant (wild) birds.

2. Results

The effects of AFB_1 on body weight and liver mass are summarized in a companion study of hepatic gene expression [17]. Sequencing produced from 9.8M to 14.2M reads per library (average 12.7 million) (Table S1). Data are deposited in the NCBI's Gene Expression Omnibus (GEO) repository as SRA BioProject 346253. Median Q scores of the trimmed and filtered reads ranged from 36.5 to 37.7 among the forward and reverse reads. The number of reads per treatment group ranged from 10.9 to 12.8M with the mean number for EW birds being slightly higher than for the DT birds (12.6M verses 11.2M). Over 90% of the quality-trimmed reads mapped to the annotated turkey gene set (NCBI Annotation 101) and the vast majority of reads (average 85.2%) mapped concordantly (Table S1). Based on mapping, the estimated mean insert size of the libraries was 195.4 ± 15.8 bp. Variation in mapped reads among the treatment groups was visualized by PCA (Figure 1). Samples (AFB_1 treatment/CNTL) generally clustered distinctly by treatment group within the space defined by the first two principal components. The exceptions were two EW AFB_1 samples (EW1C and EW3C) that clustered with the control birds. The relationships among groups was reiterated in the hierarchical clustering of groups by Euclidean distance and heat map of co-expressed genes (Figure S1). This indicates the main effect underlying this study is AFB_1 treatment.

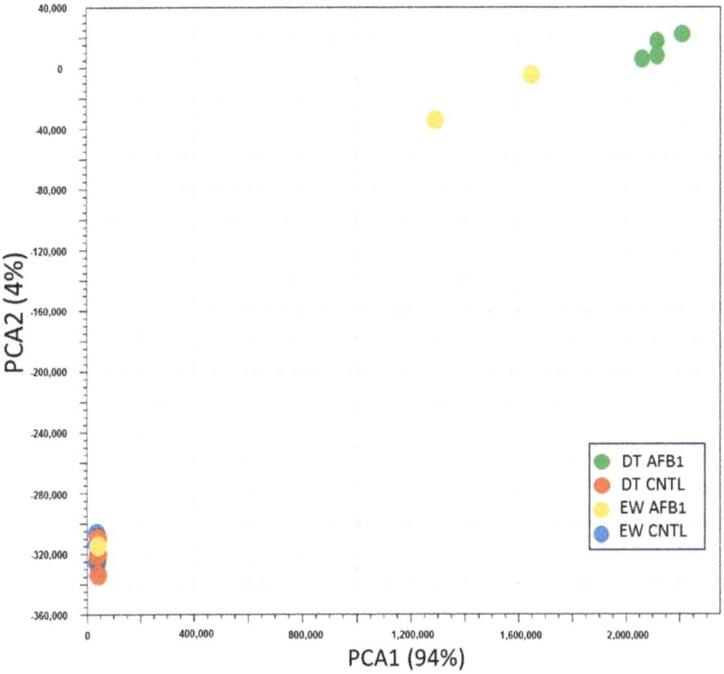

Figure 1. Principal component analysis (PCA) of by-total normalized RNAseq read counts. For each treatment group, sample to sample distances (within- and between-treatments) are illustrated on the first two principle components.

Evidence of expression (mapped reads ≥ 1.0 in at least one individual) was detected for 19,754 genes (tRNAs excluded) with an average of 17,261 genes observed per individual (Tables S1 and S2). When qualified (by-total normalized read count ≥ 3.0), the number of expressed genes averaged

16,132 per individual (76.79% of the turkey gene set) with an average of 17,877 expressed genes per treatment group. The numbers of observed and expressed genes were higher for control groups than for AFB_1-treatment groups of both EW and DT. A total of 16,097 genes (84.4%) was co-expressed among all groups and the number of co-expressed genes within the EW and DT lines was 17,833 and 16,277, respectively (Figure 2). Each treatment group had a distinct set of uniquely expressed genes, with the numbers being greater for the control groups (200 and 185) compared to the AFB_1 groups (80 and 113) (Figure 2).

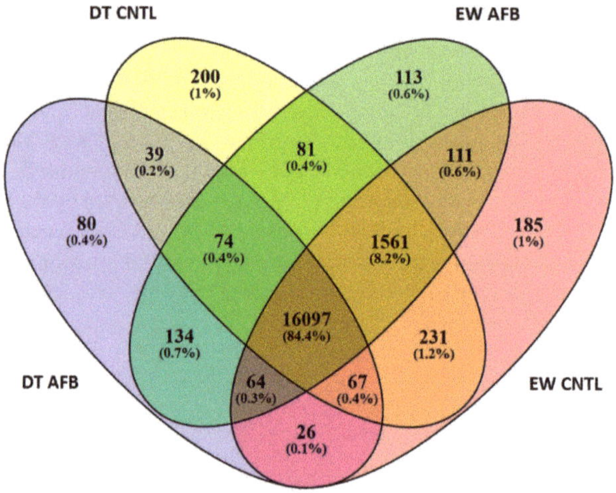

Figure 2. Distribution of expressed genes in turkey cecal tonsil by treatment group.

2.1. *Differential Gene Expression*

2.1.1. AFB_1 Treatment Effects

The full list of genes showing significant differential expression (DE) in pairwise treatment comparisons is provided in Table S3. In comparison of DT birds exposed to AFB_1 (DTAFB) with control-fed birds (CNTL) DE was observed for 11,237 genes in the cecal tonsil (FDR p-value < 0.05). Of these, 7568 had $|\log_2FC| > 1.0$ and 4515 had $|\log_2FC| > 2.0$ (Table 1). The number of DE genes was considerably fewer for the AFB_1-treated EW turkeys (703 with FDR p-value < 0.05 and 687 genes with $|\log_2FC| > 2.0$). In DT birds, the majority (65.4%) of DEGs were down regulated (Figure 3) although 48 of the 50 genes with the greatest fold change were up regulated (Table S4). In contrast, 98% of the DEGs in AFB_1-treated EW birds were up regulated. Combined, 655 DEGs were shared in comparisons for both bird types, with 3860 being unique to DT birds and 32 unique to EW birds (Figure 3). Functional interpretation of many avian genes is based on sequence and syntenic similarity with human and other model organisms and therefore many functions are necessarily posited.

Shared Transcriptome Response

Among the 655 shared genes were the two phase I enzymes important in AFB_1 metabolism (Table S3). The first, *CYP1A5* (cytochrome P450, family 1, subfamily A, polypeptide 5) was highly up regulated in both EW and DT birds treated with AFB_1 ($\log_2FC$ = 7.66 and 9.67, respectively). Secondly, *CYP3A37* (cytochrome P450 3A37) was significantly up regulated in only the DT birds ($\log_2FC$ = 2.73). Studies from our laboratory have identified these as the principal turkey hepatic cytochromes responsible for efficient epoxidation of AFB_1; CYP1A5 has highest affinity toward AFBO (low Km, high Vmax/Kcat) and bioactivates > 99% of AFB_1 in turkey liver. In turkey, CYP3A37 (high Km, low Vm, Kcat) is only active at high environmentally-irrelevant substrate (i.e., AFB_1)

concentrations [9]. Although potential biochemical activity of GSTAs in the intestine (cecal tonsil) of turkeys is unknown, expression of *GSTA4* was significantly up regulated in both the EW and DT birds with AFB_1 exposure (log_2FC = 4.53 and 5.89, respectively).

Table 1. Summary of genes with significant differential expression (DE) in pair-wise comparisons of treatment groups.

Comparison	Groups	Expressed Genes	Shared Genes	Unique Genes (Each Group)	FDR p-Value < 0.05	$\lvert log_2FC \rvert$ > 1.0	$\lvert log_2FC \rvert$ > 2.0	Up/Down Regulated
AFB_1	EW (AFB vs. CNTL)	18744	17833	402/509	703	703	687	674/13
	DT (AFB vs. CNTL)	18654	16277	304/2073	11237	7568	4515	1563/2952
Line	CNTL (EW vs. DT)	18736	17956	386/394	679	348	67	37/30
	AFB (EW vs. DT)	18447	16369	1866/212	1666	1666	1410	1308/102

For each comparison, the treatment groups, total number of expressed, shared and unique genes, genes with significant FDR p-value and the numbers of significant DE genes that also had $\lvert log_2$ fold change$\rvert$ >1.0 and >2.0 are given. For the DE genes with $\lvert log_2$ fold change$\rvert$ > 2.0 the number of genes up and down regulated are given. Genes were considered expressed in a treatment group if by-total normalized read count $\geq$ 3.0 in any individual within the group.

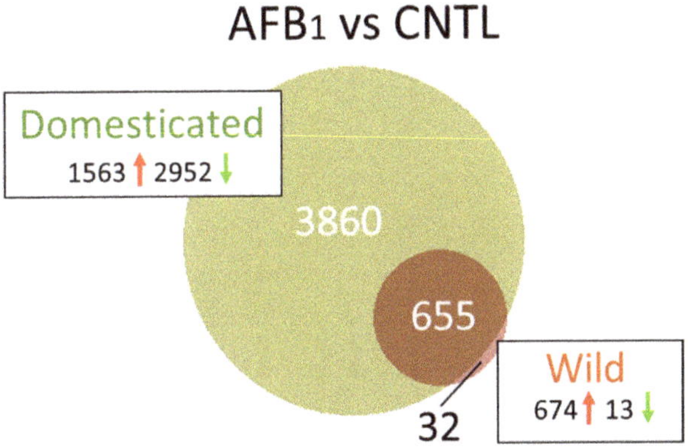

Figure 3. Distribution of differentially expressed genes in the turkey. For each comparison, the number of significant genes (FDR p-value < 0.05 and $\lvert log_2FC \rvert$ > 2.0) shared or unique to each treatment are indicated in the Venn diagram. Circle size is proportional to the number of genes and direction of expression change (↑ or ↓) is given for each group.

DE was also observed for several members of the claudin protein family. Claudins are integral components forming the backbone of the tight junctions of epithelial and endothelial cells [23]. In EW birds, *CLDN1* (claudin 1) was up regulated by AFB_1 (log_2FC = 4.55), whereas *CLDN18* was down regulated (log_2FC = −6.57) (Table S3). In DT birds, *CLDN1*, *CLDN2* and *CLDN11* were up regulated (log_2FC = 6.04, 4.01 and 2.17, respectively) and *CLDN3*, *CLDN10*, *CLDN19* and *CLDN23* were down regulated (log_2FC = −2.52, −7.17, −4.11, −8.05, respectively). Expression of other key tight-junction proteins, tricellulin (MARVEL domain-containing protein 2, *LOC104915344*) and occludin (*LOC104915505*), were also significantly altered in DT but with smaller fold changes (Table S3). Upregulation of membrane tight-junction proteins such as claudins, is indicative of an epithelial response in the gut lumen to AFB_1 and may suggest that AFB_1 could alter gut permeability and perhaps stimulate a protective response in the gut to diminish mucosal inflammation/immune defense and repair processes.

Expression differences in *CLDN1* observed in RNAseq read counts were further tested by qRT-PCR where expression of *CLDN1* transcripts was significantly higher in EW birds compared to controls regardless of AFB_1-treatment (Figure 4). Relative *CLDN1* expression was also similarly variable in other wild-type birds (Rio Grande Wild, RGW) where expression was comparable to that of EW birds and significantly elevated with AFB_1 treatment. Expression in other domestic birds (broad breasted white, BB) was more similar to that of the wild birds than the Nicholas DT suggesting that the lower *CLDN1* expression observed in the Nicholas DT birds may have a genetic component.

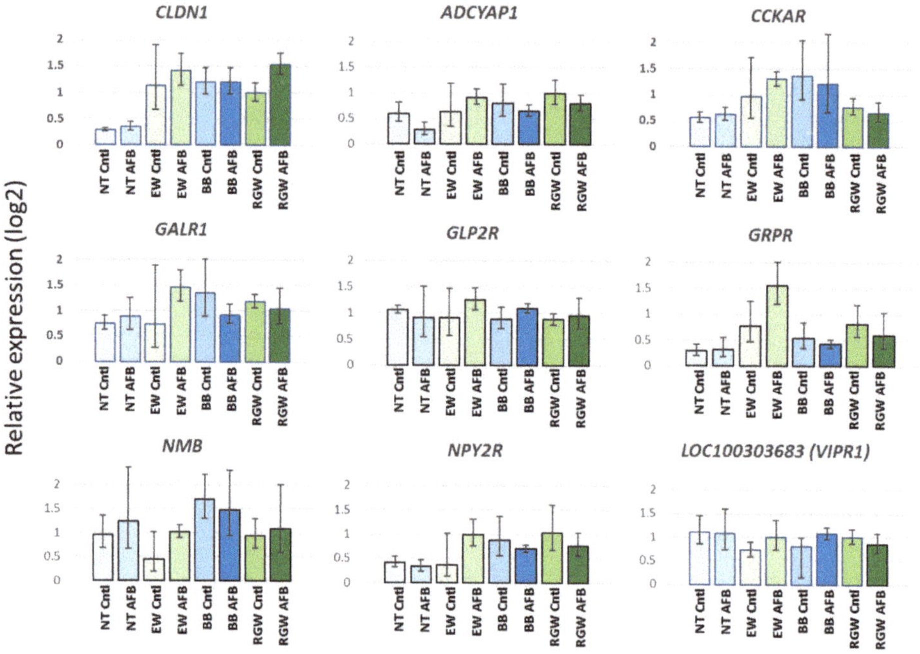

Figure 4. Effect of AFB_1 on expression of genes in the IPA canonical pathway "GPCR-Mediated Integration of Enteroendocrine Signaling Exemplified by an L Cell" in the cecal tonsil of turkeys (see Figure 5).

Only two of the 655 shared DEGs (*ATP12A* and *RSAD2*) in the RNAseq data showed differences in the directionality of expression. *ATP12A* (ATPase, H^+/K^+ transporting, non-gastric, alpha polypeptide) was down regulated ($log_2FC = -2.83$) in DT and up regulated ($log_2FC = 4.69$) in EW birds. Similarly, *RSAD2* (radical S-adenosyl methionine domain containing 2) was down regulated ($log_2FC = -3.47$) in DT and up regulated ($log_2FC = 3.23$) in EW. Two additional loci (*SCD*, stearoyl-CoA desaturase [delta-9-desaturase]) and a ncRNA (*LOC104914677*) had a similar directional expression pattern, with significant up regulation in EW with AFB_1 treatment and down regulation in DT, however the log_2FC in the DT birds was below 2.0. ATP12A is a member of the P-type cation transport ATPase family and in humans is involved in tissue-specific potassium absorption [24]. RSAD2 is an interferon inducible antiviral protein and has been shown in human cell lines to inhibit secretion of soluble proteins [25]. In mammals, SCD has a regulatory role in the expression of genes involved in lipogenesis and is important in mitochondrial fatty acid oxidation and energy homeostasis [26].

Nine of the 655 DEGs were significantly down regulated in both DT and EW with AFB_1 treatment. These included *GGT1* (gamma-glutamyltransferase 1), *OTOR* (otoraplin), *PLIN1* (perilipin 1), *RSPH14* (radial spoke head 14 homolog), *SLC34A2* (solute carrier family 34, member 2), *LOC100550279* (fatty acid-binding protein, adipocyte-like [*FABP4*-like]), *LOC104909385* (erythroblast NAD(P)(+)–arginine

ADP-ribosyltransferase pseudogene), *LOC104913555* (gamma-glutamyltranspeptidase 1-like) and *TNFRSF13C* (tumor necrosis factor receptor superfamily, member 13C). Genes of particular interest in the GI tract include Perilipin 1 and fatty acid-binding protein (*LOC100550279*) that are involved in lipid transport and metabolism in human adipocytes [27]. SLC34A2 is a sodium-dependent phosphate transporter with an inverse pH dependence [28]. It is expressed in several mammalian tissues of epithelial origin including lung and small intestine and may be the main phosphate transporter in the brush border membrane. The B-cell activating factor TNFRSF13C is known to promote survival of mammalian B-cells in vitro and is a regulator of the peripheral B-cell population [29].

Functional gene classification of the 655 shared DEGs with DAVID identified 10 enriched gene clusters (Table S5). The cluster with the highest enrichment score included members of the serpin family of protease inhibitors (*SERPINA10, SERPINC1, SERPIND1, SERPINF2* and *SERPING1*) that control many inflammation and coagulation processes. Other enriched clusters included complement components, mannan-binding lectin serine peptidase 1 and 2 (*MASP1, MASP2*), the (C4/C2 activating components) and coagulation factors F2, F7, F9 and F10. PANTHER overrepresentation tests found greatest fold enrichment for biological processes indicative of the dual absorption/immunity roles of the small intestine. Complement activation (GO:0001867) and regulation of intestinal absorption (GO:1904729, 1904478, 0030300) were significantly enriched as was cholesterol homeostasis GO:0042632) as exemplified by up regulation of several genes (*ABCG5, ABCG8, ANGPTL3, APOA1, APOA4, APOA5, CETP, EPHX2, G6PC, LIPC* and *LPL*).

Unique Transcriptome Responses

Domesticated birds showed the greatest AFB_1 gene response with 3860 unique DEGs (Figure 3). Genes showing the highest differential response (Table S4) were enriched for those encoding proteins with signal peptides and Serpins. DEGs with the greatest up regulation included *INHBC* (inhibin, beta C, $\log_2FC = 13.63$), claudin-19-like (*LOC100544298*, $\log_2FC = 12.56$), *TTC36* (tetratricopeptide repeat domain 36, $\log_2FC = 12.28$) and three ncRNAs (*LOC104913410, LOC104915491, LOC10491649*, $\log_2FC$ =12.74 to 13.15), *SMIM24* (small integral membrane protein 24, $\log_2FC = -12.48$) and *SLC10A2* (solute carrier family 10 [sodium/bile acid cotransporter], member 2, $\log_2FC = -12.07$). Expression of *GSTA3* was significantly lower in DT birds treated with AFB_1 compared to controls ($\log_2FC = -2.33$). Other αGSTs (*GSTA1* and *GSTA2*) were significantly up regulated but with lower fold change ($\log_2FC < 2.0$, Table S3).

Over 650 of the 3860 DEGs were functionally clustered (DAVID enrichment score 24.96) as having membrane or transmembrane UniProt keywords. The majority of these (518, 77.9%) were down regulated as an effect of AFB_1 treatment. Several alpha-1-antitrypsin-like loci were significantly up regulated consistent with a response to acute inflammation. Analysis of the 3860 unique genes in IPA found the most significant canonical pathways to be Axonal Guidance Signaling (-log(p-value) = 8.65), Hepatic Fibrosis / Hepatic Stellate Cell Activation (8.24), GPCR-Mediated Integration of Enteroendocrine Signaling Exemplified by an L Cell (7.33) and Calcium Signaling (7.28). DEGs in these pathways were almost exclusively down regulated in AFB_1-treated birds. This effect is dramatically illustrated for the in the IPA canonical pathway "GPCR-Mediated Integration of Enteroendocrine Signaling Exemplified by an L Cell" (Figure 5) suggesting suppression in domesticated birds of enteroendocrine cells that produce and release gastrointestinal hormones such as glucagon-like peptides, peptide YY and oxyntomodulin that participate in nutrient sensing and appetite regulation and peptides to activate nervous responses [30].

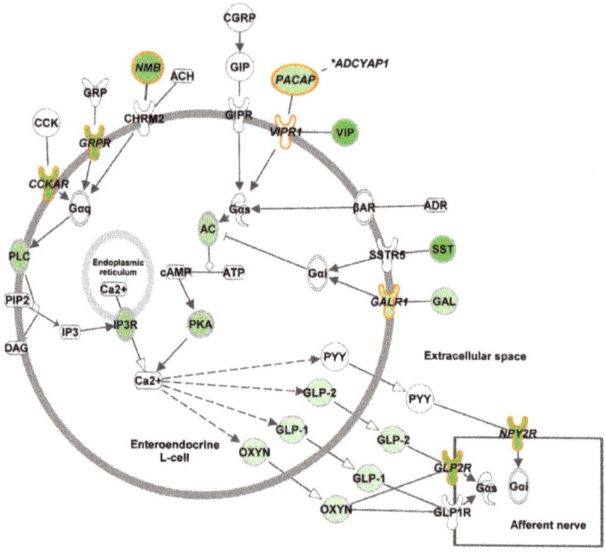

Figure 5. Differential expression of genes in the IPA canonical pathway "GPCR-Mediated Integration of Enteroendocrine Signaling Exemplified by an L Cell." Genes with significantly lower expression in domesticated turkeys relative to Eastern wild birds after AFB_1 treatment are denoted in green. Genes tested by qRT-PCR are outlined in orange (Figure 4).

Differential expression differences in genes of the "GPCR-Mediated Integration of Enteroendocrine Signaling Exemplified by an L Cell" pathway observed in RNAseq read counts were further tested in eight genes by qRT-PCR. These included *ADCYAP1* (adenylate cyclase activating polypeptide 1), *CCKAR* (cholecystokinin A receptor), *GALR1* (galanin receptor 1), *GLP2R* (glucagon-like peptide 2 receptor), *GRPR* (gastrin-releasing peptide receptor), *NMB* (neuromedin B), *NPT2R* (neuropeptide Y receptor Y2) and *VIPR1* (*LOC100303683*, vasoactive intestinal polypeptide receptor). With the exception of *VIPR1*, each of these genes showed lower expression in AFB_1-treated DT birds as compared to treated EW birds. The VIPR1 receptor was selected as it is downstream of two affected genes (*ADCYAP1* [*PACAP*] and *VIP*) in the pathway. With the exception of *NMB* and *VIPR1*, expression of the selected genes in EW birds was greater than in DT (domestic Nicholas turkey) consistent with RNAseq results (Figure 4). Disparate results between qRT experiments and RNAseq may be attributed to the higher efficiency of qRT-PCR in sampling genes with low average expression such as *NMB*. In the case of *ADCYAP1*, *CCKAR* and *GRPR* expression was also greater in the untreated EW birds relative to untreated DT birds. As expected, little variation was observed in *VIPR1*. Relative expression of these genes was also tested in the other commercial-type (broad-breasted white, BB) and wild-type birds (Rio Grande subspecies, RGW). Comparable expression results were seen for *ADCYAP1* and *GRPR*. Expression of 3 genes in the BB birds (*CCKAR*, *GALR1* and *NPY2R*) was elevated as compared to the DT group with levels more similar to the EW and RGW groups (Figure 4).

Only 32 DEGs were found unique to the wild turkey in the AFB_1 versus CNTL RNAseq comparison (Figure 3). The majority (28, 87.5%) were up regulated in the AFB_1-treated birds. Included among these are genes involved in lipid synthesis and metabolism (exemplified by *ACSBG2*, *ANGPTL4* and *SCD*) and immune response (*IRG1* [immunoresponsive 1 homolog], *PI3* [peptidase inhibitor 3]). A single annotation cluster (GO:0016021 integral component of membrane) was identified in DAVID that included 5 genes (*CLDN18*, *FAXDC2*, *PTPRQ*, *SCD* and *SLC23A1*). Interestingly, 29 of the 32 unique genes were also DE in the liver transcriptomes obtained from the same individuals [17] but showed opposite directional change in response to AFB_1.

2.2. *Wild versus Domesticated Turkey*

2.2.1. Control Birds

Comparison of the transcriptomes of EW and DT birds in the control groups found 679 DEGs (FDR p-value < 0.05, $\log_2$FC = −7.882 to 6.715, Table 1 and Table S3), with 67 having $|\log_2 FC| > 2.0$ (Figure 6, Table S6). Of the 67 genes, 13 were shared in common in the EW versus DT AFB_1 comparisons (Figure 6). The shared loci included 7 genes up regulated in EW birds; (*CAMK4* [calcium/calmodulin-dependent protein kinase IV], *LOC100548321* [Pendrin], *NEFM* [neurofilament, medium polypeptide], *LOC104914065* [pendrin-like] *LINGO2* [leucine rich repeat and Ig domain containing 2], *LOC100538933* [probable ATP-dependent RNA helicase *DDX60*] and the uncharacterized *LOC100549340* [ncRNA]). This differential expression may have implications for both epithelial function and inflammatory response. For example, as an anion exchange protein, Pendrin may function to regulate active chloride transport across epithelial membranes as a chloride-formate exchanger [31]. CAMK4 is implicated in transcriptional regulation in immune and inflammatory responses [32] and DDX60 is thought to positively regulate DDX58/RIG-I- and IFIH1/MDA5-dependent type I interferon and interferon inducible gene expression [33].

Down regulated genes among the 13 shared DE loci in the EW/DT comparison included *LOC100540418* (BPI fold-containing family C protein-like [*BPIFC*]), *LOC104915630* (3 beta-hydroxysteroid dehydrogenase/Delta 5–>4-isomerase-like [*HSD3B1*]), *LOC104917314* (14-3-3 protein gamma-B) and 3 uncharacterized ncRNA loci. Two of these genes have direct implication in gut homeostasis. BPIFC is a lipid transfer/lipopolysaccharide binding protein that may help provide defense against microorganisms [34]. In humans, HSD3B1 is an important gene in the biosynthesis of hormonal steroids as it catalyzes oxidative conversion of delta-5-3-beta-hydroxysteroid precursors. Altered expression of hormones in the gut may directly influence gene expression in the gut microbiota [35].

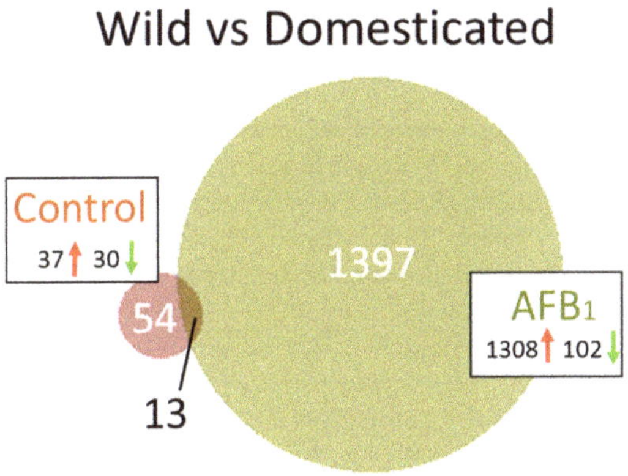

Figure 6. Distribution of differentially expressed genes between turkey types (wild and domesticated). For each comparison, the number of significant genes (FDR p-value < 0.05 and $|\log_2 FC| > 2.0$ shared or unique to each treatment group are indicated. Circle size is proportional to the number of genes and direction of expression change (↑ or ↓) is given for each group.

Of the 54 DEGs unique to the control group birds slightly more (55%) were up regulated in the EW birds compared to the DT birds (Table S6). These 54 unique DEGs included integral membrane proteins (e.g., *AQP10*), cytoplasmic enzymes (*NME8*), nuclear transcriptional regulators (*HOXB5*) and secretory proteins (*GKN2*) that are typical of intestinal epithelium but without significant enrichment for any particular biological process. Greatest differential expression was seen for claudin 18 (*CLDN18*), a membrane protein that is a component of tight junction strands with higher expression in EW

(log_2FC = 6.72) than DT. Also represented were genes with immune system roles such as *DNTT* (DNA nucleotidylexotransferase), which functions in generating antigen receptor diversity and *NOS1* (nitric oxide synthase 1), a host defense effector with antimicrobial activity.

2.2.2. AFB_1 Treatment

The greatest number gene expression differences observed between the EW and DT birds occurred in the AFB_1-treatment groups. A total of 1666 DEGs (FDR *p*-value < 0.05) were observed with 1410 having $|log_2FC| > 2.0$ (Table 1). As discussed above, 13 DEGs were shared with the control comparison and 1397 were unique (Figure 6, Table S7). Interestingly, 93% of the DEGs showed higher expression in the EW birds compared to DT. Non-coding RNAs comprised 29.4% of the down regulated genes (n = 30) and 5% of the up regulated DEGs (n = 66). Greatest differential expression (up regulation) in EW compared to DT was seen for *LOC104912821* (ovostatin homolog, log_2FC = 11.84), LOC104915655 (alpha-2-macroglobulin, *A2M*, log_2FC = 11.4) and genes such as *SLC10A2* (solute carrier family 10 [sodium/bile acid cotransporter] member 2, log_2FC = 11.06) and *FABP6* (fatty acid binding protein 6, log_2FC = 10.26). Ovostatin and A2M both have endopeptidase inhibitor activity, whereas SLC10A2 and FABP6 function in bile acid metabolism. Greatest down regulation in EW compared to DT was seen for *GYG2* (Glycogenin 2, $log_2FC = -7.19$) and *LOC104916581* (7-dehydrocholesterol reductase-like, $log_2FC = -5.56$). In humans, GYG2 is expressed mainly in the liver and heart and is involved in initiating reactions of glycogen biosynthesis; 7-dehydrocholesterol reductase is ubiquitously expressed and helps catalyze the production of cholesterol [36,37].

Functional analysis of the 1397 unique DEGs in DAVID found highest enrichment score (14.11) for the annotation cluster "Membrane" ($p = 4.1 \times 10^{-16}$), which included 284 genes (Table S7). The second annotation cluster (enrichment = 5.39) contained 50 genes with immunoglobulin-like domains or Ig-like fold (homologous superfamily IPR013783, $p = 5.7 \times 10^{-7}$). Included were several complement proteins, interleukins and Ig superfamily members (Table S7). Additional clusters identified in DAVID included "extracellular exosome" (136 DEGs, $p = 6.5 \times 10^{-3}$) and "signal" (118 DEGs, $p = 2.3 \times 10^{-8}$). Calcium signaling was the most expressively represented Kegg pathway containing 29 DEGs ($p = 1.8 \times 10^{-6}$, Figure S2), followed by "Focal adhesion" (28 DEGs, $p = 6.1 \times 10^{-4}$) and "Neuroactive ligand-receptor interaction" (28 DEGs, $p = 7.4 \times 10^{-2}$).

Among the 1397 unique DEGs were two olfactory receptor genes, *LOC100546335* (*OR51E2*-like) and *LOC1005546179* (*OR51G2*-like). Both of these loci were up regulated in the EW birds compared to DT with AFB_1-treatment (log_2FC = 8.15 and 8.46, respectively). Expression of functional taste and olfactory receptors has been observed in human enteroendocrine cells [38,39] and a survey of RNAseq data from multiple human tissues identified expressed olfactory receptors with broad and tissue-exclusive expression [40]. An interesting aspect of *LOC100546335* and *LOC1005546179* is that based on read count, expression of both loci was roughly similar. These loci are adjacent in the turkey genome and are annotated as sharing two non-coding 5′ exons (Figure 7). A total of seven transcript variants for the two genes were predicted by NCBI's automated computational analysis gene prediction method (Gnomon). Examination of RNAseq reads from 3 individuals in the present study (EW1, EW9 and NC11) found split RNAseq reads (intron spanning) that support each of the predicted variants with the exception of the variant 51E2- -X4. However, RNAseq reads did map to the non-coding upstream (5′) exon of variant 4 (Figure 7). Interestingly, split reads were also identified in each individual that indicated splicing events between the two small 5′ exons, not predicted in the NCBI models.

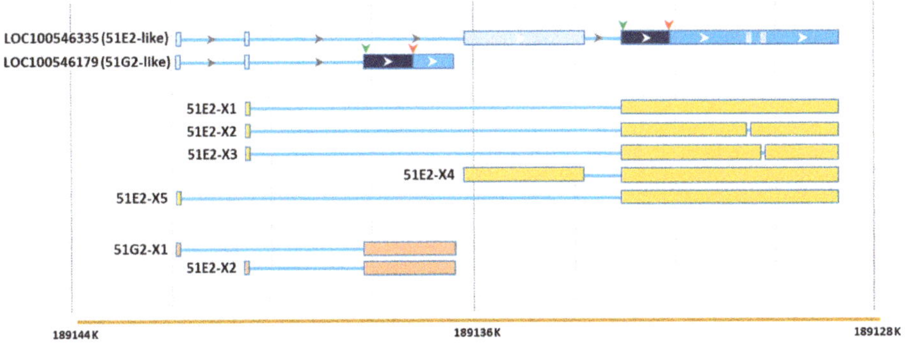

Figure 7. Alignment of NCBI predicted sequence variants to the predicted genes for two olfactory receptor loci.

3. Discussion

Naturally-occurring dietary toxins such as AFB_1 pose significant public health risk throughout the world but especially in locales characterized by high contamination levels of dietary staples such as corn. One of most significant is AFB_1 which primarily targets the liver, the organ with the highest concentration of bioactivating CYPs. Extra-hepatic metabolism and bioactivation of this mycotoxin is a much-studied topic [41] but comparatively few studies have focused on the gastrointestinal tract, even though dietary exposure is the principal route for people and animals. Conversion of AFB_1 to the AFBO epoxide has been implicated in the rat intestine [42] and even nasal mucosal cells [43]. Studies of cultured human intestinal epithelial cells (Caco-2) found AFB_1 decreases trans-epithelial electrical resistance (TEER) [44]. Similarly, Romero et al. [45] reported that AFB_1 treatment caused a reduction in TEER and mitochondrial viability and increased cell permeability. By contrast, the detoxified AFB_1 metabolite AFM_1 did not permanently compromise the integrity of Caco-2 cells grown on microporous filter supports [46]. In poultry, AFB_1 is efficiently absorbed in the upper GI tract and thus exposure of the intestinal mucosa is greater than in other organs. While we have not quantified AFB_1 bioactivation in the turkey gut, expression of the primary hepatic AFB_1-activating *CYP1A5* was highly upregulated by AFB_1 in the turkey cecum. Increased *CYP1A5* expression in AFB_1-treated turkeys was also observed in the liver [17] and is a common observation in animals, as this and other CYPs are known to be induced by AFB_1 and other foodborne and environmental toxicants [47]. Similarly, expression of GSTAs (particularly *GSTA4*), were up regulated by AFB_1. In contrast, a prior study found expression of GSTAs in the liver were oppositely affected; *GSTA1*, *GSTA2* and *GSTA4* were down regulated after 2 weeks exposure to AFB_1 and expression of *GSTA3* was significantly lower in EW birds compared to DT after AFB_1 treatment [17].

The gastrointestinal epithelium provides an important physical barrier to foreign antigens and pathogens and disruptions thereof are increasingly associated with diseases [48]. Although few studies have specifically investigated the ability of aflatoxin to compromise intestinal permeability [19,49], the potential for mycotoxins to cause dysfunction of the intestinal barrier has come under increased study. Mycotoxins modulate the composition of gut microbiota, often eliminating beneficial bacteria, which leads to increased colonization by gut pathobionts and pathogens [50,51]. Exposure to AFB_1 has been shown to induce changes in gut microbiota in rodents [52,53] and to modify barrier function in intestinal epithelial cells [49]. Probiotic gram-positive strains of *Lactobacillus*, *Propionibacterium* and *Bifidobacterium* have been proposed as feed additives to attenuate AFB_1-induced toxicity in poultry due to their ability to bind AFB_1, thereby reducing its bioavailability [54–57]. Gene expression in AFB_1-treated birds is modulated by probiotics but the negative effects of AFB_1 are not fully mitigated [15,16]. It is possible that in addition to binding AFB_1, these probiotics exert positive effects by acting to decrease gut permeability and other protective functions [58].

Of interest in the present study is the potential of AFB_1 to disrupt tight junction proteins allowing for increased translocation of substances from the lumen to the blood and lymphatic circulation [49]. Transmembrane tight junctions consist of claudins, occludin, tricellulin and a group of junction adhesion molecules that form the horizontal barrier at the apical lateral membrane [59]. Claudins are a family of transmembrane proteins that are essential components in the apical junctional complex of epithelia and endothelia cells [60], the expression of which in humans, is modulated by aflatoxins [45, 61]. Romero et al. [45] found dose-dependent down regulation in *CLDN3* and occludin in human Caco-2 cells treated with AFB_1 consistent with an observed decrease in gut barrier properties. Gao et al. [61] found decreased expression of TJ proteins (*CLDN3, CLDN4*, occludin and zonula occludens-1) and disrupted structures following exposure to aflatoxin M_1 (4-hydroxylated metabolite of AFB_1).

Dietary AFB_1 treatment in the present study elicited transcriptional changes in several claudin transcripts including up regulation of *CLDN1* in both EW and DT, down regulation of *CLDN3* in DT, down regulation of *CLDN18* in EW and up regulation of *CLDN10* and *CLDN23* in EW birds. Transcriptional modifications of claudins may indicate a response to restore impaired TJ proteins and potentially compromised gut permeability. In vivo studies in poultry have produced inconsistent results. In broilers, AFB_1 increased gut permeability as measured by the serum lactose/rhamnose ratio (dual sugar test), as well as increases in expression of *CLDN1*, multiple jejunal amino acid transporters and the translation initiation factor 4E [21]. A second study [20] found no evidence for increased gut permeability in broilers as measured by GI leakage of FITC-d following exposure to varying concentrations of AFB_1. Annotation of avian claudin genes is based on similarities to mammalian orthologs and in many cases function has not been experimentally demonstrated. Results of the present study indicate that additional studies of the effect of AFB_1 on gut permeability in turkey are needed.

Exposure to AFB_1 has widespread adverse physiologic effects. In poultry, AFB_1 adversely affects production characteristics causing poor performance, decreased growth rate, body weight, weight gain, egg production, reproductive performance and feed efficiency [62]. Humoral and cell-mediated immune functions in poultry are also impaired by AFB_1 in keeping with its well-known immunotoxicity [3,5,6,16,41,63–65]. Altered humoral response to fowl cholera and Newcastle Disease (ND) virus has been described in chickens where correlation was observed between outbreaks of ND and AFB_1-contaminated feeds (reviewed in Reference [65]). Effects on cell-mediated immunity are evident as decreased phagocytic activity in leukocytes [66–69]. Exposure to AFB_1 in turkeys causes suppression of humoral and cellular immunity resulting in compromised immune response in hatchlings making them more susceptible to disease [6]. In this respect, AFB_1 is a "force-multiplier" synergizing the adverse effects of other agents and pathogens detrimental to poultry health.

Compromised epithelial barrier is associated with increased paracellular permeability that may lead to overstimulation of the gut immune system and a non-specific systemic inflammatory response [48,70]. The cecal tonsil is the major lymphoid tissue in the avian cecum that provides important and unique immune functions. Detailed studies in poultry have demonstrated impairment of the normal function of the cecal tonsil caused by AFB_1 through depletion of lymphocytes and lesions in the absorptive cells [71]. AFB_1 significantly decreases intestinal IgA(+) cells and the expression of immunoglobulins in the intestinal mucosa [72]. Dietary AFB_1 exposure decreases cell-mediated immunity while inducing the inflammatory response. Immune activation and inflammation result in mucosal recruitment of activated cells, modulated by cytokines. Cytokine-mediated dysfunction of tight junctions is important in gastrointestinal disease [48] as cytokines and other growth factors may act to alternatively decrease (e.g., IL-10) or increase (e.g., IL-6) gut permeability [58]. In the commercial DT birds, numerous pro-inflammatory cytokines, TGF-β and EGF were significantly down regulated by AFB_1 treatment. In contrast, the interleukin 6 (*IL6R*) and interleukin 13, alpha 2 (*IL13RA2*) receptors and the interleukin 1 receptor accessory protein (*IL1RAP*) were significantly up regulated in both EW and DT birds. In humans, IL13RA2 functions to internalize the immunoregulatory cytokine IL-13. Dysregulation of IL6 impacts *CLDN2* expression (significantly up regulated by AFB_1 in DT in this study) and can undermine the integrity of the intestinal barrier [73].

In response to the luminal environment, chemical receptors of intestinal epithelial and neuroendocrine cells modulate the function of these cells and ultimately systematic metabolism and homeostasis [38,74]. For example, ingestion of food results in signaling to the brain to regulate food intake and detection of bacterial metabolites may induce host defense responses. Part of this gut-brain axis is performed by enteroendocrine L-cells with specific nutrient-sensing receptors [30]. These include intestinal olfactory receptors that recognize ingested odor compounds and alter glucose homeostasis through induced secretion of gut-peptides [75]. In pigs, the olfactory receptor OR51E1 has been localized to enteroendocrine cells along the GI tract. Expression of the gene encoding this receptor was significantly altered following modulation of the intestinal microbiota, presumably in response to microbial metabolites [76]. Differential expression of OR genes in the turkey GIT may be caused by a direct action of AFB_1 on the intestinal epithelial cells or secondarily through changes in the intestinal microbiota induced by AFB_1.

Intensive breeding and genetic selection to produce the modern domesticated turkey has dramatically affected performance metrics. For example, growth rate to market age has essentially doubled in the past 40 years and feed efficiency of contemporary tom turkeys is approximately 50% better when compared to non-growth selected birds fed modern diets [77]. Under normal conditions, commercial birds typically reach 19 lbs. by 20 weeks of age, with a feed conversion ratio of approximately 2.5 [78]. Our results suggest that selection for production traits, such as increased nutrient conversion, may have contributed to the extreme sensitivity of DT to AFB_1. In the same way, the relative resistance of WT, in addition to expression of AFB_1-detoxifying GSTAs, may also involve extra-hepatic mechanisms such as a more refractory gastrointestinal tract, in addition to the presence of functional hepatic GST-mediated AFB_1 detoxifying capability [12,13]. Possibly related to this, studies of production performance in chickens suggest that sensitivity to AFB_1 has increased since the 1980s, concomitant with industry selection for increased nutrient conversion and demands for greater metabolism (reviewed in Yunus et al. [65]). Elucidation of extra-hepatic routes of pathogenesis provides a clearer picture of the complexity of species resistance and susceptibility to this potent mycotoxin that may also suggest analogous mechanisms in humans.

4. Materials and Methods

This study used turkeys previously found to vary in AFB_1-detoxifying GST activity. Animal husbandry and the AFB_1 protocol were as described in Reed et al. [17]. Birds included AFB_1-treated and control animals from the Eastern Wild (EW, *Meleagris gallopavo silvestris*) subspecies and domesticated Nicholas turkeys (DT). Male turkey poults were subjected to a short-term AFB_1-treatment protocol in which the diet of challenge birds was supplemented beginning on day 15 of age with 320 ppb AFB_1 and continued for 14 days. Previous studies with higher AFB_1 dosing (1 ppm) caused an unacceptable mortality rate. Birds serving as experimental controls received a standard AFB_1-free diet. At the end of the trial, birds were euthanized and a section of the cecum corresponding to the cecal tonsil was removed and placed in RNAlater (ThermoFisher Scientific, Waltham, MA, USA) for RNA isolation and RNAseq analysis. All procedures were approved by Utah State University's Institutional Animal Use and Care Committee (Approval #2670, date of approve: 26 September 2016).

4.1. RNA Isolation and Sequencing

Total RNA was isolated from cecal tonsils by TRIzol extraction (ThermoFisher), treated with DNAse (Turbo DNA-freeTM Kit, ThermoFisher) and stored at −80° C. Library preparation and sequencing was performed at the University of Minnesota Genomics Center. Briefly, concentration and quality of RNA was assessed on a 2100 Bioanalyzer (Agilent Technologies) and RNA Integrity Numbers (RIN) averaged 6.7. Replicate samples (n = 4) from each treatment group were examined. Indexed libraries (n = 16) were constructed, multiplexed, pooled and sequenced (101-bp paired-end reads) on the HiSeq 2000 using v3 chemistry (Illumina, Inc., San Diego, CA, USA). Sequence reads were groomed, assessed for quality and mapped to turkey genome (UMD 5.0, NCBI Annotation 101) as described in Reed et al. [17].

4.2. Quantitative Real-Time PCR

Quantitative real-time PCR (qRT-PCR) was performed on both domesticated and wild turkeys. Samples included the Eastern Wild (EW; *M. g. silvestris*) and domesticated Nicholas turkey (DT) birds, plus domesticated Broad Breasted White (BB) and birds of the Rio Grande subspecies of wild turkey (RGW; *M. g. intermedia*) from a parallel AFB_1-challenge experiment. Of the 6 samples from the DT and EW groups used for qRT-PCR, four were in common with the RNAseq study. Synthesis of cDNA was performed on DNase-treated mRNA using Invitrogen Super Script IV First-strand synthesis kit (Invitrogen, Carlsbad, CA, USA). The iTaq Universal SYBR Green Supermix (BioRad, Hercules, CA, SA) was used for quantitative analysis of gene-specific amplicons with the CFX96 touch real time detection system (BioRad, Hercules, CA, USA). Primers were designed using the turkey genome sequence (UMD5.0) and Primer3 software [79]. Primer sets were designed so the amplicon spanned an exon/exon junction and at least one intron. Several normalizing genes were tested for uniformity and the most stable reference gene (hypoxanthine guanine phosphoribosyl transferase, *HPRT*) was determined with RefFinder [80]. Target gene reactions were conducted in triplicate and *HPRT* normalization reactions, no template and gDNA controls were run in duplicate. Disassociation curves were used to confirm single product amplification and to preclude the possibility of dimer amplification.

4.3. Statistical Analysis

For expression analysis of RNAseq data, read counts were by-total normalized and expressed as reads per 11.9M (CLC Genomics Workbench v. 8.0.2, CLC Bio, Aarhus, Denmark). Principal component analysis (PCA) and hierarchical clustering of samples based on Euclidean distance was performed (with single linkage) in CLCGWB using by-total normalization. Empirical analysis of differential gene expression (EdgeR) and ANOVA were performed in CLCGWB on mapped read counts with TMM (Trimmed Mean of M-values) normalization (Bonferroni and FDR corrected). Pair-wise comparisons between treatment groups were made following the standard workflow Wald test. Significant differentially expressed (DE) genes were used to investigate affected gene pathways with Ingenuity Pathway Analysis (IPA) (Ingenuity Systems, Redwood City, CA, USA). Gene Ontology (GO) and functional classification was performed in DAVID (v6.8, [81]) and overrepresentation tests for gene enrichment were performed with PANTHER (GO Consortium release 20150430) [82]. For analysis of qRT-PCR data, expression was normalized first to HPRT, then interpreted using the Double Delta Ct Analysis ($\Delta\Delta$Ct, [83]) and a comparative Ct approach. Expression analysis was performed using the standard $\Delta\Delta$Ct workflow within the CFX Maestro software package (Biorad, Hercules, CA, USA).

Supplementary Materials: The following are available online at http://www.mdpi.com/2072-6651/11/1/55/s1. Figure S1: Hierarchical clustering of samples based on Euclidean distance reiterated relationships shown by PCA. Figure S2: Kegg calcium-signaling pathway. Table S1: Summary of RNAseq data for turkey cecal tonsil transcriptomes. Table S2: Mean quality-trimmed RNAseq read counts for turkey cecal tonsil from two turkey types (Wild and Domesticated). Table S3: Summary of pairwise differential gene expression analysis of cecal tonsil transcriptomes. Table S4: Fifty genes showing the greatest differential expression in each pairwise comparison of treatment groups. Table S5: Functional annotation gene clusters identified in DAVID among the 655 DEGs shared between EW and DT birds in AFB_1 versus CNTL comparisons. Table S6: Significant differentially expressed genes (FDR p-values < 0.05 and $|\log_2FC| > 2.0$) identified in comparison of Eastern Wild versus domesticated turkeys in the CNTL groups. Table S7: Genes showing differential expression that were unique in the comparison of AFB_1-treated Eastern wild turkeys versus domesticated turkeys.

Author Contributions: K.M.R. and R.A.C. wrote and edited the manuscript; R.A.C. designed and performed the AFB_1-treatment experiments; K.M.R. and K.M.M. collected and analyzed data; K.M.R. and K.M.M. performed data analysis and interpretation.

Funding: This research was funded by the United States Department of Agriculture, Agriculture and Food Research Initiative, National Institute of Food and Agriculture Animal Genome Program (2013-01043), the University of Minnesota, College of Veterinary Medicine Hatch Formula Funds and the Minnesota and Utah Agricultural Experiments Stations.

Acknowledgments: The authors thank David Brown (UMN) for helpful comments on the manuscript.

Conflicts of Interest: The authors declare no conflict of interest.

Abbreviations

AFB	aflatoxin B_1
AFBO	exo-AFB1-8,9-epoxide
BB	Broad Breasted White
Ct	threshold cycle
CYP	cytochrome P450
DE	differentially expressed
DEG	differentially expressed gene
DT	domesticated turkey
EW	Eastern wild turkey (*Meleagris gallopavo silvestris*)
FC	fold change
FDR	false discovery rate
GO	gene ontology
GST	glutathione S-transferase
IPA	Ingenuity Pathway Analysis
ncRNA	non-coding RNA
PCA	principal component analysis
qRT-PCR	quantitative real-time polymerase chain reaction
RGW	Rio Grande wild turkey (*Meleagris gallopavo intermedia*)

References

1. CAST. *Mycotoxins: Risks in Plant, Animal and Human Systems*; No. 139; Council for Agricultural Science and Technology: Ames, IA, USA, 2003.
2. Blount, W.P. Turkey "X" disease. *Turkeys* **1961**, *9*, 52, 55–58, 61–71, 77.
3. Rawal, S.; Kim, J.E.; Coulombe, R., Jr. Aflatoxin B_1 in poultry: Toxicology, metabolism and prevention. *Res. Vet. Sci.* **2010**, *89*, 325–331. [CrossRef] [PubMed]
4. Monson, M.S.; Coulombe, R.A.; Reed, K.M. Aflatoxicosis: Lessons from toxicity and responses to aflatoxin B_1 in poultry. *Agriculture* **2015**, *5*, 742–777. [CrossRef]
5. Qureshi, M.A.; Brake, J.; Hamilton, P.B.; Hagler, W.M., Jr.; Nesheim, S. Dietary exposure of broiler breeders to aflatoxin results in immune dysfunction in progeny chicks. *Poult. Sci.* **1998**, *77*, 812–819. [CrossRef] [PubMed]
6. Qureshi, M.A.; Heggen, C.L.; Hussain, I. Avian macrophage: Effector functions in health and disease. *Dev. Comp. Immunol.* **2000**, *24*, 103–119. [CrossRef]
7. Williams, J.G.; Deschl, U.; Williams, G.M. DNA damage in fetal liver cells of turkey and chicken eggs dosed with aflatoxin B_1. *Arch. Toxicol.* **2011**, *85*, 1167–1172. [CrossRef] [PubMed]
8. Quist, C.F.; Bounous, D.I.; Kilburn, J.V.; Nettles, V.F.; Wyatt, R.D. The effect of dietary aflatoxin on wild turkey poults. *J. Wildl. Dis.* **2000**, *36*, 436–444. [CrossRef] [PubMed]
9. Rawal, S.; Coulombe, R.A., Jr. Metabolism of aflatoxin B_1 in turkey liver microsomes: The relative roles of cytochromes P450 1A5 and 3A37. *Toxicol. Appl. Pharmacol.* **2011**, *254*, 349–354. [CrossRef]
10. Bunderson, B.R.; Kim, J.E.; Croasdell, A.; Mendoza, K.M.; Reed, K.M.; Coulombe, R.A., Jr. Heterologous expression and functional characterization of avian mu-class glutathione S-transferases. *Comp. Biochem. Physiol. C Toxicol. Pharmacol.* **2013**, *158*, 109–116. [CrossRef]
11. Kim, J.E.; Bunderson, B.R.; Croasdell, A.; Coulombe, R.A., Jr. Functional characterization of alpha-class glutathione *S*-transferases from the turkey (*Meleagris gallopavo*). *Toxicol. Sci.* **2011**, *124*, 45–53. [CrossRef]
12. Kim, J.E.; Bunderson, B.R.; Croasdell, A.; Reed, K.M.; Coulombe, R.A., Jr. Alpha-class glutathione *S*-transferases in wild turkeys (*Meleagris gallopavo*): Characterization and role in resistance to the carcinogenic mycotoxin aflatoxin B_1. *PLoS ONE* **2013**, *8*, e60662. [CrossRef] [PubMed]
13. Klein, P.J.; Buckner, R.; Kelly, J.; Coulombe, R.A. Biochemical basis for the extreme sensitivity of turkeys to aflatoxin B_1. *Toxicol. Appl. Pharmacol.* **2000**, *165*, 45–52. [CrossRef] [PubMed]

14. Klein, P.J.; Van Vleet, T.R.; Hall, J.O.; Coulombe, R.A., Jr. Dietary butylated hydroxytoluene protects against aflatoxicosis in turkeys. *Toxicol. Appl. Pharmacol.* **2002**, *182*, 11–19. [CrossRef] [PubMed]
15. Monson, M.S.; Settlage, R.E.; McMahon, K.W.; Mendoza, K.M.; Rawal, S.; El-Nemazi, H.S.; Coulombe, R.A., Jr.; Reed, K.M. Response of the hepatic transcriptome to aflatoxin B_1 in domestic turkey (*Meleagris gallopavo*). *PLoS ONE* **2014**, *9*, e100930. [CrossRef] [PubMed]
16. Monson, M.S.; Settlage, R.E.; Mendoza, K.M.; Rawal, S.; El-Nezami, H.S.; Coulombe, R.A., Jr.; Reed, K.M. Modulation of the spleen transcriptome in domestic turkey (*Meleagris gallopavo*) in response to aflatoxin B_1 and probiotics. *Immunogenetics* **2015**, *67*, 163–178. [CrossRef] [PubMed]
17. Reed, K.M.; Mendoza, K.M.; Abrahante, J.E.; Coulombe, R.A. Comparative response of the hepatic transcriptomes of domesticated and wild turkey to aflatoxin B_1. *Toxins* **2018**, *10*, 42. [CrossRef] [PubMed]
18. Monson, M.S.; Cardona, C.C.; Coulombe, R.A.; Reed, K.M. Hepatic transcriptome responses of domesticated and wild turkey embryos to aflatoxin B_1. *Toxins* **2016**, *8*, 16. [CrossRef] [PubMed]
19. Grenier, B.; Applegate, T.J. Modulation of intestinal functions following mycotoxin ingestion: Meta-analysis of published experiments in animals. *Toxins* **2013**, *5*, 396–430. [CrossRef] [PubMed]
20. Galarza-Seeber, R.; Latorre, J.D.; Bielke, L.R.; Kuttappan, V.A.; Wolfenden, A.D.; Hernandez-Velasco, X.; Merino-Guzman, R.; Vicente, J.L.; Donoghue, A.; Cross, D.; et al. Leaky gut and mycotoxins: Aflatoxin B_1 does not increase gut permeability in broiler chickens. *Front. Vet. Sci.* **2016**, *3*, 10. [CrossRef] [PubMed]
21. Chen, X.; Naehrer, K.; Applegate, T.J. Interactive effects of dietary protein concentration and aflatoxin B_1 on performance, nutrient digestibility and gut health in broiler chicks. *Poult. Sci.* **2016**, *95*, 1312–1325. [CrossRef] [PubMed]
22. Stanley, D.; Denman, S.E.; Hughes, R.J.; Geier, M.S.; Crowley, T.M.; Chen, H.; Haring, V.R.; Moore, R.J. Intestinal microbiota associated with differential feed conversion efficiency in chickens. *Appl. Microbiol. Biotechnol.* **2012**, *96*, 1361–1369. [CrossRef] [PubMed]
23. Sasaki, H.; Matsui, C.; Furuse, K.; Mimori-Kiyosue, Y.; Furuse, M.; Tsukita, S. Dynamic behavior of paired claudin strands within apposing plasma membranes. *Proc. Natl. Acad. Sci. USA* **2003**, *100*, 3971–3976. [CrossRef] [PubMed]
24. Grishin, A.V.; Sverdlov, V.E.; Kostina, M.B.; Modyanov, N.N. Cloning and characterization of the entire cDNA encoded by ATP1AL1–a member of the human Na,K/H,K-ATPase gene family. *FEBS Lett.* **1994**, *349*, 144–150. [CrossRef]
25. Hinson, E.R.; Cresswell, P. The N-terminal amphipathic alpha-helix of viperin mediates localization to the cytosolic face of the endoplasmic reticulum and inhibits protein secretion. *J. Biol. Chem.* **2009**, *284*, 4705–4712. [CrossRef] [PubMed]
26. Wang, J.; Yu, L.; Schmidt, R.E.; Su, C.; Huang, X.; Gould, K.; Cao, G. Characterization of HSCD5, a novel human stearoyl-CoA desaturase unique to primates. *Biochem. Biophys. Res. Commun.* **2005**, *332*, 735–742. [CrossRef] [PubMed]
27. Grahn, T.H.; Zhang, Y.; Lee, M.J.; Sommer, A.G.; Mostoslavsky, G.; Fried, S.K.; Greenberg, A.S.; Puri, V. FSP27 and PLIN1 interaction promotes the formation of large lipid droplets in human adipocytes. *Biochem. Biophys. Res. Commun.* **2013**, *432*, 296–301. [CrossRef]
28. Feild, J.A.; Zhang, L.; Brun, K.A.; Brooks, D.P.; Edwards, R.M. Cloning and functional characterization of a sodium-dependent phosphate transporter expressed in human lung and small intestine. *Biochem. Biophys. Res. Commun.* **1999**, *258*, 578–582. [CrossRef] [PubMed]
29. Yan, M.; Brady, J.R.; Chan, B.; Lee, W.P.; Hsu, B.; Harless, S.; Cancro, M.; Grewal, I.S.; Dixit, V.M. Identification of a novel receptor for B lymphocyte stimulator that is mutated in a mouse strain with severe B cell deficiency. *Curr. Biol.* **2001**, *11*, 1547–1552. [CrossRef]
30. Spreckley, E.; Murphy, K.G. The L-cell in nutritional sensing and the regulation of appetite. *Front. Nutr.* **2015**, *2*, 23. [CrossRef] [PubMed]
31. Karniski, L.P.; Aronson, P.S. Chloride/formate exchange with formic acid recycling: A mechanism of active chloride transport across epithelial membranes. *Proc. Natl. Acad. Sci. USA* **1985**, *82*, 6362–6365. [CrossRef]
32. Racioppi, L.; Means, A.R. Calcium/calmodulin-dependent kinase IV in immune and inflammatory responses: Novel routes for an ancient traveler. *Trends Immunol.* **2008**, *29*, 600–607. [CrossRef]
33. Zhang, Y.; Burke, C.W.; Ryman, K.D.; Klimstra, W.B. Identification and characterization of interferon-induced proteins that inhibit alphavirus replication. *J. Virol.* **2007**, *81*, 11246–11255. [CrossRef]

34. Mulero, J.J.; Boyle, B.J.; Bradley, S.; Bright, J.M.; Nelken, S.T.; Ho, T.T.; Mize, N.K.; Childs, J.D.; Ballinger, D.G.; Ford, J.E.; et al. Three new human members of the lipid transfer/lipopolysaccharide binding protein family (LT/LBP). *Immunogenetics* **2002**, *54*, 293–300. [CrossRef] [PubMed]
35. Sperandio, V.; Torres, A.G.; Jarvis, B.; Nataro, J.P.; Kaper, J.B. Bacteria-host communication: The language of hormones. *Proc. Natl. Acad. Sci. USA* **2003**, *100*, 8951–8956. [CrossRef]
36. Prabhu, A.V.; Luu, W.; Sharpe, L.J.; Brown, A.J. Phosphorylation regulates activity of 7-dehydrocholesterol reductase (DHCR7), a terminal enzyme of cholesterol synthesis. *J. Steroid Biochem. Mol. Biol.* **2017**, *165*, 363–368. [CrossRef] [PubMed]
37. Roach, P.J.; Skurat, A.V. Self-glucosylating initiator proteins and their role in glycogen biosynthesis. *Prog. Nucl. Acid Res. Mol. Biol.* **1997**, *57*, 289–316.
38. Braun, T.; Voland, P.; Kunz, L.; Prinz, C.; Gratzl, M. Enterochromaffin cells of the human gut: Sensors for spices and odorants. *Gastroenterology* **2007**, *132*, 1890–1901. [CrossRef] [PubMed]
39. Sternini, C.; Anselmi, L.; Rozengurt, E. Enteroendocrine cells: A site of 'taste' in gastrointestinal chemosensing. *Curr. Opin. Endocrinol. Diabetes Obes.* **2008**, *15*, 73–78. [CrossRef] [PubMed]
40. Flegel, C.; Manteniotis, S.; Osthold, S.; Hatt, H.; Gisselmann, G. Expression profile of ectopic olfactory receptors determined by deep sequencing. *PLoS ONE* **2013**, *8*, e55368. [CrossRef]
41. Coulombe, R.A., Jr. Biological action of mycotoxins. *J. Dairy Sci.* **1993**, *76*, 880–891. [CrossRef]
42. Kumagai, S. Intestinal absorption and excretion of aflatoxin in rats. *Toxicol. Appl. Pharmacol.* **1989**, *97*, 88–97. [CrossRef]
43. Larsson, P.; Tjälve, H. Intranasal instillation of aflatoxin B_1 in rats: Bioactivation in the nasal mucosa and neuronal transport to the olfactory bulb. *Toxicol. Sci.* **2000**, *55*, 383–391. [CrossRef] [PubMed]
44. Gratz, S.; Wu, Q.K.; El-Nezami, H.; Juvonen, R.O.; Mykkänen, H.; Turner, P.C. *Lactobacillus rhamnosus* strain GG reduces aflatoxin B_1 transport, metabolism and toxicity in Caco-2 cells. *Appl. Environ. Microbiol.* **2007**, *73*, 3958–3964. [CrossRef] [PubMed]
45. Romero, A.; Ares, I.; Ramos, E.; Castellano, V.; Martínez, M.; Martínez-Larrañaga, M.R.; Anadón, A.; Martínez, M.A. Mycotoxins modify the barrier function of Caco-2 cells through differential gene expression of specific claudin isoforms: Protective effect of illite mineral clay. *Toxicology* **2016**, *353–354*, 21–33. [CrossRef]
46. Caloni, F.; Cortinovis, C.; Pizzo, F.; De Angelis, I. Transport of aflatoxin M_1 in human intestinal caco-2/TC7 cells. *Front. Pharmacol.* **2012**, *3*, 111. [CrossRef] [PubMed]
47. Chang, S.Y.; Voellinger, J.L.; Van Ness, K.P.; Chapron, B.; Shaffer, R.M.; Neumann, T.; White, C.C.; Kavanagh, T.J.; Kelly, E.J.; Eaton, D.L. Characterization of rat or human hepatocytes cultured in microphysiological systems (MPS) to identify hepatotoxicity. *Toxicol. In Vitro* **2017**, *40*, 170–183. [CrossRef] [PubMed]
48. Camilleri, M.; Madsen, K.; Spiller, R.; Van Meerveld, B.G.; Verne, G.N. Intestinal barrier function in health and gastrointestinal disease. *Neurogastroenterol. Motil.* **2012**, *24*, 503–512. [CrossRef]
49. Akbari, P.; Braber, S.; Varasteh, S.; Alizadeh, A.; Garssen, J.; Fink-Gremmels, J. The intestinal barrier as an emerging target in the toxicological assessment of mycotoxins. *Arch. Toxicol.* **2017**, *91*, 1007–1029. [CrossRef]
50. Liew, W.P.; Mohd-Redzwan, S. Mycotoxin: Its impact on gut health and microbiota. *Front. Cell Infect. Microbiol.* **2018**, *8*, 60. [CrossRef]
51. Robert, H.; Payros, D.; Pinton, P.; Théodorou, V.; Mercier-Bonin, M.; Oswald, I.P. Impact of mycotoxins on the intestine: Are mucus and microbiota new targets? *J. Toxicol. Environ. Health B Crit. Rev.* **2017**, *20*, 249–275.
52. Ishikawa, A.T.; Weese, J.S.; Bracarense, A.P.F.R.L.; Alfieri, A.A.; Oliveira, G.G.; Kawamura, O.; Hirooka, E.Y.; Itano, E.N.; Costa, M.C. Single aflatoxin B_1 exposure induces changes in gut microbiota community in C57Bl/6 mice. *World Mycotoxin J.* **2017**, *10*, 249–254. [CrossRef]
53. Wang, J.; Tang, L.; Glenn, T.C.; Wang, J.S. Aflatoxin B_1 induced compositional changes in gut microbial communities of male F344 rats. *Toxicol. Sci.* **2016**, *150*, 54–63. [CrossRef] [PubMed]
54. El-Nezami, H.; Kankaanpaa, P.; Salminen, S.; Ahokas, J. Ability of dairy strains of lactic acid bacteria to bind a common food carcinogen, aflatoxin B_1. *Food Chem. Toxicol.* **1998**, *36*, 321–326. [CrossRef]
55. Gratz, S.; Mykkänen, H.; El-Nezami, H. Aflatoxin B_1 binding by a mixture of *Lactobacillus* and *Propionibacterium*: In vitro versus ex vivo. *J. Food Prot.* **2005**, *68*, 2470–2474. [CrossRef] [PubMed]
56. Kankaanpää, P.; Tuomola, E.; El-Nezami, H.; Ahokas, J.; Salminen, S.J. Binding of aflatoxin B_1 alters the adhesion properties of *Lactobacillus rhamnosus* strain GG in a Caco-2 model. *J. Food Prot.* **2000**, *63*, 412–414. [CrossRef] [PubMed]

57. Oatley, J.T.; Rarick, M.D.; Ji, G.E.; Linz, J.E. Binding of aflatoxin B_1 to *Bifidobacteria* in vitro. *J. Food Prot.* **2000**, *63*, 1133–1136. [CrossRef] [PubMed]
58. Suzuki, T. Regulation of intestinal epithelial permeability by tight junctions. *Cell. Mol. Life Sci.* **2013**, *70*, 631–659. [CrossRef]
59. Tsukita, S.; Furuse, M.; Itoh, M. Multifunctional strands in tight junctions. *Nat. Rev. Mol. Cell Biol.* **2001**, *2*, 285–293. [CrossRef]
60. Tsukita, S.; Furuse, M. The structure and function of claudins, cell adhesion molecules at tight junctions. *Ann. N. Y. Acad Sci.* **2000**, *915*, 129–135. [CrossRef]
61. Gao, Y.; Songli, L.; Wang, J.; Luo, C.; Zhao, S.; Zheng, N. Modulation of intestinal epithelial permeability in differentiated Caco-2 cells exposed to aflatoxin M_1 and ochratoxin A individually or collectively. *Toxins* **2018**, *10*, 13. [CrossRef]
62. Pandey, I.; Chauhan, S.S. Studies on production performance and toxin residues in tissues and eggs of layer chickens fed on diets with various concentrations of aflatoxin AFB_1. *Br. Poult. Sci.* **2007**, *48*, 713–723. [CrossRef] [PubMed]
63. Giambrone, J.J.; Ewert, D.L.; Wyatt, R.D.; Eidson, C.S. Effect of aflatoxin on the humoral and cell-mediated immune systems of the chicken. *Am. J. Vet. Res.* **1978**, *39*, 305–308. [PubMed]
64. Hoerr, F.J. Clinical aspects of immunosuppression in poultry. *Avian Dis.* **2010**, *54*, 2–15. [CrossRef] [PubMed]
65. Yunus, A.W.; Razzazi-Fazeli, E.; Bohm, J. Aflatoxin B_1 in affecting broiler's performance, immunity and gastrointestinal tract: A review of history and contemporary issues. *Toxins* **2011**, *3*, 566–590. [CrossRef] [PubMed]
66. Chang, C.F.; Hamilton, P.B. Impaired phagocytosis by heterophils from chickens during aflatoxicosis. *Toxicol. Appl. Pharmacol.* **1979**, *48*, 459–466. [CrossRef]
67. Chang, C.F.; Hamilton, P.B. Impairment of phagocytosis in chicken monocytes during aflatoxicosis. *Poult. Sci.* **1979**, *58*, 562–566. [CrossRef] [PubMed]
68. Ghosh, R.C.; Chauhan, H.V.; Jha, G.J. Suppression of cell-mediated immunity by purified aflatoxin B_1 in broiler chicks. *Vet. Immunol. Immunopathol.* **1991**, *28*, 165–172. [CrossRef]
69. Neldon-Ortiz, D.L.; Qureshi, M.A. Effects of AFB_1 embryonic exposure on chicken mononuclear phagocytic cell functions. *Dev. Comp. Immunol.* **1992**, *16*, 187–196. [CrossRef]
70. König, J.; Wells, J.; Cani, P.D.; García-Ródenas, C.L.; MacDonald, T.; Mercenier, A.; Whyte, J.; Troost, F.; Brummer, R.J. Human intestinal barrier function in health and disease. *Clin. Transl. Gastroenterol.* **2016**, *7*, e196. [CrossRef]
71. Liu, C.; Zuo, Z.; Zhu, P.; Zheng, Z.; Peng, X.; Cui, H.; Zhou, Y.; Ouyang, P.; Geng, Y.; Deng, J.; et al. Sodium selenite prevents suppression of mucosal humoral response by AFB_1 in broiler's cecal tonsil. *Oncotarget* **2017**, *8*, 54215–54226.
72. Jiang, M.; Fang, J.; Peng, X.; Cui, X.; Yu, Z. Effect of aflatoxin B_1 on IgA+ cell number and immunoglobulin mRNA expression in the intestine of broilers. *Immunopharmacol. Immunotoxicol.* **2015**, *37*, 450–457. [CrossRef] [PubMed]
73. Suzuki, T.; Yoshinaga, N.; Tanabe, S. Interleukin-6 (IL-6) regulates claudin-2 expression and tight junction permeability in intestinal epithelium. *J. Biol. Chem.* **2011**, *286*, 31263–31271. [CrossRef] [PubMed]
74. Kaji, I.; Karaki, S.; Kuwahara, A. Taste sensing in the colon. *Curr. Pharm. Des.* **2014**, *20*, 2766–2774. [CrossRef] [PubMed]
75. Kim, K.S.; Lee, I.S.; Kim, K.H.; Park, J.; Kim, Y.; Choi, J.H.; Choi, J.S.; Jang, H.J. Activation of intestinal olfactory receptor stimulates glucagon-like peptide-1 secretion in enteroendocrine cells and attenuates hyperglycemia in type 2 diabetic mice. *Sci. Rep.* **2017**, *7*, 13978. [CrossRef] [PubMed]
76. Priori, D.; Colombo, M.; Clavenzani, P.; Jansman, A.J.; Lallès, J.P.; Trevisi, P.; Bosi, P. The olfactory receptor OR51E1 is present along the gastrointestinal tract of pigs, co-localizes with enteroendocrine cells and is modulated by intestinal microbiota. *PLoS ONE* **2015**, *10*, e0129501. [CrossRef] [PubMed]
77. Havenstein, G.B.; Ferket, P.R.; Grimes, J.L.; Qureshi, M.A.; Nestor, K.E. Comparison of the performance of 1966- versus 2003-type turkeys when fed representative 1966 and 2003 turkey diets: Growth rate, livability and feed conversion. *Poult. Sci.* **2007**, *86*, 232–240. [CrossRef] [PubMed]
78. Swalander, M. Aspects of feed efficiency and feeding behaviour in turkeys. *Aviagen Turk. Manag.* **2015**, *4*, 9.
79. Untergasser, A.; Cutcutache, I.; Koressaar, T.; Ye, J.; Faircloth, B.C.; Remm, M.; Rozen, S.G. Primer3-new capabilities and interfaces. *Nucleic Acids Res.* **2012**, *40*, e115. [CrossRef]

80. Xie, F.; Xiao, P.; Chen, D.; Xu, L.; Zhang, B. miRDeepFinder: A miRNA analysis tool for deep sequencing of plant small RNAs. *Plant Mol. Biol.* **2012**, *80*, 75–84. [CrossRef]
81. Huang, D.W.; Sherman, B.T.; Lempicki, R.A. Systematic and integrative analysis of large gene lists using DAVID bioinformatics resources. *Nat. Protoc.* **2009**, *4*, 44–57. [CrossRef]
82. Mi, H.; Muruganujan, A.; Thomas, P.D. PANTHER in 2013: Modeling the evolution of gene function and other gene attributes, in the context of phylogenetic trees. *Nucleic Acids Res.* **2013**, *41*, D377–D386. [CrossRef] [PubMed]
83. Schmittgen, T.D.; Livak, K.J. Analyzing real-time PCR data by the comparative C(T) method. *Nat. Protoc.* **2008**, *3*, 1101–1108. [CrossRef] [PubMed]

toxins

MDPI

Article

Time-Dependent Changes in the Intestinal Microbiome of Gilts Exposed to Low Zearalenone Doses

Katarzyna Cieplińska [1], Magdalena Gajęcka [2,*], Michał Dąbrowski [2], Anna Rykaczewska [2], Sylwia Lisieska-Żołnierczyk [3], Maria Bulińska [4], Łukasz Zielonka [2] and Maciej T. Gajęcki [2]

1 Microbiology Laboratory, Non-Public Health Care Centre, Limanowskiego 31A, 10-342 Olsztyn, Poland; kasiacieplinska@gmail.com

2 Department of Veterinary Prevention and Feed Hygiene, Faculty of Veterinary Medicine, University of Warmia and Mazury in Olsztyn, Oczapowskiego 13, 10-718 Olsztyn, Poland; michal.dabrowski@uwm.edu.pl (M.D.); anna.rykaczewska@uwm.edu.pl (A.R.); lukasz.zielonka@uwm.edu.pl (Ł.Z.); gajecki@uwm.edu.pl (M.T.G.)

3 Independent Public Health Care Centre of the Ministry of the Interior and Administration, and the Warmia and Mazury Oncology Centre in Olsztyn, Wojska Polskiego 37, 10-228 Olsztyn, Poland; lisieska@wp.pl

4 Department of Discrete Mathematics and Theoretical Computer Science, Faculty of Mathematics and Computer Science, University of Warmia and Mazury in Olsztyn, Słoneczna 34, 10-710 Olsztyn, Poland; bulma@uwm.edu.pl

* Correspondence: mgaja@uwm.edu.pl; Tel.: +48-89-523-3773; fax: +48-89-523-3618

Received: 26 March 2019; Accepted: 22 May 2019; Published: 24 May 2019

Abstract: Zearalenone is a frequent contaminant of cereals and their by-products in regions with a temperate climate. This toxic molecule is produced naturally by *Fusarium* fungi in crops. The aim of this study was to determine the influence of low zearalenone doses (LOAEL, NOAEL and MABEL) on the intestinal microbiome of gilts on different days of exposure (days 7, 21 and 42). Intestinal contents were sampled from the duodenal cap, the third part of the duodenum, jejunum, caecum and the descending colon. The experiment was performed on 60 clinically healthy gilts with average BW of 14.5 ± 2 kg, divided into three experimental groups and a control group. Group ZEN5 animals were orally administered ZEN at 5 μg /kg BW, group ZEN10—10 μg ZEN/kg BW and group ZEN15—15 μg ZEN/kg BW. Five gilts from every group were euthanized on analytical dates 1, 2 and 3. Differences in the log values of microbial counts, mainly *Escherichia coli* and *Enterococcus faecalis*, were observed between the proximal and distal segments of the intestinal tract on different analytical dates as well as in the entire intestinal tract. Zearalenone affected the colony counts of intestinal microbiota rather than microbiome diversity, and its effect was greatest in groups ZEN10 and ZEN15. Microbial colony counts were similar in groups ZEN5 and C. In the analysed mycobiome, ZEN exerted a stimulatory effect on the log values of yeast and mould counts in all intestinal segments, in particular in the colon, and the greatest increase was noted on the first analytical date.

Keywords: zearalenone; doses; intestinal microbiome; intestinal mycobiome; pre-pubertal gilts

Key Contribution: The study demonstrated that MABEL doses stimulate the growth of selected intestinal microbiota in pre-pubertal gilts.

1. Introduction

Plant materials and their by-products are used in feed production, which increases the risk of mycotoxin (undesirable substance) poisoning in humans [1] and livestock, pigs in particular. Exposure to high doses of mycotoxins, including zearalenone (ZEN), has been well documented [2,3].

However, extensive research conducted in the last decade indicates that health problems resulting from exposure to small doses of the parental compound [4–6] without modified mycotoxins [7] can be equally important. The above is confirmed by the hormesis paradigm [7,8]. Doses below LOAEL values (lowest observed adverse effect level) [9–11] which induce pathological changes without clinical symptoms (sub-clinical states) are referred to as NOAEL doses (no observed adverse effect level) [12].

The minimal anticipated biological effect level (MABEL) dose enters into positive interactions with macroorganisms in different stages of their life cycle [13]. However, this observation contradicts the low-dose hypothesis, which plays an important role in relation to natural and hormonally active compounds [14] such as ZEN. In animals, the variations in the dose-response relationship induce differences in the interpretation of clinical symptoms and laboratory tests evaluating the risk of contamination with low doses of mycosteroids, such as ZEN, in plant materials [15]. In biomedical practice, an accurate determination of low mycotoxin doses in plant material would support a more reliable interpretation of the final effects [16].

Our findings indicate that the duodenum and the jejunum play the most important role in ZEN absorption [17,18]. The above can be attributed to the anatomical structure of the proximal segments of the small intestine, in particular differences in the quality and quantity of mucus glycoproteins. The discussed segments of the small intestine are characterized by very small quantities of strongly adhering mucus; therefore, digested nutrients have easy access to the intestinal wall [19]. Dietary sources of energy are also highly available in the proximal segments of the small intestine [20]. In animals exposed to mycotoxins, the energy derived from the diet promotes biotransformation processes that are essential for porcine health [13]. In the first week of exposure, a physiological deficiency of endogenous steroids inhibits biotransformation, and mycosteroids become deposited in intestinal tissues only in successive weeks [10,21,22].

Initially, ZEN is accumulated mainly in the duodenum. The above is observed until the end of the third week of exposure to the parental compound. In the fifth week of exposure, the accumulation of ZEN was highest in the descending colon [13].

The changes induced by exposure to low mycotoxin doses have been insufficiently investigated in the literature. In view of the hormesis paradigm, the variations in clinical symptoms or the absence of such symptoms lead to doubt in clinical evaluations. These doubts result not only from the dose, but also from the time of exposure [23]. There are three possible causes of the above. The first is the body's failure to recognise the threat [24], which is consistent with the T-regs theory [25]. The second is the compensatory effect, namely increased absorption to compensate for the physiological deficiency of endogenous steroids [26,27].

A review of the literature indicates that diet also influences the type and severity of physiological responses to ZEN in the porcine digesta. Diet and exposure to ZEN determine the specific composition of intestinal microbiome [28]. According to some researchers, due to its ecological complexity, the microbiome should be regarded as a "microbiological organ" which enters into dynamic interactions with the host and digesta [29] throughout the host's life. Intestinal microbiome stimulates the production of vitamins and cofactors, enhances digestion, eliminates feed toxins, creates an inner microbiological layer in the intestine that physically removes pathogens, produces natural antibiotics and fungicidal compounds, maintains intestinal barrier function and promotes the anti-inflammatory response [30]. Microbiome composition significantly affects gut health, nutrient utilization and bodily functions in pigs [31]. For this reason, the presence of ZEN in digesta can induce changes in ecological homeostasis and lead to dysbiosis in gut microbiota [4,32]. The above can promote local adhesion of pathogenic bacteria and the development of intestinal inflammations [33,34].

A well-balanced gut microbiome with a stable qualitative and quantitative composition is required for healthy bodily function in animals [23,35]. Intestinal bacteria stimulate the immune response and produce metabolites which are important for the host's well-being. Gut microflora facilitate nutrient absorption, deliver protective effects, stimulate the immune system, promote fermentation processes and prevent pathogen colonization. Intestinal bacteria are also used in the prevention and treatment of inflammatory bowel diseases (IBD) [36].

Despite those benefits, microorganisms can also exert negative effects on animals [37]. Pathogens produce toxic metabolites and faecal enzymes which can promote the generation of carcinogenic substances [38,39]. In the literature, the influence of gut bacteria has been analysed mainly in the context of intestinal microflora's ability to remove mycotoxins. The mechanisms by which ZEN can induce quantitative changes in bacterial microflora have not been fully elucidated [4,32,40,41].

The existing knowledge about the gut microbiome has been derived mainly from analyses of the isolated microorganisms and their phenotypic identification. Genotyping methods, including analyses of the highly conserved regions of the 16S rRNA gene, revealed that 20% to 60% of microorganisms (gut microbiome) cannot be cultured in vitro. Genotyping also demonstrated that the qualitative composition of the gut microbiome is far more complex and individually varied than initially believed. The gut microbiome is modified by age, environment, diet/feed type, genetic factors, animal welfare standards and the presence of undesirable substances. In human medicine, newly identified sequences of the 16S rRNA gene from various ecological niches were compared with known sequences to detect and identify (to the species level) microorganisms that cannot be cultured or are difficult to culture in vitro. However, the properties and functions of the bacteria identified in a given ecosystem are not always easy to determine. Genetic analyses are carried out to elucidate the potential roles of such microorganisms. Metagenomics (population genomics of environmental microorganisms) tools have been used to analyse the collective genome of gut microbiota based on DNA acquired directly from environmental samples [41,42]. In contemporary research, the aim of quantitative and qualitative analyses is not only to identify the sequences of the 16S rRNA gene, but also to identify the genes encoding specific traits and to generate comprehensive information about the gut microbiome. The most popular analytical techniques are denaturing gradient gel electrophoresis, real-time PCR, microarray analyses, cloning and sequencing, including pyrosequencing [29]. However, phenotypic identification of microbiota produces more comprehensive results that are easier to apply in clinical practice.

The aim of this study was to determine the effect (dose, variability of microbiota) of low doses of ZEN (MABEL, NOAEL and LOAEL) on microbial counts in the porcine gut on different days of exposure with the use of conventional analytical methods.

2. Results and Discussion

2.1. Experimental Feed

The analysed feed did not contain mycotoxins, or its mycotoxin content was below the sensitivity of the method (VBS). The concentrations of modified mycotoxins were not analysed [5,6].

2.2. Clinical Observations

Clinical signs of ZEN mycotoxicosis were not observed throughout the experiment. However, changes in specific tissues or cells were frequently noted in analyses of selected biochemical parameters in samples collected from the same animals and in those animals' growth performance. The results of these analyses were published in a different paper [5,6].

2.3. Evaluation of the Gut Microbiome

2.3.1. General Information

The evaluated microbiota was discussed in the following order: Enterobacteriaceae—Escherichia, Citrobacter, Salmonella, Yersinia and Klebsiella; Enterococcaceae—Enterococcus; Staphylococcaceae—Staphylococcus; Clostridiaceae—Clostridium; Incertae sedis—Candida; Nectriaceae—Fusarium.

Bacteria of the genera *Citrobacter*, *Salmonella*, *Klebsiella* and *Yersinia* were not identified in microbiological analyses on date D1.

Bacteria of the genera *Citrobacter* ad *Salmonella* were not detected on date D2. In group ZEN15, bacteria of the genus *Yersinia* were detected at 0.8 to 6.0 log CFU/g in the third part of the duodenum and the caecum, respectively. In group ZEN5, bacteria of the genus *Klebsiella* were identified in all evaluated intestinal segments at 0.4, 0.4, 3.4, 9.0 and 3.0 log CFU/g, respectively. *Klebsiella* pathogens were detected at 3.0 log CFU/g in the caecum in group ZEN10, and at 9.0 and 3.0 log CFU/g in the caecum and the descending colon, respectively, in group ZEN15.

Bacteria of the genera *Citrobacter*, *Salmonella* and *Yersinia* were not identified on date D3. *Klebsiella* pathogens colonised the third part of the duodenum at 3.0 log CFU/g in group ZEN10 and successive intestinal segments (6.0, 3.0, 6.0 and 6.0 log CFU/g), excluding the descending colon, in group ZEN15.

The overgrowth of the small intestinal microbiome, including changes in microbial counts and/or microbial types, was not observed. In the proximal segment of the small intestine, the counts of non-pathogenic bacterial strains exceeded 105 log CFU due to colonisation by bacterial strains that are ubiquitous in the colon. Only the results where significant differences were noted are presented in the figures.

Significant differences were not observed in the presented results.

2.3.2. Microbiome Analysis in Different Intestinal Segments (Dose Effect)

This subsection analyses the effects of the applied ZEN doses on quantitative changes in microbiota in different groups on different analytical dates, in the same segment of intestinal tract.

Duodenal Cap

The duodenal cap is the proximal segment of the duodenum which ends in the major duodenal papilla [43]. This segment has a specific anatomical structure, and in some respects, it resembles the stomach more than the intestine [44]. The duodenal cap receives blood from two different sources. In pre-pubertal gilts, the muscular layer is not yet fully developed, which can lead to the retention of digesta. The local microbiome is not highly diverse due to gastric acid secretions. In the experiment, the counts of *Enterococcus faecalis* were fairly stable at up to 18 log CFU/g throughout the experiment (see Figure 1A). However, considerable differences were observed between groups (5 to 18 log CFU/g) on selected dates.

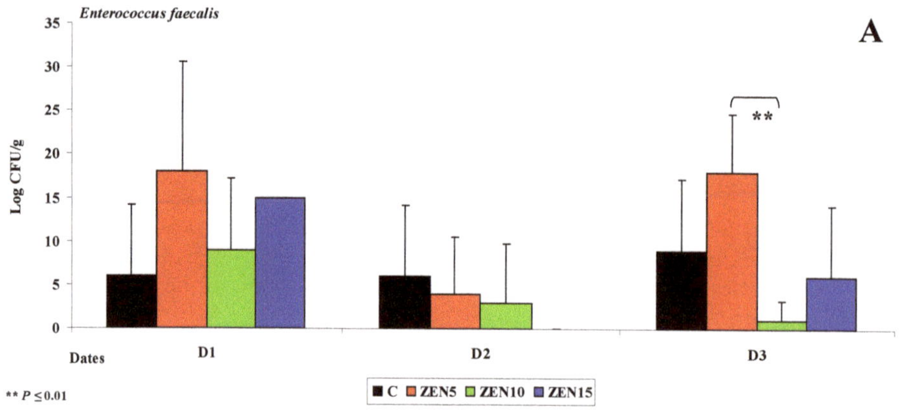

Figure 1. *Cont.*

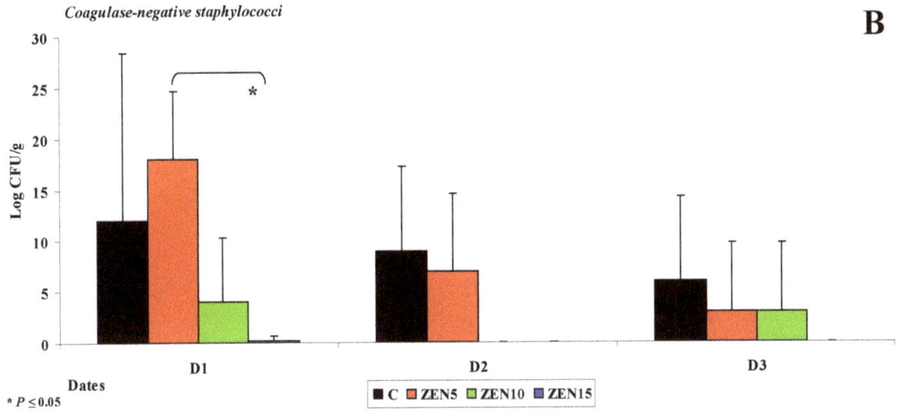

Figure 1. The dose effect of ZEN on functional diversity in the microbiome in the duodenal cap: (**A**,**B**) arithmetic means ($\overline{x}$) and standard deviation (SD) in five samples collected on each analytical date (D1, D2 and D3) in the evaluated groups (C, ZEN5, ZEN10 and ZEN15); Statistically significant differences: * at $p \leq 0.05$ and ** $p \leq 0.01$.

Variations were also noted in the counts of coagulase-negative *Staphylococci* (see Figure 1B). The highest microbial counts (log CFU/g) on selected analytical dates were found in group ZEN5. *Enterococcus faecalis* are ubiquitous in the gastrointestinal tract, and they maintain intestinal homeostasis [31], excluding selected pathogenic strains which are classified based on their virulence [45]. These strains are conditional pathogens [46]. In this experiment, bacterial counts were inversely proportional to ZEN dose (see Figure 1). Coagulase-negative *Staphylococci* occupy an ecological niche in animal farms, and their pathogenic effects have not yet been fully investigated [47]. These opportunistic bacteria participate in endogenous infections [48].

Third Part of the Duodenum

A significant decrease in the counts (log CFU/g) of *Escherichia coli* (see Figure 2A), *Enterococcus faecalis* (see Figure 2B) and coagulase-negative *Staphylococci* (see Figure 2C) was noted in groups ZEN10 and ZEN15 on all analytical dates relative to group C. The differences in the counts of coagulase-negative *Staphylococci* were highly significant on date D1. An analysis of differences in bacterial counts (log CFU/g) between analytical dates revealed the greatest variations in group ZEN5 in the mean counts of *Enterococcus faecalis* and coagulase-negative *Staphylococci* (3 to 16 CFU/g and 15 to 19 log CFU/g, respectively; see Figure 3C,D) on date D1 in the mean counts of *Escherichia coli* (26 to 43 log CFU/g; see Figure 2B) on date D3.

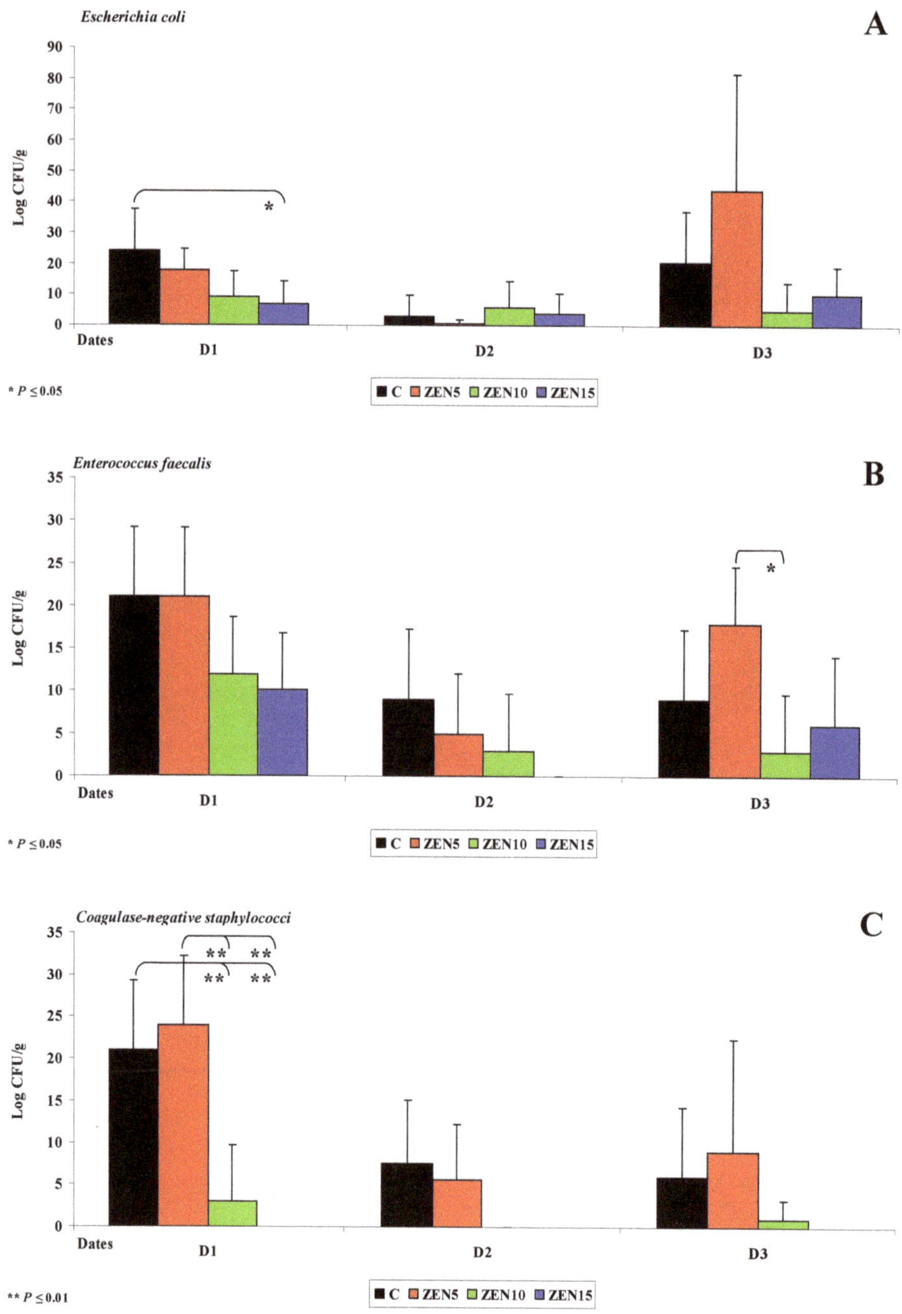

Figure 2. The dose effect of ZEN on functional diversity in the microbiome in the third part of duodenum: (**A–C**) Arithmetic means ($\overline{x}$) and standard deviation (SD) in five samples collected on each analytical date (D1, D2 and D3) in the evaluated groups (C, ZEN5, ZEN10 and ZEN15). Statistically significant differences: * at $p \leq 0.05$ and ** $p \leq 0.01$.

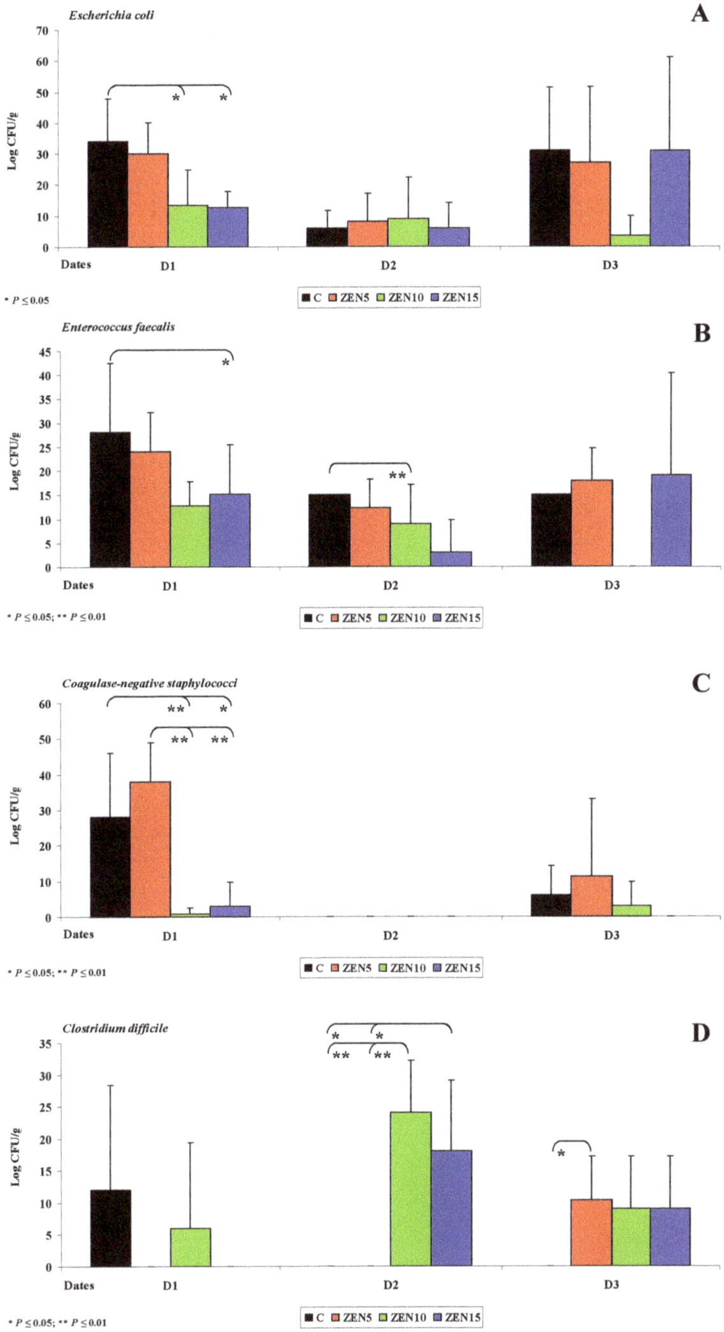

Figure 3. The dose effect of ZEN on functional diversity in the jejunal microbiome: (**A–D**) arithmetic means ($\bar{x}$) and standard deviation (SD) in five samples collected on each analytical date (D1, D2 and D3) in the evaluated groups (C, ZEN5, ZEN10 and ZEN15). Statistically significant differences: * at $p \leq 0.05$ and ** $p \leq 0.01$.

In group C, the average counts of coagulase-negative *Staphylococci* (15 and 13 log CFU/g) on date D1 also differed most significantly (by 15 and 13 log CFU/g) relative to the remaining analytical dates. Highly similar results were reported in a study where antibiotics were used as growth promoters in pigs [49]. Sub-therapeutic doses of antibiotics induced similar changes in the intestinal ecosystem [30] to the NOAEL doses of ZEN (group ZEN10) in this experiment. In turn, MABEL doses (group ZEN5) increased the counts of saprophytic bacteria which inhibited the adhesion of pathogenic cells to the intestinal epithelium. Therefore, a question arises whether low doses of ZEN can induce eubiotic effects [50].

On date D2, bacterial counts (log CFU/g) in the duodenum decreased relative to dates D1 and D3. The average differences in the abundance of *Enterococcus faecalis* ranged from 15 to 18 log CFU/g in group ZEN5 in the duodenal cap (see Figure 1A,B) and the third part of the duodenum (*Escherichia coli* was not identified in the duodenum in group ZEN15 on date D2). The average difference in *Escherichia coli* counts was estimated at 44 log CFU/g in group ZEN5 (see Figure 2A). The above observations validate our previous findings [4] as well as the results presented by Gajęcka et al. [10] which indicate that ZEN has bacteriostatic or even bactericidal effects [49].

Jejunum

Similar results were noted in the jejunum. On date D2 (see Figure 3A), *Escherichia coli* counts (log CFU/g) decreased in all groups, and significant differences were observed only between dates in group C. The decrease in *Escherichia coli* counts was directly proportional to the increase in ZEN dose (from 34 and 30 log CFU/g to 13 and 12 log CFU/g, respectively), and significant differences were observed between group C vs. groups ZEN10 and ZEN 15 (see Figure 3A).

Differences were also observed in the counts (log CFU/g) of *Enterococcus faecalis* (Figure 3B) and coagulase-negative *Staphylococci* (see Figure 3C). Coagulase-negative *Staphylococci* were not detected on date D2 (see Figure 3C). Considerable functional variations were noted in *Clostridium difficile* (see Figure 3D) on all dates and in all groups. These findings suggest that ZEN decreases the counts of mesophilic aerobes [49], *Clostridium difficile* (obligate anaerobes), *Escherichia coli* and other bacteria of the family *Staphyococaceae* during and after 42 days of exposure. The above could indicate that prolonged exposure to LOAEL (group ZEN15) or NOAEL (group ZEN10) doses eliminates bacteria or significantly decreases their counts. Similar results were reported by Piotrowska et al. [4] where the mycotoxin dose was 40 ug/kg BW. Bacterial abundance (log CFU/g) was maintained at a higher level only under exposure to the MABEL dose (group ZEN5). The above could suggest that high doses of ZEN exert bacteriostatic or bactericidal effects [49], whereas the lowest dose of ZEN has stimulating properties [10]. Similar results were observed in a study evaluating the genotoxicity of caecal water in the same gilts [5] where genotoxic processes of various intensity were noted in groups ZEN10 and ZEN15. Genotoxicity was not reported in group ZEN5. It should be noted, however, that ZEN is absorbed mainly in the duodenum (65%) [51]. In hypoestrogenic gilts, ZEN is directly used in steroidogenesis or is converted to α-zearalenol [10]. The resulting modified mycotoxin [7,51] is more toxic and/or more metabolically active [6], depending on the dose of the parental compound.

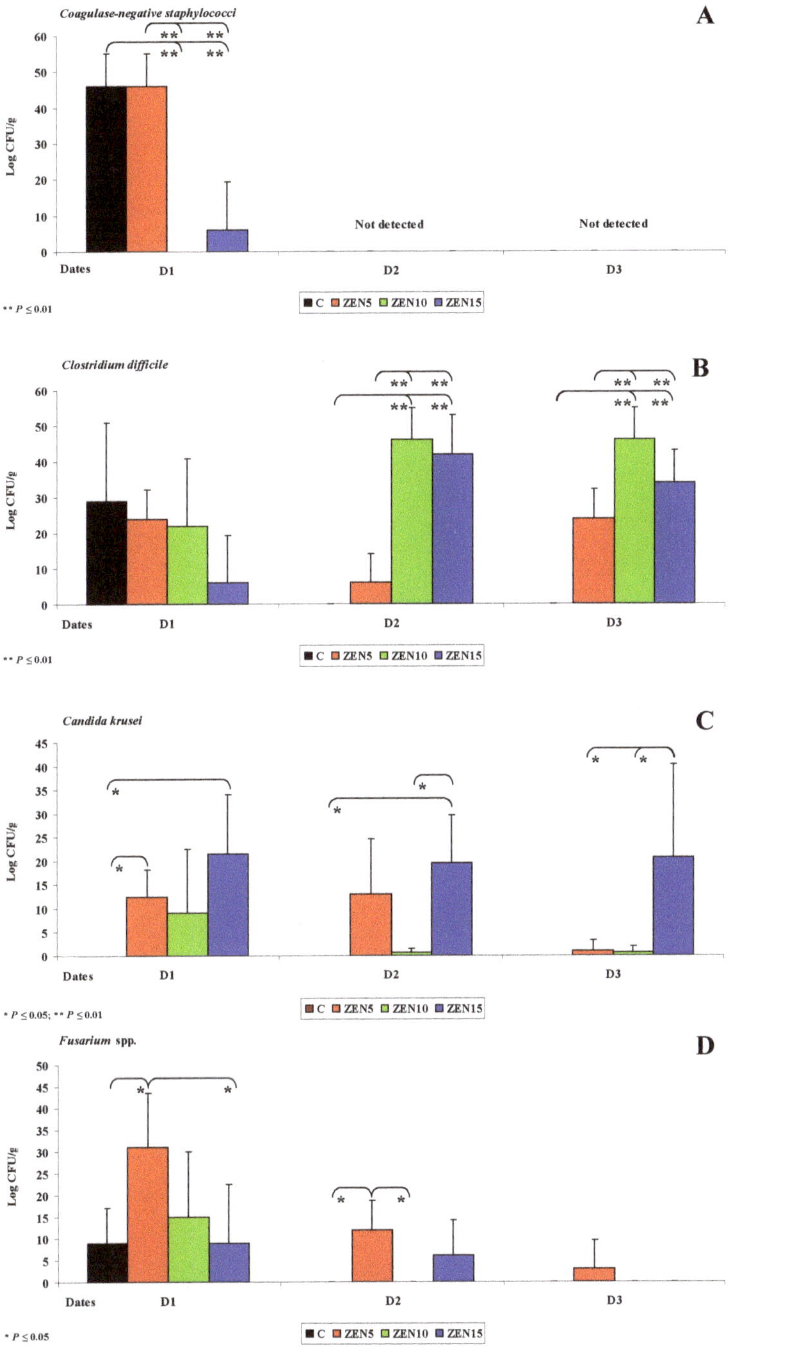

Figure 4. The dose effect of ZEN on functional diversity in the caecal microbiome: (**A–D**) arithmetic means ($\overline{x}$) and standard deviation (SD) in five samples collected on each analytical date (D1, D2 and D3) in the evaluated groups (C, ZEN5, ZEN10 and ZEN15). Statistically significant differences: * at $p \leq 0.05$ and ** $p \leq 0.01$.

Caecum

The following sampled segment of the intestinal tract was the caecum. In pre-pubertal gilts, the caecum is not yet fully developed, and intestinal dysfunctions often originate in this segment of the digestive system [29]. Resistant starch (RS) is not degraded by digestive enzymes in proximal segments of the intestinal tract, and it can be fermented by residual microbiota in the colon [30]. *Enterobacteria* and other bacterial species decompose RS into short-chain fatty acids (SCFAs) which promote the proliferation of caecal cells, increase the expression of genes that participate in intestinal development and acidify the local ecosystem [52]. An acidic environment inhibits the growth of pathogenic microbiota and selectively promotes the growth of selected beneficial microorganisms. Therefore, RS contributes to intestinal health by modifying and stabilizing the populations of intestinal microorganisms and boosting immunity [53]. At the same time, exposure to ZEN inhibits the production of SCFAs [49]. These observations explain the absence of bacteria of the genera *Citrobacter*, *Salmonella*, *Klebsiella* and *Yersinia* and selected coagulase-negative *Staphylococci* on dates D1-D3 (see Figure 4A). In turn, *Escherichia coli* and *Enterococcus faecalis* play a less important role in the fermentation process, which is why their counts (log CFU/g) were similar in the experimental groups and in group C in all intestinal segments [54].

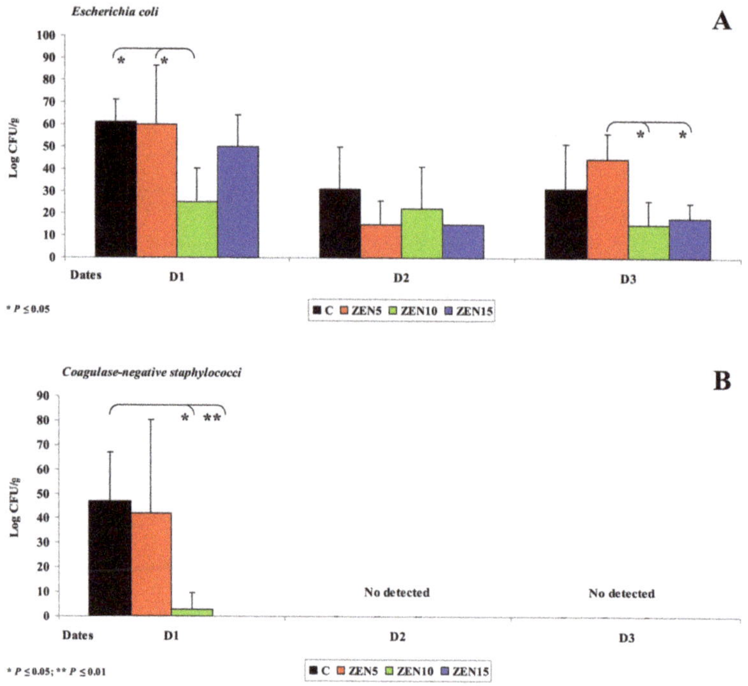

Figure 5. *Cont.*

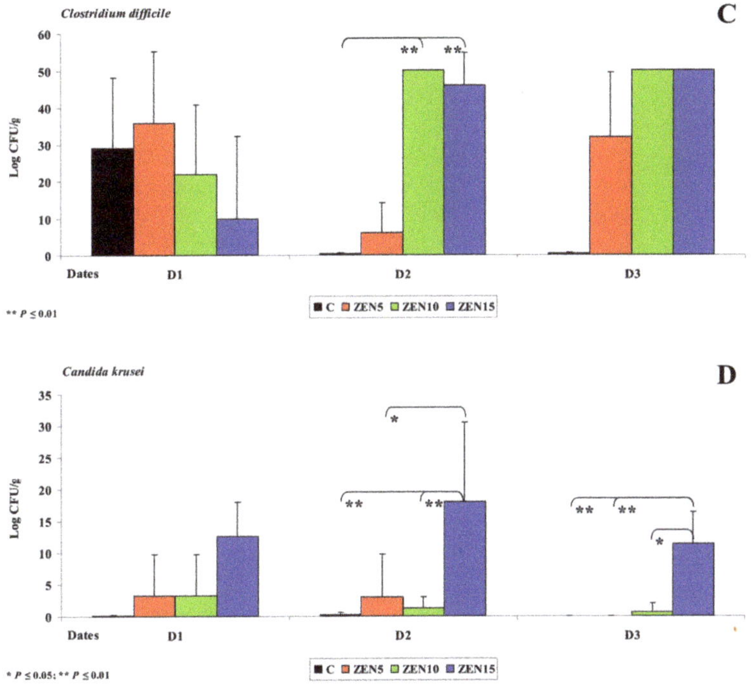

Figure 5. The dose effect of ZEN on functional diversity in the descending colon microbiome: (**A–D**) arithmetic means ($\overline{x}$) and standard deviation (SD) in five samples collected on each analytical date (D1, D2 and D3) in the evaluated groups (C, ZEN5, ZEN10 and ZEN15). Statistically significant differences: * at $p \leq 0.05$ and ** $p \leq 0.01$.

An analysis of Figure 4A,B indicates that bacterial counts (log CFU/g) in the caecum were lower in the experimental groups than in group C on day D1 (see Figure 4A,B). Coagulase-negative *Staphylococci* were not detected on successive sampling dates (D2 and D3) (see Figure 4A), which could be attributed to ongoing fermentation processes in the caecum [31] and exposure to ZEN. The observed processes create a closed-loop system: ZEN decreases microbial counts, which inhibits SCFA synthesis and, consequently, leads to dysbiosis in the caecum [5,55].

On date D1, the counts (log CFU/g) of coagulase-negative *Staphylococci* and *Clostridium difficile* were higher in group ZEN5 than in groups ZEN10, ZEN15 and C, but the observed differences were not statistically significant (see Figure 4A,B). Coagulase-negative *Staphylococci* (see Figure 4A) were not detected on dates D2 and D3 (see Figure 7A,B). This is a desirable situation from the perspective of animal health, but it should be noted that these pathogens are frequently undetected in laboratory analyses [56,57]. The population of *Clostridium difficile* (see Figure 4B) increased proportionally with a rise in ZEN dose. These observations suggest that LOAEL and NOAEL doses of ZEN contribute to subclinical pathological states, in particular those caused by opportunistic strains such as *Clostridium difficile* [58]. This bacterial strain is responsible for intestinal inflammations [59] in piglets and grower-finishing pigs and causes substantial losses in commercial farms [60,61].

Descending Colon

The descending colon was the last analysed segment of the intestinal tract. The presented values of $\overline{x}$ and SD indicate that the counts (log CFU/g) of *Escherichia coli* (see Figure 5A) and coagulase-negative *Staphylococci* (see Figure 5B) decreased over time. The results are nearly identical to those noted in the caecum. Significant differences ($p \leq 0.05$) in *Escherichia coli* counts (log CFU/g) were observed between group ZEN5 and group ZEN10 and between group C and group ZEN10 on date D1, and between group ZEN5 and groups ZEN10 and ZEN15 on date D3 (35, 36, 29.6 and 26.6 log CFU/g, respectively). *Staphylococcaceae* counts differed between group C and group ZEN10 (44 log CFU/g) and between group C and group ZEN15 (47 log CFU/g) on date D1, and similarly to the caecum, *Staphylococcaceae* were not detected on dates D2 and D3. However, ZEN exerted powerful antimicrobial effects on date D1 (see Figure 5B). The decrease in microbial counts (log CFU/g) indirectly suggests that ZEN does not promote the proliferation of *Staphylococcus* bacteria [47]. It appears that ZEN's biological effects on digesta were similar to those observed in the caecum in at least two aspects.

Microbiological fermentation of RS [31] leads to the production of SCFAs, cell proliferation, acidification and other beneficial changes [53]. In hypoestrogenic gilts, the bacteriostatic effects of ZEN in distal intestinal segments were manifested on successive analytical dates because ZEN biotransformation occurs in the proximal segments of the gastrointestinal tract [13]. Similarly to the caecum, a closed-loop system was created where ZEN decreased microbial counts, which inhibited SCFA synthesis and, consequently, led to dysbiosis in the descending colon [23,57]. However, the absence of clinical symptoms indicates that eubiosis was not significantly compromised.

The counts of *Clostridium difficile* in the descending colon were also highly similar to those noted in the caecum. Significant differences ($p \leq 0.01$) were observed only on date D2 between group C and groups ZEN10 and ZEN15 (difference 49.5 and 45.5 log CFU/g, respectively) (see Figure 5C). These findings confirm that the growth of *Clostridium difficile* is stimulated proportionally to the applied ZEN dose. According to recent research [61], this opportunistic strain can lead to intestinal inflammations in piglets and grower-finishing pigs and generate substantial losses in commercial farms [60]. Low doses of ZEN could inhibit *m*RNA expression of both nitric oxide synthases, which decreases nitric oxide levels and suppresses inflammatory processes in the digestive tract, in particular the colon. These processes can contribute to the growth of selected gut bacteria [62]. Therefore, exposure to ZEN stimulates intestinal barrier function, enhances nutrient and protein synthesis, and improves the utilization of energy from substrates that are difficult to degrade (RS), while minimizing the harmful consequences of inflammations and subclinical pathological states [33].

Microbial activity was intensified on date D1 relative to the remaining analytical dates, which could be attributed to the fact that the biological (toxic) effects of ZEN are most pronounced in the first seven days of exposure [13]. Functional variations in the gut microbiome indicate that the intestinal system begins to tolerate ZEN on successive days of exposure [10].

2.3.3. Mycobiome Analysis in Different Intestinal Segments

This is the first study to demonstrate significant differences in yeast and mould counts in the caecum (see Figure 4C,D). Proximal segments of the intestinal tract were also characterised by variations in the counts of mycobiome components, but the noted differences were not statistically significant and were observed only in the experimental groups. In the caecum, *Candida krusei* counts differed significantly on all analytical dates. Yeasts were not detected in group C, which could suggest that ZEN stimulates the growth of yeasts in the digesta. Yeasts were determined on all analytical dates only in group ZEN15 (19.4 to 21.4 log CFU/g) (see Figure 4C). Yeast counts tended to decrease in the remaining experimental groups. In the descending colon, *Candida krusei* counts were very low in group C (see Figure 5D), and this yeast species was not detected on date D3 (average counts were determined at 0.1, 0.2 and 0.0 log CFU/g on successive dates). The abundance of *Candida krusei* was also low in groups ZEN5 and ZEN10. In group ZEN15, *Candida krusei* counts were relatively high on successive dates (12.6, 18.0 and 11.4 log CFU/g, respectively). Significant differences were observed only between dates D2 and D3 in group ZEN15.

Interestingly, only *Fusarium* spp. was detected in the caecum in group C on date D1 (see Figure 4D). Significant differences ($p \leq 0.05$ and $p \leq 0.01$) were observed between group C vs. groups ZEN5 and ZEN15 on date D1.

These results imply that both opportunistic mycobiota can cause intestinal mucosa infections, but unlike in other bodily tissues and systems, the difference between fungal overgrowth and fungal infection is difficult to capture [63,64].

2.3.4. Changes in Microbiome and Mycobiome under Exposure to ZEN (Variability of Microbiota)

This subsection analyses quantitative changes in all groups on a given analytical date, in all segments of intestinal tract.

Under exposure to ZEN, significant differences in the counts of five out of the six analysed microbiota were observed on date D1 (see Figure 6). The variations in the abundance of *Escherichia coli* (see Figure 6A) and *Enterococcus faecalis* (see Figure 6B) were similar in all groups during the experiment.

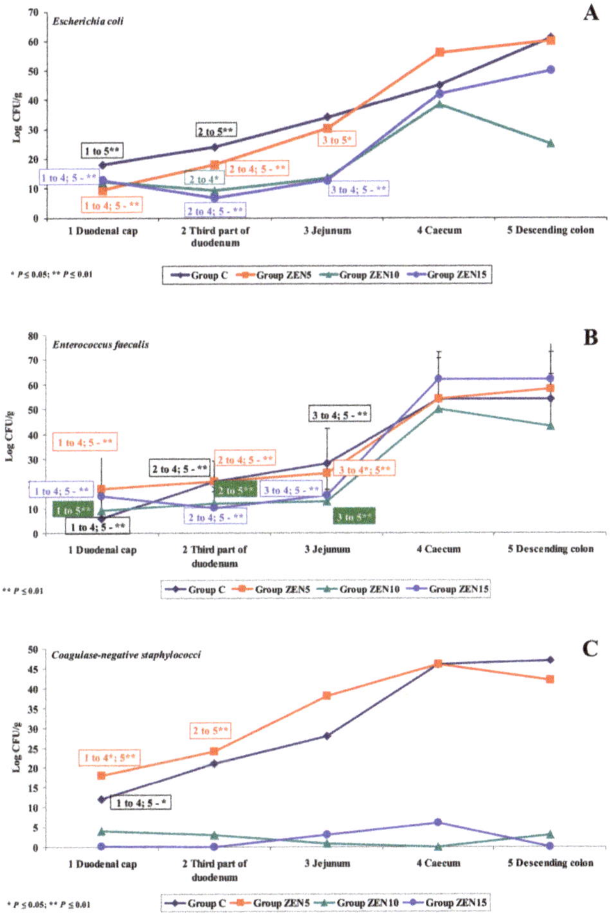

Figure 6. *Cont.*

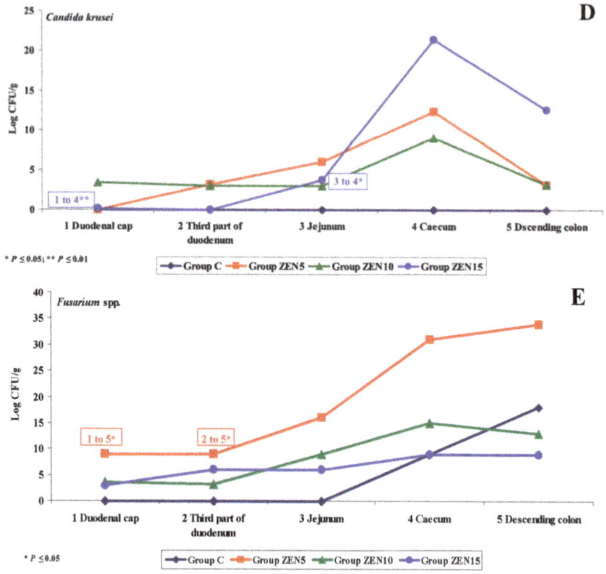

Figure 6. Variability of microbiota. Variations in the counts of selected microbiota and mycobiota under exposure to ZEN on the first analytical date (D1): (**A–E**) arithmetic means ($\overline{x}$) in five samples of selected bacterial strains (Groups C, ZEN5, ZEN10 and ZEN15). Statistically significant differences: * at $p \leq 0.05$ and ** $p \leq 0.01$.

The counts of *Escherichia coli* and *Enterococcus faecalis* (log CFU/g) were low in the first three segments of the intestine. In the caecum and the descending colon, the respective values were two or three times higher, and the differences were statistically significant ($p \leq 0.05$ and $p \leq 0.01$). The above findings suggest that ZEN has no effect on *Escherichia coli* or *Enterococcus faecalis*. The dysbiosis index suggests that the biological activity of *Escherichia coli* decreased in the experimental groups relative to group C, but a gradual increase in activity was noted in distal segments of the intestine. According to Youssef and Kamphues [55], *Escherichia coli* counts decrease in response to enhanced fermentation processes and increasing acidification of intestinal digesta. In contrast, the dysbiosis index of *Enterococcus faecalis* was equal to (eubiosis) or higher than 1.0 (dysbiosis) in nearly all intestinal segments (excluding the jejunum) in group ZEN5. The value of the dysbiosis index reached 3.0 in the duodenal cap. These results indicate that ZEN creates a supportive environment for the proliferation of *Enterococcus faecalis* in the first, fourth and fifth segment of the intestine with low pH values [23].

Similar observations were made in metabolomic research [6] which demonstrated that ZEN's initial stimulatory effect in gilts is neutralised over time by compensatory or adaptive mechanisms, which leads to considerable energy and protein loss in the metabolome. These findings can be used to formulate two hypotheses: (i) feed conversion is more effective, and it contributes to detoxification processes (biotransformation), and (ii) body weight gains increase even under exposure to a MABEL dose. These hypotheses suggest that exposure to low ZEN doses leads to the initiation of compensatory and/or adaptive mechanisms. However, these processes require substantial amounts of energy [55], and they are significantly influenced by the gut microbiome [23].

Similar variations in the counts of coagulase-negative *Staphylococci* were noted in groups C and ZEN5 (see Figure 6C). Significant differences were found between the analysed segments of the duodenum, caecum and the descending colon. In the remaining groups, bacterial counts (log CFU/g) were very low in all intestinal segments, and significant differences were not observed. Interestingly, the values of the dysbiosis index reached 1.0 (eubiosis) in group ZEN5, and were significantly higher than 1.0 in the first three intestinal segments. These findings could suggest that unlike the remaining doses, the MABEL dose stimulates the evaluated bacteria.

On date D1, *Candida krusei* was not detected in any intestinal segments in group C or in the first two segments in group ZEN15. For this reason, the dysbiosis index could not be calculated. On the remaining analytical dates, bacterial counts were higher in the experimental groups by up to 24 log CFU/g, in particular in two distal sampling sites. The above could indicate that ZEN stimulates the proliferation of yeasts in the colon, which may pose health risks to the host. Exposure to ZEN is probably negatively correlated with a diet rich in amino acids, fatty acids and proteins [64]. *Fusarium* spp. counts were also low (see Figure 6E), but in group C, moulds were detected only in the last two intestinal segments. In those segments, the dysbiosis index in group ZEN5 exceeded 3.0, which is indicative of dysbiosis and points to a strong synergistic interaction between ZEN and *Fusarium* spp. in the caecum and a somewhat weaker response in the descending colon.

On date D2, weaker interactions were noted between ZEN and *Escherichia coli* (see Figure 7A) and *Enterococcus faecalis* (see Figure 7B). In the caecum and descending colon, the respective bacterial counts decreased from 60 and 65 log CFU/g to 40 and 45 log CFU/g. Significant differences were also observed between the first three and the last two intestinal segments. The dysbiosis index of *Escherichia coli* in the duodenum increased by 1.0, in particular in groups C/ZEN10 and C/ZEN15. The said increase is indicative of a decrease in pH, which can occur in the initial stages of carbohydrate fermentation [53]. The dysbiosis index of *Enterococcus faecalis* decreased from more than 1.0 on date D1 to below 1.0 on date D2. On date D2, *Clostridium difficile* (see Figure 7C): (i) was not detected in group C; (ii) was detected in the colon at 6 log CFU/g in group ZEN5 and at 42-50 CFU/g in groups ZEN10 and ZEN15. The noted differences were statistically significant, but the dysbiosis index could not be determined in group C. However, it could be hypothesised that LOAEL/NOAEL doses are capable of stimulating the proliferation of *Clostridium difficile* and could exert opposite effects than those suggested in other studies where the examined ZEN doses were several times higher [65]. Our findings indicate that low ZEN doses, in particular NOAEL and smaller doses, exert antibiotic-like effects [29,31]. The above is consistent with the low dose hypothesis [10], whereby high ZEN doses exert toxic effects, whereas low doses can stimulate the development of the macroorganism as well as organisms that do not recognise its presence [66]. *Fusarium* spp. was not detected in group C (see Figure 7D), and the relevant dysbiosis index could not be calculated. In groups ZEN5 and ZEN15, mould counts increased from 0 to 12 log CFU/g (synergistic interaction) with the passage of digesta into more distal intestinal segments. In group ZEN10, *Fusarium* spp. was identified only in the jejunum at 6 log CFU/g.

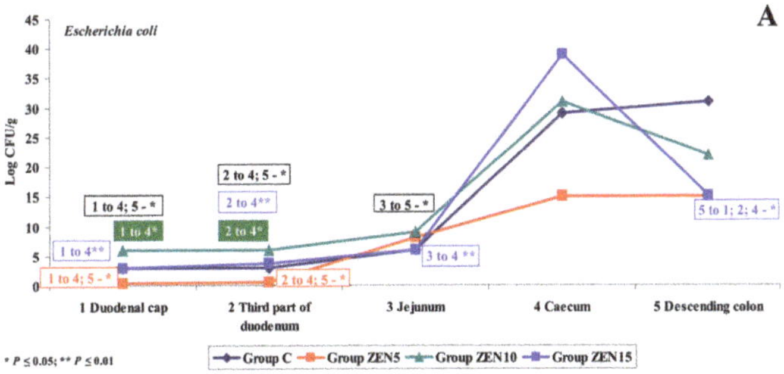

Figure 7. *Cont.*

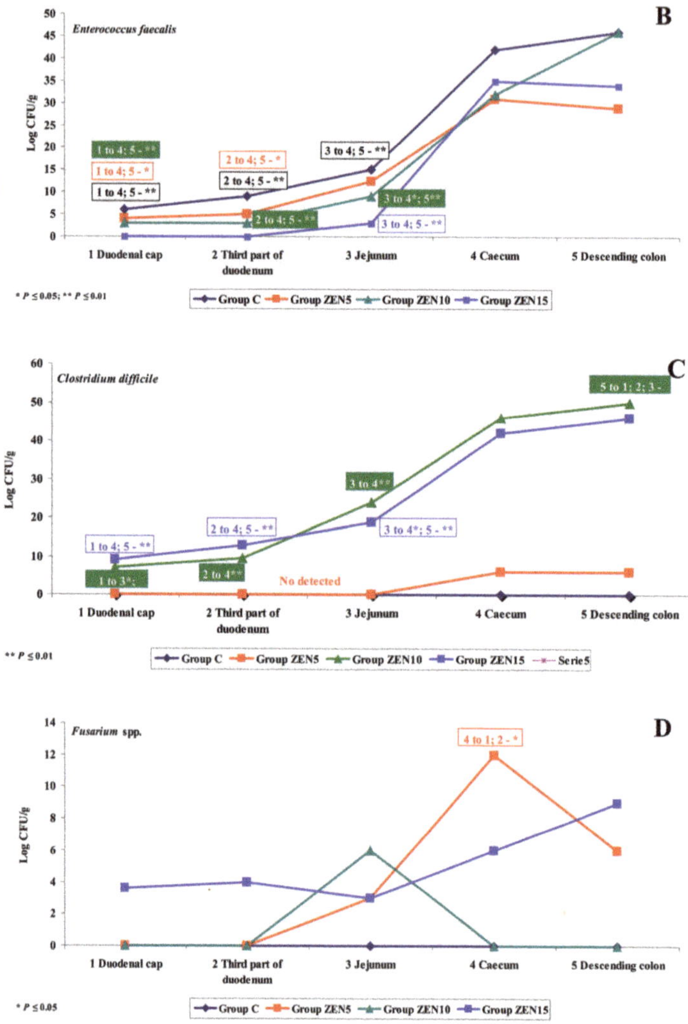

Figure 7. Variability of microbiota. The effect of ZEN on functional diversity in selected microbiota and mycobiota on analytical date D2: (**A–D**) arithmetic means ($\bar{x}$) in five samples of selected bacterial strains on (Groups C, ZEN5, ZEN10 and ZEN15). Statistically significant differences: * at $p \leq 0.05$ and ** $p \leq 0.01$.

On date D3, significant functional variations in the microbiome were noted only in *Escherichia coli* (see Figure 8A), *Enterococcus faecalis* (see Figure 8B) and *Clostridium difficile* (see Figure 8C). The microbiome was stabilised relative to dates D1 and D2. *Escherichia coli* counts decreased by approximately 10 log CFU/g on date D2 and were maintained at a similar level on date D3 (see Figure 8A). A different pattern of functional variations was noted in group ZEN5 where microbial counts in the duodenal cap were nearly 40 log CFU/g higher relative to other groups and dates. In the remaining tissues and groups, functional variations were similar to the previous dates, and microbial counts (CFU/g) increased considerably in the caecum and descending colon. Considerable differences were also observed in the values of the dysbiosis index which increased to 2.0 or even 2.5 in group ZEN5 and decreased to 1.0 or less in group ZEN10. Similar results were noted in group ZEN 15, and the highest value of the dysbiosis index (1.5) was noted in the caecum. The functional variations in *Enterococcus faecalis* (see Figure 8B) were nearly identical to those noted on date D2 and similar to those observed in group C. Functional differences were noted between the small intestine and the colon, which can probably be attributed to a local increase in bacterial fermentation [52]. In group ZEN5, the dysbiosis index in the duodenum increased considerably (to 0.65 on date D2 and 2.0 on date D3) relative to group ZEN10 and, partly, in group ZEN15 where similar values (below 1.0) were noted in the colon on date D2. On date D3, the presence of *Clostridium difficile* (see Figure 8C) was observed already in the duodenal cap, whereas on date D2, the caecum was the first intestinal segment colonised by the above microbiota. *Clostridium difficile* was not detected in group C, and its dysbiosis index could not be calculated. These findings suggest that ZEN could promote the development of this bacterial group [31].

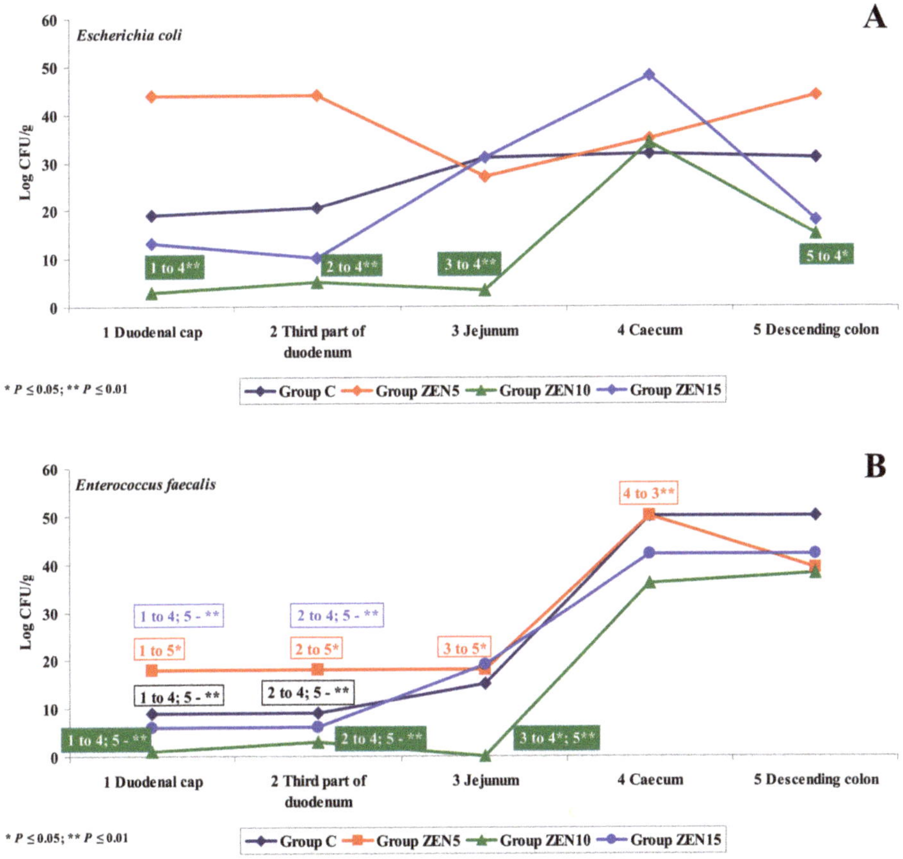

Figure 8. *Cont.*

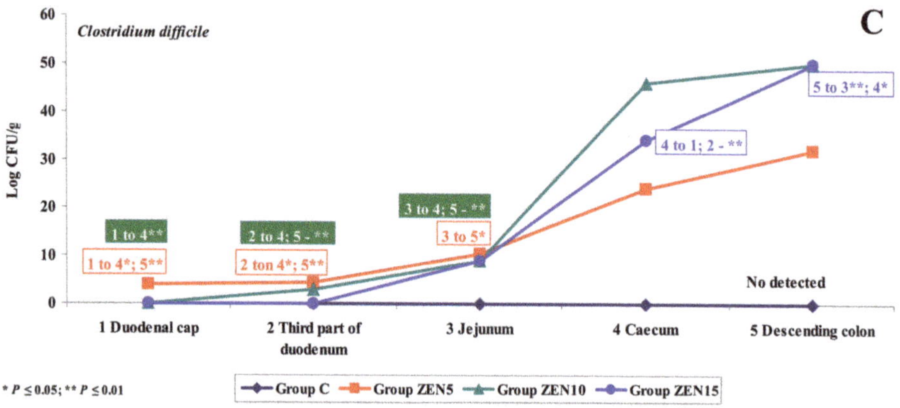

Figure 8. Variability of microbiota. The effect of ZEN on functional diversity in the microbiome on analytical date D3: (**A–C**) arithmetic means ($\bar{x}$) in five samples of selected bacterial strains (Groups C, ZEN5, ZEN10 and ZEN15). Statistically significant differences: * at $p \leq 0.05$ and ** $p \leq 0.01$.

2.3.5. Summary

The following observations were made in the intestinal tract of animals exposed to low doses of ZEN in feed:

(i) Differences in the dose effect) and variability of microbiota (differences in microbial counts, log CFU/g), mainly in *Escherichia coli* and *Enterococcus faecalis*, were noted between the proximal (microbial counts were lowest in the duodenum) and the distal (microbial counts were highest in the colon) segments of the intestinal tract;

(ii) The smallest differences in microbial counts (log CFU/g) were observed in group ZEN5, in particular in proximal intestinal segments (values of the dysbiosis index);

(iii) The counts of coagulase-negative *Staphylococci* decreased significantly over time in the evaluated intestinal segments, and these microbiotas were not detected in the colon;

(iv) In analyses of the variability of microbiota, *Clostridium difficile* colonies were not identified in group C, but they were detected already in the jejunum and in more distal segments of the intestines in the experimental groups, and microbial counts increased rapidly with an increase in ZEN dose on successive analytical dates (the lowest increase was noted in group ZEN5);

(v) ZEN affected the colony counts of intestinal microbiota rather than microbiome diversity, and its effect was greatest in groups ZEN10 and ZEN15. Microbial colony counts were similar in groups ZEN5 and C.

In the analysed mycobiome, ZEN exerted a stimulatory effect on the log values of yeast and mould counts in all intestinal segments, in particular in the colon, and the greatest increase was noted on the first analytical date. Yeast and mould colonies were not detected in group C, excluding on date D1 when they were detected from the jejunum to the descending colon.

The results of this study and our previous findings suggest that the MABEL dose could exert preventive and stimulatory effects on pre-pubertal gilts.

3. Materials and Methods

3.1. In Vivo Study

3.1.1. General Information

All experimental procedures involving animals were carried out in compliance with Polish regulations setting forth the terms and conditions of animal experimentation (Opinions No. 12/2016 and 45/2016/DLZ of the Local Ethics Committee for Animal Experimentation of 27 April 2016 and 30 November 2016) [5,6].

3.1.2. Experimental Animals and Feed

The in vivo experiment was performed at the Department of Veterinary Prevention and Feed Hygiene of the Faculty of Veterinary Medicine at the University of Warmia and Mazury in Olsztyn on 60 clinically healthy pre-pubertal gilts (grower-finisher crossbred pigs) with initial BW (body weight) of 14.5 ± 2 kg. The animals were housed in pens with free access to water. All groups of gilts received the same feed throughout the experiment. They were randomly assigned to three experimental groups (group ZEN5, group ZEN10 and group ZEN15; n = 15) and a control group (group C; n = 15) [5,6,67,68]. Group ZEN5 gilts were orally administered ZEN (Sigma-Aldrich Z2125-26MG, Saint Louis, MO, USA) at 5 µg ZEN/kg BW, group ZEN10 pigs—10 µg ZEN/kg BW, and group ZEN15 pigs—15 µg ZEN/kg BW. Analytical samples of ZEN were dissolved in 96 µL of 96% ethanol (SWW 2442-90, Polskie Odczynniki SA, Poland) in weight-appropriate doses. Feed containing different doses of ZEN in an alcohol solution was placed in gel capsules. The capsules were stored at room temperature before administration in order to evaporate the alcohol. In the experimental groups, ZEN was administered daily in gel capsules before morning feeding. The animals were weighed at weekly intervals, and the results were used to adjust individual mycotoxin doses. Feed was the carrier, and group C pigs were administered the same gel capsules, but without mycotoxins [5,6].

The feed administered to all experimental animals was supplied by the same producer. Friable feed was provided ad libitum twice daily, at 8:00 a.m. and 5:00 p.m., throughout the experiment. The composition of the complete diet, as declared by the manufacturer, is presented in Table 1 [5,6].

Table 1. Declared composition of the complete diet.

Parameters	Composition Declared by the Manufacturer (%)
Soybean meal	16
Wheat	55
Barley	22
Wheat bran	4.0
Chalk	0.3
Zitrosan	0.2
Vitamin-mineral premix [1]	2.5

[1] Composition of the vitamin-mineral premix per kg: vitamin A—500.000 IU; iron—5000 mg; vitamin D3—100.000 IU; zinc—5000 mg; vitamin E (alpha-tocopherol)—2000 mg; manganese—3000 mg; vitamin K—150 mg; copper ($CuSO_4{\cdot}5H_2O$)—500 mg; vitamin B_1—100 mg; cobalt—20 mg; vitamin B_2—300 mg; iodine—40 mg; vitamin B_6—150 mg; selenium—15 mg; vitamin B_{12}—1500 µg; L-lysine—9.4 g; niacin—1200 mg; DL-methionine+cystine—3.7 g; pantothenic acid—600 mg; L-threonine—2.3 g; folic acid—50 mg; tryptophan—1.1 g; biotin—7500 µg; phytase+choline—10 g; ToyoCerin probiotic+calcium—250 g; antioxidant+mineral phosphorus and released phosphorus—60 g; magnesium—5 g; sodium and calcium—51 g.

The proximate chemical composition of diets fed to pigs in groups C, ZEN5, ZEN10, and ZEN15 was determined using the NIRS™ DS2500 F feed analyser (FOSS, Hillerød, Denmark), a monochromator-based NIR reflectance and transflectance analyser with a scanning range of 850–2500 nm [5,6].

3.1.3. Toxicological Analysis

Feed was analysed for the presence of ZEN and DON by high-performance liquid chromatography with UV—vis detection (HPLC-UV). The obtained values did not exceed the limits of quantitation (LOQ) of 2 ng/g for ZEN and 5 ng/g for DON based on the validation of chromatographic methods for the determination of ZEN and DON levels in feed materials and feeds, which was performed at the Department [5,6,69]. This study investigated ZEN and DON which are the most ubiquitous feed contaminants that enter into synergistic interactions [4,18,70,71].

3.2. *In Vitro Study*

3.2.1. Sampling for in Vitro Tests

Five pre-pubertal gilts from every group were euthanized on analytical date 1 (D1—exposure day 7), date 2 (D2—exposure day 21) and date 3 (D3—exposure day 42) by the intravenous administration of pentobarbital sodium (Fatro, Ozzano Emilia BO, Italy) and bleeding. Samples were collected from the gastrointestinal tract of pre-pubertal gilts immediately after cardiac arrest and were prepared for analyses [5,6]. Samples for in vitro analysis were collected from a 10-cm-long intestinal fragment resected from different intestinal segments. Resected fragments were cut from: the duodenum—the first portion (duodenal cup) and the horizontal or third portion; the jejunum, ileum and from the descending colon—from the middle portion. Intestinal segments were tied at both ends before resection to avoid tissue damage. The studied material consisted of sterile digesta samples which were delivered to the microbiological laboratory under refrigerated conditions. A total of 300 samples were collected (20 gilts × 5 intestinal segments × 3 sampling dates).

3.2.2. Microbiological Tests

Microbiological tests were performed at the Microbiological Laboratory of the Non-Public Health Care Centre in Olsztyn, Poland.

Samples of intestinal contents were analysed microbiologically by the culture method according to the relevant ISO standards (PN-EN ISO 18416:2009; PN-EN ISO 21149:2009; PN-EN ISO 22718:2010; PN-EN ISO 22717:2010; PN-EN ISO 21150:2010; PN-EN ISO 16212:2011).

Bacteriological tests. Members of the family *Enterobacteriaceae*, including *Escherichia coli*, *Citrobacter freundii* and *Klebsiella pneumoniae*, were cultured on Biomerieux®-France Mac Conkey Agar (MCK) at 37 °C for 24–48 h. *Yersinia enterocolitica* was cultured on Biomerieux®-France Yersinia agar (CIN) at 20–25 °C for 3–4 days. *Salmonella* spp. were cultured on Biomerieux®-France SS Agar (SS) at 37 °C for 24–48 h. Members of the family *Enterococcaceae*, including faecal strepotococci (Enterococcus), and family *Staphylococcaceae*, including coagulase-negative staphylococci, were cultured on Biomerieux®-France Columbia ANC agar + 5% sheep blood (CNA) at 37 °C for 24–48 h. *Clostridium difficile* of the family *Clostridiaceae* was cultured on Biomerieux®-France Schaedler agar + 5% sheep blood (SCS) at 37 °C for 48 h.

Fungal tests. *Candida krusei* of the family *Saccharomycetaceae* was cultured on Chrom Agar Candida with a chromogenic mixture, peptone and chloramphenicol (GRASO-Poland) at 37 °C for up to 10 days. *Fusarium* spp. moulds of the family *Nectriaceae* were cultured on Biomerieux®-France Dermatophyte agar (DERM) at 20–25 °C for 3–4 weeks.

3.2.3. Microbial Identification

The isolated pure bacterial and fungal cultures were identified in the VITEK 2 system for microbial identification and antibiotic susceptibility testing (Biomerieux®, bioMérieux, Craponne, France). Bacteria were additionally identified with the use of standard culture methods based on their morphological features, Gram staining, oxidase production (OXI Gel Polish, Puławy, Poland, Diagnostics Slovakia), coagulase production (Staphytect Plus, Oxoid, Thermo Fisher Microbiology Sale, Hampshire, UK) and the Salmonella Latex agglutination test (Biomex-Kraków, Kraków, Poland).

Yeasts were identified based on macroscopic and microscopic characteristics in the VITEK 2 system (Biomerieux®-France). Identification tests were performed for the prevalent microflora.

3.2.4. Evaluation of Dysbiosis

The dysbiosis of intestinal microflora was evaluated to determine quantitative differences in bacterial counts between intestinal segments. The dimensionless dysbiosis index was determined based on the ratio of bacterial counts (log CFU/g) in group C and the experimental groups. Values equal to 1.0 were regarded as normal, and values higher or lower than 1.0 were indicative of dysbiosis.

3.2.5. Statistical Analysis

Changes in the log CFU/g values of different bacteria in different sections of the intestine in group C were evaluated under exposure to three doses of ZEN. Data were obtained on three analytical dates, and they were processed separately for each date. The log CFU/g values of each type of bacteria were divided into groups based on two factors: (a) ZEN dose, and (b) the analysed intestinal segment (variability of microbiota). Two-way ANOVA could not be performed because bacteria were not detected in all groups or log CFU/g values were identical (zero variance). Therefore, the following analyses were carried out: (i) differences in log CFU/g values in the same intestinal segment in the control group were determined under exposure to three doses of ZEN, and (ii) differences in log CFU/g values in different intestinal segments in the control group were determined under exposure to the same dose of ZEN. In both scenarios, the observed differences between groups (1—ZEN dose/2—section of the intestine) were processed by one-way ANOVA. Differences between pairs of means were determined with Tukey's multiple comparison test. If no bacterial colonies were observed or if all log CFU values were identical in any of the compared groups, one-way ANOVA was performed for the remaining groups, and group means were compared against zero or against the value of an excluded group with the use of Student's *t*-test. Data were processed in Statistica v. 13 (TIBCO Software Inc., 2017, Warsaw, Poland).

Author Contributions: The experiments were conceived and designed by M.G. and M.T.G. The experiments were performed by K.C., A.R. and M.D. Data were analysed and interpreted by K.C., M.D., M.B., S.L.-Ż. and M.G. The manuscript was drafted by K.C. and M.G. and critically edited by Ł.Z. and M.T.G.

Funding: The study was supported by the "Healthy Animal—Safe Food" Scientific Consortium of the Leading National Research Centre (KNOW) pursuant to a decision of the Ministry of Science and Higher Education No. 05-1/KNOW2/2015.

Conflicts of Interest: The authors declare no conflict of interest.

References

1. Montanha, F.Z.; Anater, A.; Burchard, J.F.; Luciano, F.B.; Meca, G.; Manyes, L.; Pimpão, C.T. Mycotoxins in dry-cured meats: A review. *Food Chem. Toxicol.* **2018**, *111*, 494–502. [CrossRef] [PubMed]
2. Zachariasova, M.; Dzumana, Z.; Veprikova, Z.; Hajkovaa, K.; Jiru, M.; Vaclavikova, M.; Zachariasova, A.; Pospichalova, M.; Florian, M.; Hajslova, J. Occurrence of multiple mycotoxins in European feeding stuffs, assessment of dietary intake by farm animals. *Anim. Feed Sci. Technol.* **2014**, *193*, 124–140. [CrossRef]
3. Knutsen, H.-K.; Alexander, J.; Barregård, L.; Bignami, M.; Brüschweiler, B.; Ceccatelli, S.; Cottrill, B.; Dinovi, M.; Edler, L.; Grasl-Kraupp, B.; et al. Risks for animal health related to the presence of zearalenone and its modified forms in feed. *EFSA J.* **2017**, *15*, 4851. [CrossRef]
4. Piotrowska, M.; Sliżewska, K.; Nowak, A.; Zielonka, Ł.; Żakowska, Z.; Gajęcka, M.; Gajęcki, M. The effect of experimental fusarium mycotoxicosis on microbiota diversity in porcine ascending colon contents. *Toxins* **2014**, *6*, 2064–2081. [CrossRef]
5. Cieplińska, K.; Gajęcka, M.; Nowak, A.; Dąbrowski, M.; Zielonka, Ł.; Gajęcki, M.T. The gentoxicity of caecal water in gilts exposed to low doses of zearalenone. *Toxins* **2018**, *10*, 350. [CrossRef]

6. Rykaczewska, A.; Gajęcka, M.; Dąbrowski, M.; Wiśniewska, A.; Szcześniewska, J.; Gajęcki, M.T.; Zielonka, Ł. Growth performance, selected blood biochemical parameters and body weight of pre-pubertal gilts fed diets supplemented with different doses of zearalenone (ZEN). *Toxicon* **2018**, *152*, 84–94. [CrossRef]
7. Freire, L.; Sant'Ana, A.S. Modified mycotoxins: An updated review on their formation, detection, occurrence, and toxic effects. *Food Chem. Toxicol.* **2018**, *111*, 189–205. [CrossRef] [PubMed]
8. Calabrese, E.J. Paradigm lost, paradigm found: The re-emergence of hormesis as a fundamental dose response model in the toxicological sciences. *Environ. Pollut.* **2005**, *138*, 378–411. [CrossRef]
9. Gajęcka, M.; Zielonka, Ł.; Gajęcki, M. The effect of low monotonic doses of zearalenone on selected reproductive tissues in pre-pubertal female dogs—A review. *Molecules* **2015**, *20*, 20669–20687. [CrossRef] [PubMed]
10. Gajęcka, M.; Zielonka, Ł.; Gajęcki, M. Activity of zearalenone in the porcine intestinal tract. *Molecules* **2017**, *22*, 18. [CrossRef] [PubMed]
11. Stopa, E.; Babińska, I.; Zielonka, Ł.; Gajęcki, M.; Gajęcka, M. Immunohistochemical evaluation of apoptosis and proliferation in the mucous membrane of selected uterine regions in pre-pubertal bitches exposed to low doses of zearalenone. *Pol. J. Vet. Sci.* **2016**, *19*, 175–186. [CrossRef]
12. Kramer, H.J.; van den Ham, W.A.; Slob, W.; Pieters, M.N. Conversion Factors Estimating Indicative Chronic No-Observed-Adverse-Effect Levels from Short-Term Toxicity Data. *Regul. Toxicol. Pharmacol.* **1996**, *23*, 249–255. [CrossRef]
13. Zielonka, Ł.; Waśkiewicz, A.; Beszterda, M.; Kostecki, M.; Dąbrowski, M.; Obremski, K.; Goliński, P.; Gajęcki, M. Zearalenone in the Intestinal Tissues of Immature Gilts Exposed per os to Mycotoxins. *Toxins* **2015**, *7*, 3210–3223. [CrossRef] [PubMed]
14. Vandenberg, L.N.; Colborn, T.; Hayes, T.B.; Heindel, J.J.; Jacobs, D.R.; Lee, D.-H.; Shioda, T.; Soto, A.M.; vom Saal, F.S.; Welshons, W.V.; et al. Hormones and endocrine-disrupting chemicals: Low-dose effects and nonmonotonic dose responses. *Endocr. Rev.* **2012**, *33*, 378–455. [CrossRef] [PubMed]
15. Grenier, B.; Applegate, T.J. Modulation of intestinal functions following mycotoxin ingestion: Meta-analysis of published experiments in animals. *Toxins* **2013**, *5*, 396–430. [CrossRef] [PubMed]
16. Hickey, G.L.; Craig, P.S.; Luttik, R.; de Zwart, D. On the quantification of intertest variability in ecotoxicity data with application to species sensitivity distributions. *Environ. Toxicol. Chem.* **2012**, *31*, 1903–1910. [CrossRef] [PubMed]
17. Gajęcka, M.; Jakimiuk, E.; Zielonka, Ł.; Obremski, K.; Gajęcki, M. The biotransformation of chosen mycotoxins. *Pol. J. Vet. Sci.* **2009**, *12*, 293–303. [PubMed]
18. Gajęcka, M.; Waśkiewicz, A.; Zielonka, Ł.; Goliński, P.; Rykaczewska, A.; Lisieska-Żołnierczyk, S.; Gajęcki, M.T. Mycotoxin levels in the digestive tissues of immature gilts exposed to zearalenone and deoxynivalenol. *Toxicon* **2018**, *153*, 1–11. [CrossRef] [PubMed]
19. Bakhru, S.H.; Furtado, S.; Morello, A.P.; Mathiowitz, E. Oral delivery of proteins by biodegradable nanoparticles. *Adv. Drug Deliv. Rev.* **2013**, *65*, 811–821. [CrossRef] [PubMed]
20. Carlson, S.J.; Chang, M.I.; Nandivada, P.; Cowan, E.; Puder, M. Neonatal intestinal physiology and failure. *Semin. Pediatr. Surg.* **2013**, *22*, 190–194. [CrossRef]
21. Hueza, I.M.; Raspantini, P.C.F.; Raspantini, L.E.R.; Latorre, A.O.; Górniak, S.L. Zearalenone, an estrogenic mycotoxin, is an immunotoxic compound. *Toxins* **2014**, *6*, 1080–1095. [CrossRef]
22. Lupescu, A.; Bissinger, R.; Jilani, K.; Lang, F. In vitro induction of erythrocyte phosphatidyloserine translocation by the natural Naphthoquinone Shikonin. *Toxins* **2014**, *6*, 1559–1574. [CrossRef]
23. Celi, P.; Verlhac, V.; Pérez, C.E.; Schmeisser, J.; Kluenter, A.M. Biomarkers of gastrointestinal functionality in animal nutrition and health. *Anim. Feed Sci. Technol.* **2018**. [CrossRef]
24. Dąbrowski, M.; Obremski, K.; Gajęcka, M.; Gajęcki, M.; Zielonka, Ł. Changes in the subpopulations of porcine peripheral blood lymphocytes induced by exposure to low doses of zearalenone (ZEN) and deoxynivalenol (DON). *Molecules* **2016**, *21*, 557. [CrossRef]
25. Silva-Campa, E.; Mata-Haro, V.; Mateu, E.; Hernández, J. Porcine reproductive and respiratory syndrome virus induces $CD4^{+}CD8^{+}CD25^{+}$Foxp3+ regulatory T cells (Tregs). *Virology* **2012**, *430*, 73–80. [CrossRef]
26. Zielonka, Ł.; Jakimiuk, E.; Obremski, K.; Gajęcka, M.; Dąbrowski, M.; Gajęcki, M. An evaluation of the proliferative activity of immunocompetent cells in the jejunal and iliac lymph nodes of prepubertal female wild boars diagnosed with mixed mycotoxicosis. *B. Vet. I. Pulawy* **2015**, *59*, 197–203. [CrossRef]

27. Bryden, W.L. Mycotoxin contamination of the feed supply chain: Implications for animal productivity and feed security. *Anim. Feed Sci. Technol.* **2012**, *173*, 134–158. [CrossRef]
28. Alassane-Kpembi, I.; Pinton, P.; Oswald, I.P. Effects of Mycotoxins on the Intestine. *Toxins* **2019**, *11*, 159. [CrossRef]
29. Putignani, L.; Dallapiccola, B. Foodomics as part of the host-microbiota-exposome interplay. *J. Proteom.* **2016**, *147*, 3–20. [CrossRef]
30. Sun, X.; Jia, Z. Microbiome modulates intestinal homeostasis against inflammatory diseases. *Vet. Immunol. Immunop.* **2018**, *205*, 97–105. [CrossRef]
31. Liao, S.F.; Nyachoti, M. Using probiotics to improve swine gut health and nutrient utilization. *Anim. Nutr.* **2017**, *3*, 331–343. [CrossRef]
32. Liew, W.P.P.; Mohd-Redzwan, S. Mycotoxin: Its impact on gut health and microbiota. *Front. Cell. Infect. Microbiol.* **2018**, *8*, 60. [CrossRef]
33. Robert, H.; Payros, D.; Pinton, P.; Théodorou, V.; Mercier-Bonin, M.; Oswald, I.P. Impact of mycotoxins on the intestine: Are mucus and microbiota new targets? *J. Toxicol. Environ. Health B* **2017**, *20*, 249–275. [CrossRef]
34. Pluske, J.R.; Turpin, D.L.; Kim, J.C. Gastrointestinal tract (gut) health in the young pig. *Anim. Nutr.* **2018**, *4*, 187–196. [CrossRef]
35. Giang, H.H.; Viet, T.Q.; Ogle, B.; Lindberg, J.E. Growth performance, digestibility, gut environment and health status in weaned piglet s fed a diet supplemented with potentially probiotic complexes of lactic acid bacteria. *Livest. Sci.* **2010**, *129*, 95–103. [CrossRef]
36. Embry, M.R.; Bachman, A.N.; Bell, D.R.; Boobis, A.R.; Cohen, S.M.; Dellarco, M.; Dewhurst, I.C.; Doerrer, N.G.; Hines, R.N.; Moretto, A.; et al. Risk assessment in the 21st century: Roadmap and matrix. *Crit. Rev. Toxicol.* **2014**, *44*, 6–16. [CrossRef]
37. Guevarra, R.B.; Hong, S.H.; Cho, J.H.; Kim, B.R.; Shin, J.; Lee, J.H.; Kang, B.N.; Kim, Y.H.; Wattanaphansak, S.; Isaacson, R.E.; et al. The dynamics of the piglet gut microbiome during the weaning transition in association with health and nutrition. *J. Anim. Sci. Biotechnol.* **2018**, *9*, 54. [CrossRef]
38. Gajęcki, M.; Gajęcka, M.; Zielonka, Ł.; Jakimiuk, E.; Obremski, K. Zearalenone as a potential allergen in the alimentary tract—A review. *Pol. J. Food Nutr. Sci.* **2006**, *15/56*, 263–268.
39. Rovers, M. Healthy pigs with less use of antibiotics—A nutritional approach in three steps. *Int. Pigs Top.* **2012**, *27*, 15–17.
40. Franco, T.S.; Garcia, S.; Hirooka, E.Y.; Ono, Y.S.; dos Santos, J.S. Lactic acid bacteria in the inhibition of *Fusarium graminearum* and deoxynivalenol detoxification. *J. Appl. Microbiol.* **2011**, *111*, 739–748. [CrossRef]
41. Vignal, C.; Djouina, M.; Pichavant, M.; Caboche, S.; Waxin, C.; Beury, D.; Hot, D.; Gower-Rousseau, C.; Body-Malapel, M. Chronic ingestion of deoxynivalenol at human dietary levels impairs intestinal homeostasis and gut microbiota in mice. *Arch. Toxicol.* **2018**, *92*, 2327–2338. [CrossRef]
42. Binek, M. Human microbiome—Health and disease. *Post. Mikrobiol.* **2012**, *51*, 27–36.
43. Gliński, Z.; Kostro, K. Microbiome—Its characteristics and the role. *Życie Wet.* **2015**, *90*, 446–450. (In Polish)
44. Shames, B. Chapter 68—Anatomy and Physiology of the Duodenum. *Shackelford's Surg. Aliment. Tract* **2019**, *2*, 786–803. [CrossRef]
45. Brisola, M.C.; Crecencio, R.B.; Bitner, D.S.; Frigo, A.; Rampazzo, L.; Stefani, L.M.; Faria, G.A. *Escherichia coli* used as a biomarker of antimicrobial resistance in pig farms of Southern Brazil. *Sci. Total Environ.* **2019**, *647*, 362–368. [CrossRef]
46. De Jong, A.; Simjee, S.; El Garch, F.; Moyaert, H.; Rose, M.; Youala, M.; Dry, M. Antimicrobial susceptibility of enterococci recovered from healthy cattle, pigs and chickens in nine EU countries (EASSA Study) to critically important antibiotics. *Vet. Microbiol.* **2018**, *216*, 168–175. [CrossRef]
47. Schoenfelder, S.M.K.; Dong, Y.; Feßler, A.T.; Schwarz, S.; Schoen, C.; Köck, R.; Ziebuhr, W. Antibiotic resistance profiles of coagulase-negative staphylococci in livestock environments. *Vet. Microbiol.* **2017**, *200*, 79–87. [CrossRef]
48. Heilmann, C.; Ziebuhr, W.; Becker, K. Are coagulase-negative staphylococci virulent? *Clin. Microbiol. Infec.* **2018**. [CrossRef]
49. Zheng, W.; Ji, X.; Zhang, Q.; Yao, W. Intestinal microbiota ecological response to oral administrations of hydrogen-richwater and lactulose in female piglets fed a fusarium toxin-contaminated diet. *Toxins* **2018**, *10*, 246. [CrossRef]

50. Bajagai, Y.S.; Klieve, A.V.; Dart, P.J.; Bryden, W.L. Probiotics in animal nutrition e production, impact and regulation. In *FAO Animal Production and Health Paper No. 179*; Makkar, H.P.S., Ed.; Food and Agriculture Organization of the United Nation: Rome, Italy, 2016.
51. Lewczuk, B.; Przybylska-Gornowicz, B.; Gajęcka, M.; Targońska, K.; Ziółkowska, N.; Prusik, M.; Gajęcki, M. Histological structure of duodenum in gilts receiving low doses of zearalenone and deoxynivalenol in feed. *Exp. Toxicol. Pathol.* **2016**, *68*, 157–166. [CrossRef]
52. Panasiuk, Ł.; Piątkowska, M.; Pietruszka, K.; Jedziniak, P.; Posyniak, A. Modified mycotoxins—A hidden threats beyond official control. *Życie Wet.* **2018**, *93*, 54–547.
53. Regassa, A.; Nyachotim, C.M. Application of resistant starch in swine and poultry diets with particular reference to gut health and function. *Anim. Nutr.* **2018**, *4*, 305–310. [CrossRef]
54. Metzler-Zebeli, B.U.; Trevisi, P.; Prates, J.A.M.; Tanghe, S.; Bosi, P.; Canibe, N.; Montagne, L.; Freire, J.; Zebeli, Q. Assessing the effect of dietary inulin supplementation on gastrointestinal fermentation, digestibility and growth in pigs: A meta-analysis. *Anim. Feed Sci. Technol.* **2017**, *233*, 120–132. [CrossRef]
55. Youssef, I.M.I.; Kamphues, J. Fermentation of lignocellulose ingredients in vivo and in vitro via using fecal and caecal inoculums of monogastric animals (swine/turkeys). *Beni-Suef Univ. J. Basic Appl. Sci.* **2018**, *7*, 407–413. [CrossRef]
56. Yu, W.; Kim, H.K.; Rauch, S.; Schneewind, O.; Missiakas, D. Pathogenic conversion of coagulase-negative staphylococci. *Microbes Infect.* **2017**, *19*, 101–109. [CrossRef]
57. Davis, M.F.; Pisanic, N.; Rhodes, S.M.; Brown, A.; Keller, H.; Nadimpalli, M.; Christ, A.; Ludwig, S.; Ordak, C.; Spicer, K.; et al. Occurrence of Staphylococcus aureus in swine and swine workplace environments on industrial and antibiotic-free hog operations in North Carolina, USA: A One Health pilot study. *Environ. Res.* **2018**, *163*, 88–96. [CrossRef]
58. Drew, M.D.; Van Kessel, A.G.; Estrada, A.E.; Ekpe, E.D.; Zijlstra, R.T. Effect of dietary cereal on intestinal bacterial populations in weaned pigs. *Can. J. Anim. Sci.* **2002**, *82*, 607–609. [CrossRef]
59. Dowarah, R.; Verma, A.K.; Agarwal, N.; Patel, B.H.M.; Singh, P. Effect of swine based probiotic on performance, diarrhoea scores, intestinal microbiota and gut health of grower-finisher crossbred pigs. *Livest. Sci.* **2017**, *195*, 74–79. [CrossRef]
60. Baker, A.A.; Davis, E.; Rehberger, T.; Rosener, D. Prevalence and Diversity of Toxigenic Clostridium perfringens and Clostridium difficile among Swine Herds in the Midwest. *Appl. Environ. Microb.* **2010**, *76*, 2961–2967. [CrossRef]
61. Krutova, M.; Zouharova, M.; Matejkova, J.; Tkadlec, J.; Krejčí, J.; Faldyna, M.; Nyc, O.; Bernardy, J. The emergence of *Clostridium difficile* PCR ribotype 078 in piglets in the Czech Republic clusters with Clostridium difficile PCR ribotype 078 isolates from Germany, Japan and Taiwan. *Int. J. Med. Microbiol.* **2018**, *308*, 770–775. [CrossRef]
62. Gajęcka, M.; Stopa, E.; Tarasiuk, M.; Zielonka, Ł.; Gajęcki, M. The expression of type-1 and type-2 nitric oxide synthase in selected tissues of the gastrointestinal tract during mixed mycotoxicosis. *Toxins* **2013**, *5*, 2281–2292. [CrossRef]
63. Forero-Reyes, C.M.; Alvarado-Fernández, A.M.; Ceballos-Rojas, A.M.; González-Carmona, L.C.; Linares-Linares, M.Y.; Castañeda-Salazar, R.; Pulido-Villamarín, A.; Góngora-Medina, M.E.; Cortés-Vecino, J.A.; Rodríguez-Bocanegra, M.X. Evaluation of *Fusarium* spp. pathogenicity in plant and murine models. *Rev. Argent. Microbiol.* **2018**, *50*, 90–96. [CrossRef]
64. Otašević, S.; Momčilović, S.; Petrović, M.; Radulović, O.; Stojanović, N.M.; Arsić-Arsenijević, V. The dietary modification and treatment of intestinal Candida overgrowth—A pilot study. *J. De Mycol. Méd.* **2018**, *28*, 623–627. [CrossRef]
65. Reddy, K.E.; Jeong, J.Y.; Song, J.; Lee, Y.; Lee, H.J.; Kim, D.W.; Jung, H.Y.; Kim, K.H.; Kim, M.; Oh, Y.K.; et al. Colon microbiome of pigs fed diet contaminated with commercial purified deoxynivalenol and zearalenone. *Toxins* **2018**, *10*, 347. [CrossRef]
66. Zhabinskii, V.N.; Khripach, N.B.; Khripach, V.A. Steroid plant hormones: Effects outside plant kingdom. *Steroids* **2015**, *97*, 87–97. [CrossRef]
67. Heberer, T.; Lahrssen-Wiederholt, M.; Schafft, H.; Abraham, K.; Pzyrembel, H.; Henning, K.J.; Schauzu, M.; Braeunig, J.; Goetz, M.; Niemann, L.; et al. Zero tolerances in food and animal feed-Are there any scientific alternatives? A European point of view on an international controversy. *Toxicol. Lett.* **2007**, *175*, 118–135. [CrossRef]

68. Smith, D.; Combes, R.; Depelchin, O.; Jacobsen, S.D.; Hack, R.; Luft, J.; Lammens, L.; von Landenberg, F.; Phillips, B.; Pfister, R.; et al. Optimising the design of preliminary toxicity studies for pharmaceutical safety testing in the dog. *Regul. Toxicol. Pharmacol.* **2005**, *41*, 95–101. [CrossRef]
69. Gajęcki, M. The effect of experimentally induced *Fusarium* mycotoxicosis on selected diagnostic and morphological parameters of the porcine digestive tract. In Proceedings of the Final Report for the National Centre for Research and Development in Warsaw, Poland, Development Project NR12-0080-10 entitled, Warsaw, Poland, 30 November 2013; pp. 1–180.
70. Bensassi, F.; Gallerne, C.; Sharaf el dein, O.; Hajlaoui, M.R.; Lemaire, C.; Bacha, H. In vitro investigation of toxicological interactions between the fusariotoxins deoxynivalenol and zearalenone. *Toxicon* **2014**, *84*, 1–6. [CrossRef]
71. Ji, J.; Wang, Q.; Wu, H.; Xia, S.; Guo, H.; Blaženović, I.; Zhang, Y.; Sn, X. Insights into cellular metabolic pathways of the combined toxicity responses of Caco-2 cells exposed to deoxynivalenol, zearalenone and Aflatoxin B1. *Food Chem. Toxicol.* **2019**, *126*, 106–112. [CrossRef] [PubMed]

toxins

MDPI

Article

Gut Microbiota Profiling of Aflatoxin B1-Induced Rats Treated with *Lactobacillus casei* Shirota

Winnie-Pui-Pui Liew [1], Sabran Mohd-Redzwan [1,*] and Leslie Thian Lung Than [2]

[1] Department of Nutrition and Dietetics, Faculty of Medicine and Health Sciences, Universiti Putra Malaysia, 43400 Serdang, Selangor, Malaysia; liew.winnie@outlook.com

[2] Department of Medical Microbiology and Parasitology, Faculty of Medicine and Health Sciences, Universiti Putra Malaysia, 43400 Serdang, Selangor, Malaysia; leslie@upm.edu.my

* Correspondence: mohdredzwan@upm.edu.my or mohd.redzwan.sabran@gmail.com; Tel.: +3-8947-2766

Received: 20 December 2018; Accepted: 10 January 2019; Published: 17 January 2019

Abstract: Aflatoxin B1 (AFB1) is a ubiquitous carcinogenic food contaminant. Gut microbiota is of vital importance for the host's health, regrettably, limited studies have reported the effects of xenobiotic toxins towards gut microbiota. Thus, the present study aims to investigate the interactions between AFB1 and the gut microbiota. Besides, an AFB1-binding microorganism, *Lactobacillus casei* Shirota (Lcs) was tested on its ability to ameliorate the changes on gut microbiota induced by AFB1. The fecal contents of three groups of rats included an untreated control group, an AFB1 group, as well as an Lcs + AFB1 group, were analyzed. Using the MiSeq platform, the PCR products of 16S rDNA gene extracted from the feces were subjected to next-generation sequencing. The alpha diversity index (Shannon) showed that the richness of communities increased significantly in the Lcs + AFB1 group compared to the control and AFB1 groups. Meanwhile, beta diversity indices demonstrated that AFB1 group significantly deviated from the control and Lcs + AFB1 groups. AFB1-exposed rats were especially high in *Alloprevotella* spp. abundance. Such alteration in the bacterial composition might give an insight on the interactions of AFB1 towards gut microbiota and how Lcs plays its role in detoxification of AFB1.

Keywords: Aflatoxin B1; *Lactobacillus casei* Shirota; Alloprevotella; metagenomic sequencing; microbiota

Key Contribution: These findings implied that AFB1 could alter the gut microbiota composition. In addition, data also showed that Lcs treatment reduced the AFB1-induced dissimilarities in the gut microbiota profile.

1. Introduction

Mycotoxins, a structurally diverse group of poisonous fungal secondary metabolites that contaminate agricultural crops during pre-harvest or post-harvest storage in the hot and humid climate regions [1]. Among the well-known mycotoxins, aflatoxin B1 (AFB1) is the most ubiquitous and poisonous mycotoxins, which has been categorized as group I carcinogen [2]. Moreover, AFB1 also causes significant economic losses of crops globally [3]. Several studies have produced conclusive evidence that the carcinogenicity of aflatoxins operates via a mutagenic mechanism. The process involves the cytochrome (CYP-450) enzyme metabolism systems, the formation of genotoxic metabolite (AFB1-8,9-epoxide), the generation of DNA adducts, as well as the alteration of tumor suppressor (TP53) gene [4]. In addition to its carcinogenic properties, AFB1 also induces a number of health problems, such as gastrointestinal (GI) pain, diarrhea, as well as affects the growth and development in both animals and human beings, as demonstrated in numerous studies reviewed by Gong et al. [5].

The negative impacts of AFB1 towards GI tract is of high concern since AFB1 commonly enter the host via food contamination [6]. Diet contaminated with AFB1 influences the GI tract, subsequently causes epithelial injuries in the stomach and intestine, primarily, intestinal inflammation in animal models included rat, pig, and chicken [7]. Both in vitro and in vivo studies have demonstrated that AFB1 induces intestinal damages via perturbation of the intestinal barrier and activation of immune system, cell apoptosis, and cell proliferation [7]. At the same time, AFB1 exposure can cause gut dysbiosis and disrupt the gut microbiota balance by increasing the growth of non-beneficial and pathogenic bacteria as discussed by Liew and Mohd-Redzwan [8]. Moreover, gut dysbiosis can affect the health condition of the host as reported in numerous studies [9].

The gastrointestinal tract is colonized by the largest community of bacterial members of the microbiota which made up of a rich variety of microorganisms [10]. Substantial progress in the gut microbiota research has discovered the vital role of gut microbiota in maintaining health status [11]. Such metagenomic studies were made possible with the improvement of currently available next-generation sequencing (NGS) technologies, which reduce the cost and increase the throughput of bases sequenced/run concurrently [12]. The involvement of gut microbiota on host physiological functions and metabolic activities, such as through the activation of the immunity, excretion of fermentation products, and inhibition of colonization by pathogens has been well recognized [13].

An altered gut microbiota composition is affected by several factors including genetics [14], stressful experiences [14], dietary changes [15], as well as the development of disorders and diseases [16]. Recently, the gut microbiota dysbiosis has frequently been associated with the development of various diseases [16]. A vast range of gut microbiota-related diseases have been discovered, such as food allergies, asthma, obesity, cardiovascular disease, diabetes, eczema, autism, irritable bowel syndrome, Crohn's Disease, colon cancer, hepatic encephalopathy, and mental disorders [17]. A study demonstrated that metabolism products and enzymes from pathogenic microorganisms lead to higher level of carcinogenic compounds [18]. However, studies on the reactions of AFB1 towards the gut microbiota are limited.

Probiotics are well recognized for their vital roles in maintaining wellbeing, especially gut health and microbiota restoration [17]. Probiotics are defined as "live micro-organisms which, when administered in adequate amounts, confer a health benefit on the host" [19]. Among all probiotics, the most conventional bacteria used in both human and animal are lactic acid bacteria (LAB), especially *Lactobacillus* spp. [20]. *Lactobacillus* spp. have recently become the focus of health-promoting bacteria research in diarrhea, lactose intolerance, allergies, infections, cholesterol reduction, eczema, immune function, as well as central nervous system dysfunctions [21]. Additionally, some species of *Lactobacillus* have aflatoxin-reducing activities [22]. Studies revealed that 2×10^{10} CFU/mL of *Lactobacillus* sp. is able to reduce the AFB1 level to 0.1–13% [23]. It appears that the surface components of probiotic bacteria are involved in AFB1-binding [24]. It is worth to mention that probiotic intervention is potentiated to alleviate AFB1-induced toxicity [25].

In the present study, *Lactobacillus casei* Shirota (Lcs) was selected for the AFB1 removal purpose. Lcs is notable for its status in the healthcare industry, especially in maintaining gastrointestinal health [26]. Lcs has previously exhibited high affinity for binding AFB1 in animal [27], as well as in human [28]. Despite this, further studies are necessary in order to evaluate the possible effects of Lcs towards microbiota at the intestinal level under chronic AFB1 exposure. This research involves the investigation of the gut microbiota changes by Lcs in the AFB1 detoxification process. Such knowledge may discover novel approaches for both the treatment, as well as prevention, of mycotoxin contamination and mycotoxicosis. Predicated upon that, it is hypothesized that the gut microbiota composition of rat would be influenced by the toxic effects of AFB1. Besides, the AFB1-altered gut microbiota composition can be recovered upon Lcs treatment.

2. Results and Discussion

2.1. Sequencing and Bacterial Abundance

The filtered rRNA sequences obtained from the colon contents of the control, AFB1, and Lcs + AFB1 dietary groups, resulted in a total of 703,616 sequences, with read lengths averaging 450 nucleotides and GC contents of 53%. Among all, 218,312 sequences belonged to control feces, while 240,975 and 244,329 represented AFB1 and Lcs + AFB1 feces respectively. The number of rRNA sequences from individual control samples ranged from 49,957 to 61,517; those from AFB1-treated samples ranged from 52,567 to 69,055 while those from Lcs + AFB1-treated samples ranged from 49,161 to 74,075. Normalization was performed on the number of operational taxonomic units (OTUs) by subsampling 45,771 sequences from each individual sample.

All rRNA sequences from the fecal contents were grouped into known phyla. The phyla Bacteroidetes and Firmicutes were dominant and they were represented by 81.99% and 13.51% of all rRNA sequences, respectively, as shown in Figure 1A. Proteobacteria, which was represented by 3.27% of the total sequences was the third highly abundant phylum. Some of the phyla were each represented by <2.00% of all rRNA sequences. The phyla Actinobacteria and Saccharibacteria were represented by 1.7% and 1.0% of all rRNA sequences, respectively. Whereas, the remaining phyla constituted <0.3% of the total rRNA sequences. The minorities were represented by Cyanobacteria (~0.01%) and Spirochaetae (~0.01%).

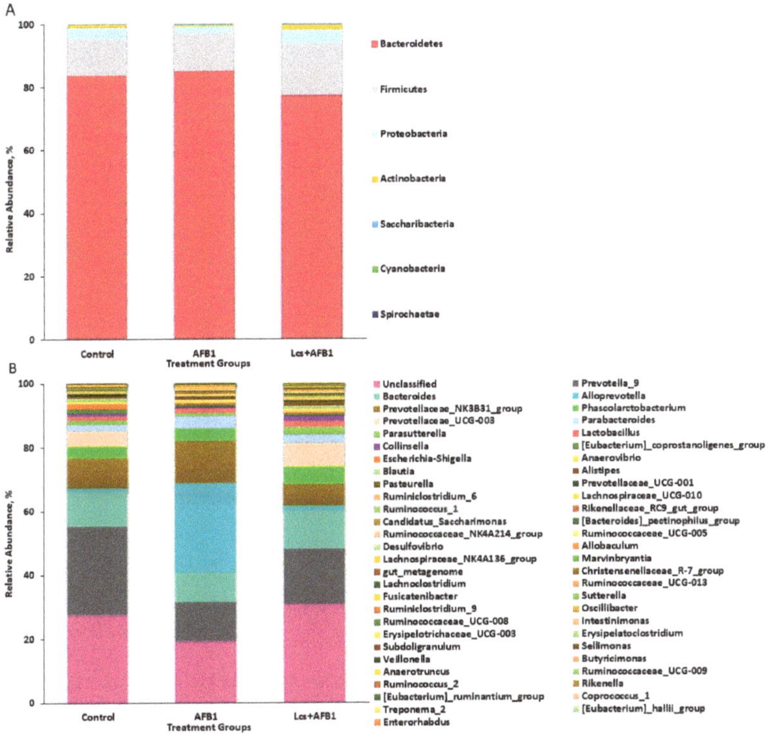

Figure 1. Microbial taxonomic profiles from the fecal contents of the three treatment groups at the phylum (**A**) and genus (**B**) levels, classified by the representation of >1% of the total sequences. The X-axis is the sample name or group name, and the Y-axis is the relative abundance (taxon reads/total reads in the gut microbiota) of different species. The legend is the name of the taxonomic classification of the species.

At the genus level (Figure 1B), Prevotella was highly abundant, comprised 19.35% (106,271) of the total rRNA sequences. There was a group of taxa showing high abundance at the phylum level, which includes Firmicutes and Bacteroidetes, but were not classified at the genus level. Meanwhile, some genera were each represented around 10% of the total sequences, such as *Bacteroides* (10.82%), *Alloprevotella* (10.05%), and *Prevotellaceae*_NK3B31_group (9.93%). Other genera, represented more than 0.5% of the total sequences, were *Phascolarctobacterium* (4.19%), *Prevotellaceae*_UCG-003 (4.03%), *Parabacteroides* (2.95%), *Parasutterella* (1.65%), *Lactobacillus* (1.36%), *Collinsella* (0.98%), *Eubacterium_coprostanoligenes*_group (0.97%), *Escherichia-Shigella* (0.88%), *Anaerovibrio* (0.85%), and *Blautia* (0.72%). A phylogenetic tree in Figure 2 infers approximately-maximum-likelihood phylogenetic relationship from the alignments of the top 30 most abundant OTU sequences.

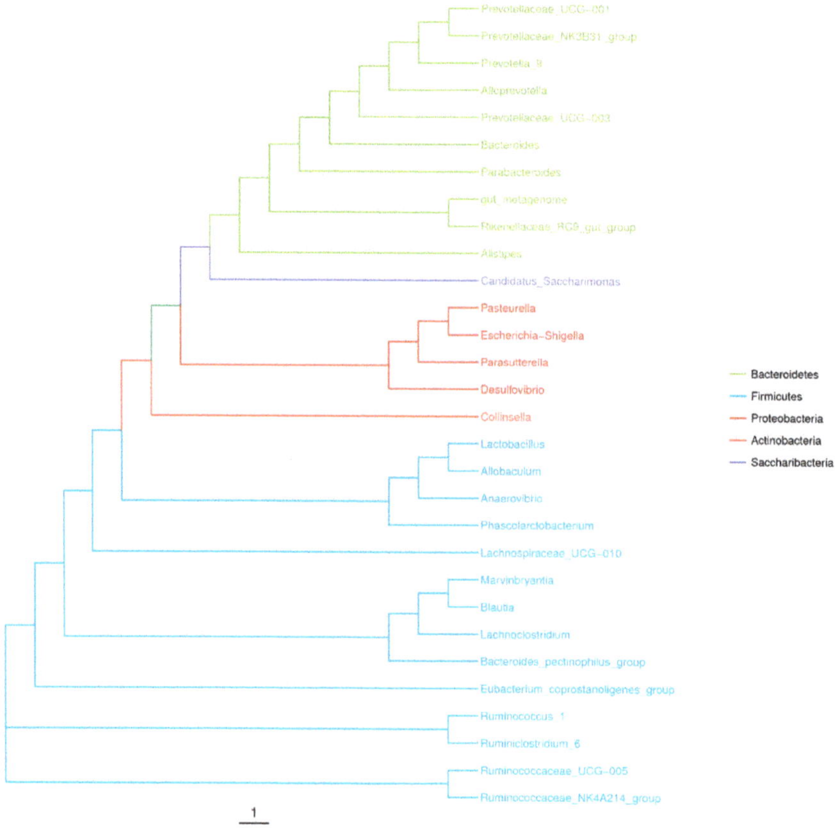

Figure 2. Phylogenetic tree of the top 30 most abundant operational taxonomic unit (OTU) sequences. The color of the branch indicates its corresponding phylum, different colors represents different phylum.

Generally, the gut microbiota of human and laboratory animals, such as rat and mice are dominated by two major phyla, Bacteroidetes and Firmicutes [29]. As shown in this study, Bacteriodetes and Firmicutes are the dominant phyla followed by other major phyla, such as Proteobacteria, Actinobacteria, and Saccharibacteria. The fecal contents from all the treatment groups consisted of similar phyla. The phyla found in the rats' gut microbiota are commonly reported in previous rat microbiota studies [30,31]. In this study, rats were chosen as study subjects due to rats are a better representative of the human gut microbiota compared to other animals [32]. The gut bacterial communities of rats are comparable to the gut microbiota of human. Most of the genera obtained from this study are common microbiota found in rat's fecal content [30,31]. Based on the microbial taxonomic profiles at phylum and genus levels, a different distribution pattern can be observed. Therefore, the clustered OTUs of each sample were subjected to analysis on their alpha and beta diversity.

2.2. Alpha and Beta Diversity

According to the results of OTU cluster analysis using the sequences obtained, Venn diagram (Figure 3A), as well as the alpha diversity indices (Chao1 and Shannon diversity index), were analyzed (Figure 3B,C). Chao index indicates the richness of the community, the estimated number of species/features per sample; and Shannon index indicates community diversity [33]. The Chao index showed that all the treatment groups were not significantly different from each other in term of microbiota richness, although the mean value of control group and Lcs+AFB1 were higher compared to AFB1-treated group (Figure 3B). For a better understanding of the shared richness among each group, a Venn diagram was illustrated to display the overlaps between groups [34]. OTU Venn diagram plotted indicates the common and unique OTUs among the three treatment groups (control, AFB1, and Lcs + AFB1). This analysis showed that the core microbiota consisted of 161 OTUs (Figure 3A). Results showed that there were only 17 unique OTUs found. Among the three treatment groups, the microbiota of Lcs + AFB1 treated rats had significantly higher Shannon diversity index compared to control and AFB1-treated groups (Figure 3C). Furthermore, the Good's coverage estimator is evaluated to calculate the percentage of diversity captured by the devoted sequencing effort. In this study, the average Good's coverage was 100% for all samples, indicating that the true number of OTUs was adequately represented [35].

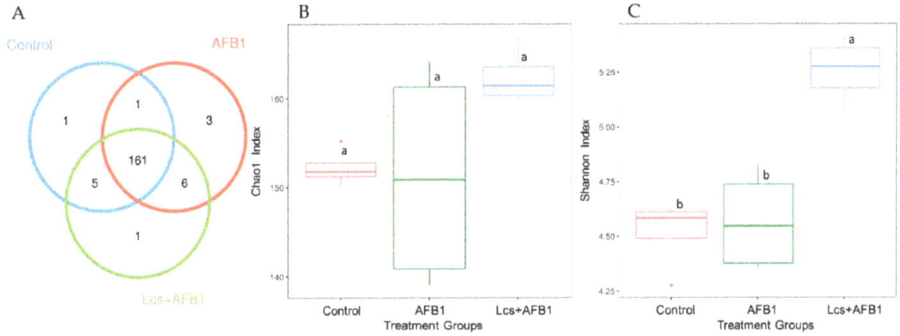

Figure 3. OTU Venn diagram (**A**) and alpha diversity indices (Chao1; (**B**) and Shannon index: (**C**)). The circles of different colors in the Venn diagram represent different treatment groups, and the numbers in the figure represent the numbers of OTUs unique or common to each treatment group. In the petal diagram, each petal represents a treatment group. The numbers on the petals represent the number of OTUs unique to the treatment group, and the white circle in the middle represents the number of OTUs shared by all groups. The chao1 index showed boxplot of each group. The X-axis indicates the names of the groups and Y-axis indicates the Chao 1 index. Each box diagram shows the minimum, first quartile, medium, third quartile and maximum values of the chao1 index of the corresponding treatment groups. Graph C is the Shannon index boxplot of each group. Means between different treatment groups with different superscript letters (a and b) are significantly different ($p < 0.05$).

In order to measure the extent of similarity between microbial communities in the treatment groups, their beta diversity was calculated by unweighted/ weighted UniFrac (Figure 4), and principal coordinate analysis (PCA) (Figure 5A) was performed [36]. PCA analysis is a statistical method to determine the key variables in a multidimensional data set that is most responsible for the differences in the observations and thus is commonly used to simplify complex data analysis [37]. PCA and UniFrac distance heat maps showed that gut microbial communities in AFB1 group and Lcs + AFB1 group were different from that of untreated control rats. It was shown that gut microbiota in the control group of normal rats and in rats that were challenged by AFB1 was distributed in different regions. This result indicated that AFB1 ingestion altered the microbiota composition. Based on the beta diversity distance matrix, the non-metric multidimensional scaling (NMDS) plot showed a clear clustering of the AFB1 samples from the control and Lcs-AFB1 samples. The stress value of NMDS obtained is <0.2 (0.079) which indicates the results can accurately reflect the difference between the samples [38]. These results indicate that diet with AFB1 and Lcs, both influence mammal gut bacterial diversity. Subsequently, the differences were estimated using the unweighted pair group method with arithmetic mean (UPGMA) tree cluster analysis, which uses evolutionary information derived from sample sequences to calculate whether samples in a specific environment is significantly different from an evolutionary lineage in microbial communities [39]. The results in Figure 6 indicated that the phylogenetic relationship of the AFB1 group was relatively far from the control group. In contrast, the AFB1-induced rat which received Lcs treatment was phylogenetically close to the control group. Overall, the results from the beta diversity index demonstrated that gut microbiota in the AFB1-treated rat was normalized to the microbiota diversity of untreated rat after Lcs probiotic treatment.

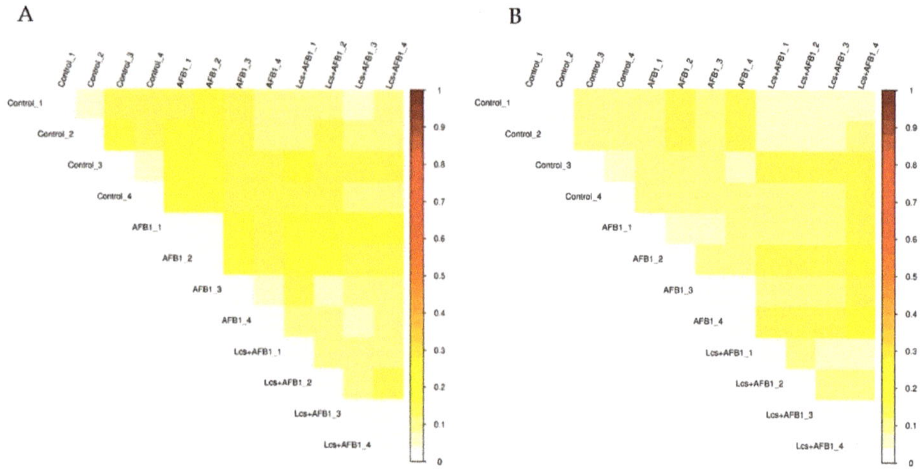

Figure 4. Heatmap of Unweighted Unifrac (phylogenetic distance; **A**), and Weighted Unifrac (phylogenetic distance weighted by abundance counts; **B**). The color scheme in the heatmap represents the degree of difference between the two samples. The lighter the color, the smaller the coefficient between the two samples, and the smaller the difference in species diversity.

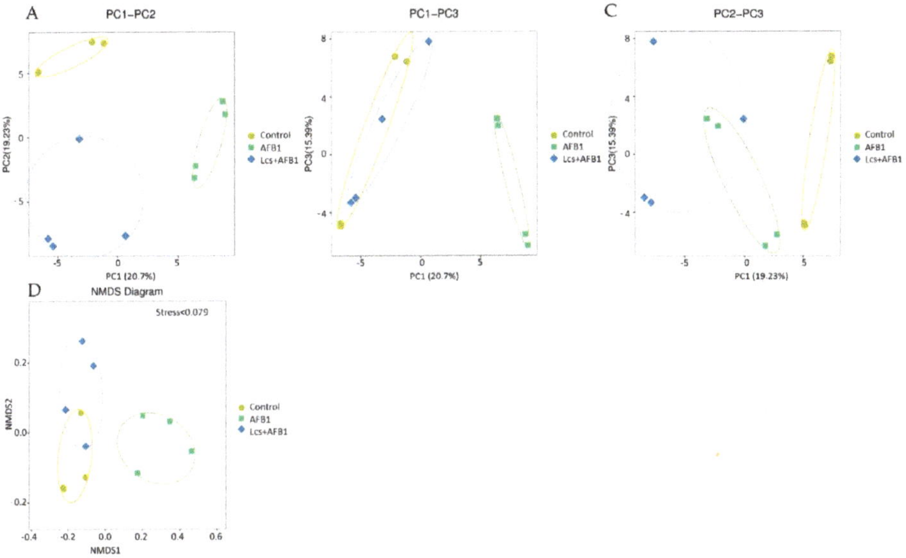

Figure 5. Beta diversity measures using Bray-Curtis (counts; **A–C**), and non-metric multidimensional scaling (NMDS) diagram (**D**). PC1, PC2, PC3 represent the first, second and third principal components, respectively. The percentage after the principal component represents the contribution rate of this component to sample difference and measures how much information the principal component can extract from the original data. The distance between samples indicates the similarity of the distribution of functional classifications in the sample. The closer the distance, the higher the similarity. NMDS diagram accurately reflects the difference between the samples with a stress value <0.2.

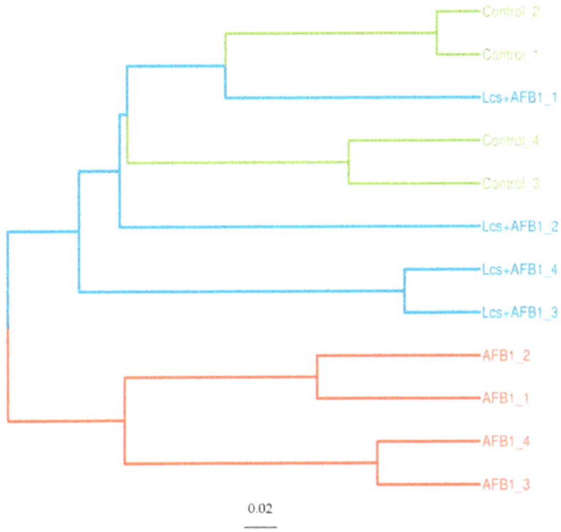

Figure 6. Unweighted pair group method with arithmetic mean (UPGMA)-Tree Cluster Analysis. Each branch in the figure represents a sample. Different colors representing different groups.

2.3. Variation Analysis Between Groups

Analysis of similarities (ANOSIM) and linear discriminant analysis effect size (LEfSe) were used to further confirm the differences between the control, AFB1, and Lcs-AFB1 groups. The ANOSIM statistic examines the mean of ranked dissimilarities between groups to the mean of ranked dissimilarities within groups [40]. It is used to determine whether the grouping is meaningful. An R-value near to 1.0 indicates dissimilarity between groups, whereas an R-value near to 0 indicates an even distribution of high and low ranks within and between groups [41]. There is a significant separation of bacterial composition was observed between control and AFB1 group (ANOSIM $R = 0.292$; Table 1) with p-value < 0.05. After Lcs treatment, the difference between the control group was significantly increased to R-value of 0.87 with p-value < 0.094. Such dramatic changes revealed the efficiency of Lcs in removing AFB1, and thus reducing AFB1-induced microbiota changes in the rat.

Table 1. Group difference evaluation by analysis of similarities (ANOSIM).

Factor	*R*-Value	*p*-Value
Control vs AFB1	1	0.025
Control vs Lcs + AFB1	0.292	0.094
AFB1 vs Lcs + AFB1	0.87	0.025

Note: The value of *R* ranges from 0 to 1. The closer it is to 0, the less significant the between-group difference is compared to within-group difference; the closer it is to 1, the more significance the between-group difference compared to within-group difference.

Lastly, the taxa that best characterized each population was determined using LEfSe with default parameters on species-level OTU tables [42]. In the present study, LEfSe was calculated to identify bacterial taxa differentially distributed between control, AFB1, and Lcs-AFB1 group (Figure 7A–C). The evolutionary relationships of the differential taxa in all the tested groups were plotted using cladograms (Figure S1A–C). In Figure 7A, 2 genera were differentially represented in the control and AFB1 group. Alloprevotella was found dramatically high in the AFB1 group compared to the control group. In contrast, the abundance of Prevotella_9 reduced significantly after AFB1 ingestion. It is worth to note that the distinct difference which distinguished AFB1-induced rats from the untreated control rats is the reduction of a group of unclassified microorganisms at the genus level (Figure 1B).

A total of 16 bacterial taxa were differentially represented among the control and Lcs + AFB1 groups, with 8 more abundant bacterial taxa with increasing trends (g_Christensenellaceae_R_7_group, g_Ruminiclostridium_9, g_Lachnospiraceae_NK4A136_group, o_Burkholderiales, c_Betaproteobacteria, f_Alcaligenaceae, f_Christensenellaceae, o_Clostridiales, c_Clostridia, p_Firmicutes, and g_Anaerotruncus) in the Lcs + AFB1 group. Similar to AFB1 group, the abundance of Prevotella_9 in Lcs + AFB1 group was reduced tremendously compared to the control group. Such results indicate Prevotella_9 is one of the key changes after AFB1 ingestion. Besides, c_Bacteroidia, p_Bacteroidetes, o_Bacteroidales, and g_Ruminococcaceae_UCG_013 were depleted in the Lcs+AFB1 group, in relation to the control group.

Comparing both AFB1 and Lcs + AFB1 groups, g_Anaerotruncus, p_Actinobacteria, g_Collinsella, o_Coriobacteriales, f_Coriobacteriaceae, c_Coriobacteria, c_Betaproteobacteria, p_Proteobacteria, o_Bukholderiales, f_Alcaligenaceae, f_Lachnospiraceae, g_Eubacterium_hallii_group, p_Firmicutes, f_Bacteroidales_S24_7_group were overrepresented in the Lcs + AFB1 group in an increasing order. On the other hand, p_Cyanobacteria, c_Melainabacteria, o_Gastranaerophilales, o_Bacteroidales, c_Bacteroidia, g_Prevotellaceae_NK3B31_group, p_Bacteroidetes, f_Prevotellaceae, g_Alloprevotella were depleted in the Lcs + AFB1 compared to AFB1 group.

Such bacterial composition alteration might give an insight into the interactions of AFB1 towards gut microbiota. In this study, *Alloprevotella* spp. was found present abundantly in the feces of AFB1-treated rats. *Alloprevotella* spp. belongs to the order Bacteroidales. In a study conducted by Wang et al. [43], the bacterial compositions of Bacteroidales was found significantly increased in a dose-dependent manner of AFB1. *Alloprevotella* spp. has been related to the high production of succinic acid and acetic acid as end products [44,45]. Succinic acid at a high level can cause pathological conditions includes inflammation, tissue injury and malignant transformation [46,47]. Acetic acid, on the other hand, may induce colitis at high concentration and frequently used to produce ulcerative colitis animal model [48]. These microbial products from *Alloprevotella* spp. may induce damages to the GI tract.

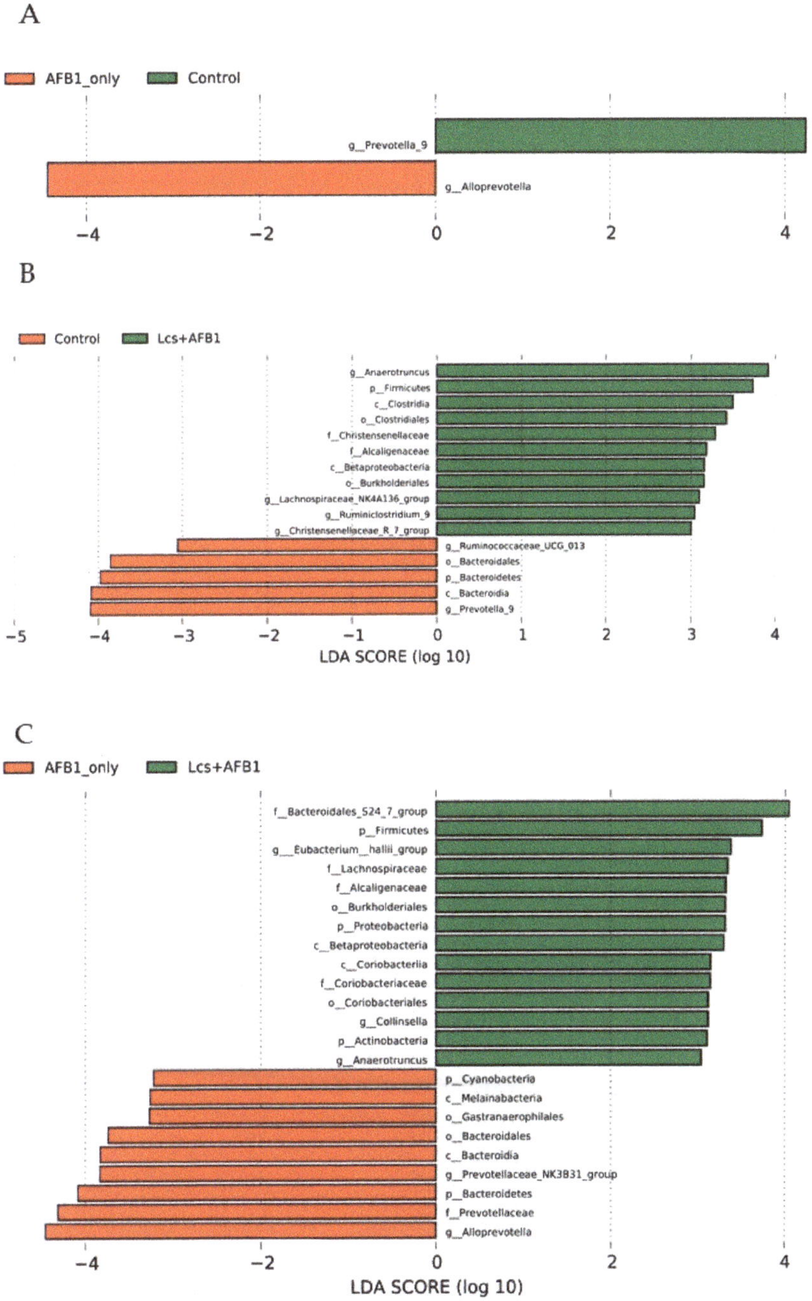

Figure 7. The figure shows the categories of species that are significantly different between the two groups (AFB1 group vs Control group, (**A**) Control group vs Lcs + AFB1 group, (**B**) AFB1 groupvs Lcs + AFB1 group, (**C**) as well as the LDA score from LDA analysis.

The current study is an extension of previous work where we found that AFB1 exerted harmful effects towards small intestine and colon [27]. In the AFB1-exposed rat, lymphocytes accumulation was observed in both small intestine and colon, moreover, large carcinoma was detected in the small intestine. Abundant accumulation of lymphocytes implies localized inflammation [49]. Similar findings have been reported in another study by Nurul Adilah et al. [50] where AFB1 exerted damaging effects towards GI tracts especially in the small intestine. The GI tract, specifically small intestine is the main absorption site of ingested aflatoxin [28]. AFB1 may induce intestinal damages directly via the generation of the genotoxic metabolite. The intestinal epithelial cells produce CYPs which convert AFB1 into the reactive epoxide and subsequently into AFB1-DNA adducts. The negative reactions on the gut from AFB1 exposure include the disruption of the intestinal barrier, cell proliferation, cell apoptosis, and immune system [51]. Indirectly, AFB1 may impair the gut health through gut microbiota perturbation as revealed in this study. Such alteration in gut microbiota profiles may lead to gut dysbiosis. Following that, gut dysbiosis may cause the disruption of intestinal barrier function and bacterial overgrowth. In this study, AFB1-induced gut dysbiosis which leads to overgrowth of *Alloprevotella* spp. A high abundance of this genus has been associated with the carcinogenic process [52]. The alteration in gut microbiota balance could be one of the pathways exploited by AFB1 to induce gut damages. AFB1 perturbates the gut microbiota balance and leads to gut dysbiosis. Without the protection from a healthy gut microbiota, AFB1 can induce intestinal inflammation and carcinoma.

Surprisingly, the increased abundance of *Alloprevotella* spp. was not observed in the Lcs + AFB1 group (Figure 7B,C). On the other hand, previous works on histopathological analysis of Lcs + AFB1 group's intestinal tissues revealed that Lcs can alleviate the detrimental effects induced by AFB1 [27,50]. The result is correlated with this study where the overgrowth of *Alloprevotella* spp. was inhibited by Lcs. Therefore, the study demonstrated that Lcs treatment can protect the GI tracts of the studied animal against AFB1 toxicity. Probiotic Lcs has been demonstrated to protect the gut via various mechanisms. Apart from the direct removal of AFB1, Lcs also produces metabolic byproducts which offer health-promoting effects for the host [53]. Several studies also revealed that Lcs treatment can positively modulate the gut microbiota profile of the host, which eventually improves the health status of the host [54,55]. Lcs colonized the GI tracts and suppress the growth of pathogenic microorganisms via production of antimicrobial agents or competitive exclusion [56]. Moreover, Lcs can control the intestinal immunity and modulate the reactions of the intestinal epithelia and immune cells towards the microorganisms in the intestinal lumen [54]. Beside its AFB1-binding ability, Lcs may alleviate AFB1-induced toxicity via gut microbiota modulation.

Even though the current knowledge on gut microbiota is inadequate, however, their roles in maintaining and influencing the host health have been frequently reported. As mentioned previously, various important immune and metabolic disorders are known to be affected by the imbalanced gut microbiota. Therefore, it is crucial to maintaining the balance of gut microbiota for the health maintenance of the host. The findings in this study revealed that AFB1 caused substantial gut microbiota alteration. However, Lcs was able to ameliorate the gut microbiota composition alteration induced by AFB1. The results from beta diversity and UPGMA-Tree Cluster Analysis demonstrated that the Lcs treatment reversed the aberrant gut microbiota profile and shifted the gut microbiota composition of the AFB1 group to be substantially like that of the control group.

3. Conclusions

In conclusion, the intestinal bacterial flora was significantly affected by AFB1 and Lcs. Particularly, the AFB1 group demonstrated a high abundance of *Alloprevotella spp.* among all the groups, possibly suggesting its role in aflatoxicosis induced by AFB1 via production of short chain fatty acids (SCFAs), such as succinic acid and acetic acid. It is therefore recommended to pay attention to the concentration of SCFAs in the feces for future relevant study. Meanwhile, Lcs significantly modulated the AFB1-induced gut microbiota fluctuations back to normal level. It is suggested that these changes will eventually influence the toxic effects of the xenobiotic agent. Extensive in-depth studies are required to investigate the microbial products in the gut which may affect the AFB1 toxicity level.

Such future studies may reveal potential relationships between AFB1, Lcs, and the gut microbiota, to develop an alternative therapy for aflatoxicosis occurrences.

4. Materials and Methods

AFB1 was acquired from Trilogy Analytical Laboratory, Inc. (Vossbrink Drive, WA, USA). The bacterial culture media were Man deRogosa (MRS) broth (Himedia, Bombay, India), MRS agar (Himedia, Bombay, India), and glycerol solution (Sigma-Aldrich, St. Louis, MO, USA). Phosphate-buffered saline was purchased from Merck (Darmstadt, Germany).

4.1. Ethics Statement

The use of animal in the present experiment was subjected to review and approved by the Institutional Animal Care and Use Committee of Universiti Putra Malaysia on 1 March 2017 (UPM/IACUC/AUP-R098/2016).

4.2. Bacterial Culture

The bacterial culture of Lcs was isolated from Yakult® fermented milk product. In order to confirm the identity of the bacteria, the bacterial 16s RNA sequence was analysed by First BASE Laboratories Sdn. Bhd (Seri Kembangan, Malaysia). Using the BLASTN program (http://www.ncbi.nlm.nih.gov/), the sequences were found to have 100% similarity index with Lcs 16s RNA sequence. Lcs was cultured at 37 °C using MRS agar. The bacterial concentration was standardized at an optical density of 1.0 using UV–VIS spectrophotometer (UV-1800, Shimadzu, Kyoyo, Japan) at 600 nm wavelength. Using plate counting, the bacteria was then measured at 10^9 cells in MRS agar [57]. The bacterial stock cultures were maintained at −20 °C in 10 % (v/v) glycerol after centrifugation (5417, Eppendorf, Barkhausenweg, Germany) at 3500 rpm for 15 min. Meanwhile, the working cultures were kept in MRS agar at 4 °C [58]. Prior to the oral administration, the glycerol liquid was removed and replaced with 200 µL PBS solution [59].

4.3. Experimental Animals

A total of twenty-four (N = 24) 7–8 weeks old Sprague Dawley (SD) rats (male, 250–300g) were used in this study [60]. The animals were supplied by Animal Resource Unit (ARU), Faculty of Veterinary Medicine, University Putra Malaysia (UPM). The protocol was carried out in the animal research house of Comparative Medicine and Technology Unit (COMeT), Institute of Bioscience UPM. The cages with wood shavings were used for housing the rats in groups of two or three. The rats are acclimatized for one week prior to the experiment under regulated temperature (20–22 °C), 12 h light-dark cycle (0700–1900 h), and feed on a normal diet and water *ad-libitum* [60]. The weight and feed intake of the rats in all groups were measured and monitored every week.

4.4. Experimental Protocol

The rats were separated into three different groups randomly (n = 8): Control, AFB1, and Lcs + AFB1. Control: Oral gavaged with 1× PBS buffer at pH 7.4; AFB1 group: Fed with AFB1 only via oral gavage; Lcs + AFB1 group: Supplemented daily with 10^9 CFU Lcs by oral gavage. After five days of probiotic treatment, the rats were fed with AFB1 daily 4 h after Lcs treatment. The complete dosage given to the rats were 25 µg AFB1/kg body weight (b.w.) for five days per week [61]. The concentration of AFB1 fed on rats in the present study was chosen according to the AFB1 level (30–450 ng/mL) found in the diet of developing countries [62]. Throughout the experiment, the animals were given *ad libitum* access to food and water. The health status of rats was monitored every week. After a treatment period of four weeks, rats were subjected to anaesthesia using ketamine-xylazine.

4.5. Gut Microbiome Modulation via Administration of *Lactobacillus casei* Shirota on AFB1-Induced Rat

4.5.1. Fecal Sample Collection

At the end of the study, the rats were kept in metabolic cages for feces collection [63]. The feces were sampled using sterile tweezers to avoid cross-contamination [63]. In order to protect the quality of the samples, the samples were kept at −80 °C.

4.5.2. Extraction of Fecal Sample DNA

Based on the manufacturer's protocol, the fecal samples were subjected to bacterial DNA extraction at the same time using fecal QiaAmp DNA Stool Mini Kit (Qiagen, Hilden, Germany) [64].

4.5.3. Metagenomic Sequencing of Gut Microbiota

Metagenomic sequencing was performed based on the protocol used in a study by Kelly et al. [65]. The library preparations of next-generation sequencing and Illumina MiSeq sequencing were both performed at GENEWIZ, Inc. (Suzhou, China). The DNA samples extracted were measured using Qubit 2.0. Fluorometer (Invitrogen, Grand Island, NY, USA). Approximately 30-50 ng DNA was used to generate amplicons using a MetaVx™ Library Preparation kit (GENEWIZ, Inc., South Plainfield, NJ, USA). The hypervariable regions of V3 and V4 in bacterial 16S rDNA were amplified and subjected to subsequent taxonomic analysis. The conserved regions bordering the V3 and V4 regions were amplified using forward primers "CCTACGGRRBGCASCAGKVRVGAAT" and reverse primers "GGACTACNVGGGTWTCTAATCC". Next, the products from the first polymerase chain reaction (PCR) were amplified in a second round of PCR. For the generation of indexed libraries, the indexed adapters were connected to the 16S rDNA amplicons for NGS sequencing steps using Illumina Miseq. The DNA libraries generated were validated using Agilent 2100 Bioanalyzer (Agilent Technologies, Santa Clara, CA, USA), and measured using Qubit 2.0 Fluorometer [66]. Next, the DNA libraries were multiplexed and inserted into an Illumina MiSeq instrument based on manufacturer's instructions (Illumina, San Diego, CA, USA). Lastly, the sequencing was completed using a 2 × 300 paired-end (PE) configuration. MiSeq Control Software (MCS, 2.6.2, Illumina, Inc., San Diego, CA, USA, 2016) embedded in the MiSeq instrument carried out the image analysis and base calling [67].

4.5.4. Data Analysis

The data analysis of 16S rRNA was performed using Quantitative Insight Into Microbial Ecology (QIIME) open-source software package version 1.9.1 [68]. Based on barcode, the forward and reverse reads were merged and designated to samples. The sequences were trimmed by removing the barcode and primer sequence. Following that, quality filtering on the joined sequences was conducted based on the following criteria: No ambiguous bases, sequence length <200 bp, mean quality score ≥ 20. A reference database (RDP Gold database) was used to detect chimeric sequence via UCHIME algorithm. The sequences that did not fulfill the criteria were removed, therefore the final analysis only involved the effective sequences.

Using the clustering program VSEARCH(1.9.6) against the Silva 119 database pre-clustered at 97% sequence identity, the sequences were clustered into OTUs. Next, all OTUs were assigned into taxonomic category up to the species level at a confidence threshold of 0.8 based on Silva 123 database using Ribosomal Database Program (RDP) classifier [69]. The phylogenetic tree of the top 30 OTU sequences was plotted using R software version 3.3.1 (https://www.r-project.org/, Lucent Technologies, Inc., Murray Hill, NJ, USA, 2014) [70]. The core gut microbiota's Venn diagram (OTU overlapping) was generated by the VennDiagram package in R software [70]. The sequences were subjected to the alpha and beta diversity analysis in QIIME after rarefying steps. Alpha diversity indexes include the richness indicated by Chao1 index and the for diversity indicated by Shannon index [33]. On the other hand, beta diversity was evaluated from weighted and unweighted UniFrac, PCA, NMDS, and clustered using UPGMA [36,71].

4.6. Statistical Analysis

Each sample was analyzed with four replicates for three different group combinations (Control vs AFB1; Control vs Lcs + AFB1; and AFB1 vs Lcs + AFB1). The statistical difference between-groups vs the difference within-group was analyzed by ANOSIM analysis using R software [40]. For the variation analysis between groups, LEfSe (LDA Effect Size) was performed to reveal taxonomic characteristics and to characterize the differences between the two groups [42]. LEfSE was performed using online available software Galaxy version 1.0 (http://galaxyproject.org/) [72] and STAMP version 2.1.3. Significance difference was determined based on p-value < 0.05.

Supplementary Materials: The following are available online at http://www.mdpi.com/2072-6651/11/1/49/s1, Figure S1: Cladograms that indicate the evolutionary relationships of different species between the two groups (AFB1 group vs Control group, A; Control group vs Lcs + AFB1 group, B; AFB1 groupvs Lcs + AFB1 group, C).

Author Contributions: W.-P.-P.L., S.M.-R., and L.T.L.T. conceived and designed the experiments; W.-P.-P.L. performed the experiments; W.-P.-P.L., S.M.-R., and L.T.L.T. analyzed the data; S.M.-R., and L.T.L.T. contributed reagents/materials/analysis tools; W.-P.-P.L. and S.M.-R. wrote the paper. S.M.-R. and W.-P.-P.L. revised the article and approved the final version to be published.

Funding: Research grant GP-IPS/2018/9613100 from Universiti Putra Malaysia.

Acknowledgments: The authors would like to acknowledge financial support through research grant GP-IPS/2018/9613100. W.-P.-P.L. is the recipient of Graduate Research Fellowship (GRF) from School of Graduate Studies, Universiti Putra Malaysia, Malaysia. W.-P.-P.L. would like to thank the Ministry of Higher Education Malaysia (MoHE) for the MyBrain15 Program Scholarship.

Conflicts of Interest: The authors confirmed that there is no known conflict of interest associated with this publication.

References

1. Neme, K.; Mohammed, A. Mycotoxin occurrence in grains and the role of postharvest management as a mitigation strategies. A review. *Food Control* **2017**, *78*, 412–425. [CrossRef]
2. Dai, Y.; Huang, K.; Zhang, B.; Zhu, L.; Xu, W. Aflatoxin B1-induced epigenetic alterations: An overview. *Food Chem. Toxicol.* **2017**, *109*, 683–689. [CrossRef] [PubMed]
3. Bhatnagar-Mathur, P.; Sunkara, S.; Bhatnagar-Panwar, M.; Waliyar, F.; Sharma, K.K. Biotechnological advances for combating aspergillus flavus and aflatoxin contamination in crops. *Plant Sci.* **2015**, *234*, 119–132. [CrossRef] [PubMed]
4. Marchese, S.; Polo, A.; Ariano, A.; Velotto, S.; Costantini, S.; Severino, L. Aflatoxin B1 and M1: Biological properties and their involvement in cancer development. *Toxins* **2018**, *10*, 214. [CrossRef] [PubMed]
5. Gong, Y.Y.; Watson, S.; Routledge, M.N. Aflatoxin exposure and associated human health effects, a review of epidemiological studies. *Food Saf.* **2016**, *4*, 14–27. [CrossRef]
6. Prakash, B.; Kedia, A.; Mishra, P.K.; Dubey, N. Plant essential oils as food preservatives to control moulds, mycotoxin contamination and oxidative deterioration of agri-food commodities–potentials and challenges. *Food Control* **2015**, *47*, 381–391. [CrossRef]
7. Robert, H.; Payros, D.; Pinton, P.; Théodorou, V.; Mercier-Bonin, M.; Oswald, I.P. Impact of mycotoxins on the intestine: Are mucus and microbiota new targets? *J. Toxicol. Environ. Health Part B* **2017**, *20*, 249–275. [CrossRef]
8. Liew, W.-P.-P.; Mohd-Redzwan, S. Mycotoxin: Its impact on gut health and microbiota. *Front. Cell. Infect. Microbiol.* **2018**, *8*, 60. [CrossRef]
9. Lynch, S.V.; Pedersen, O. The human intestinal microbiome in health and disease. *N. Engl. J. Med.* **2016**, *375*, 2369–2379. [CrossRef]
10. Palm, N.W.; de Zoete, M.R.; Flavell, R.A. Immune–microbiota interactions in health and disease. *Clin. Immunol.* **2015**, *159*, 122–127. [CrossRef]
11. Jandhyala, S.M.; Talukdar, R.; Subramanyam, C.; Vuyyuru, H.; Sasikala, M.; Reddy, D.N. Role of the normal gut microbiota. *World J. Gastroenterol. WJG* **2015**, *21*, 8787. [CrossRef] [PubMed]
12. D'Argenio, V.; Salvatore, F. The role of the gut microbiome in the healthy adult status. *Clin. Chim. Acta* **2015**, *451*, 97–102. [CrossRef] [PubMed]

13. Schroeder, B.O.; Bäckhed, F. Signals from the gut microbiota to distant organs in physiology and disease. *Nat. Med.* **2016**, *22*, 1079. [CrossRef]
14. Ussar, S.; Griffin, N.W.; Bezy, O.; Fujisaka, S.; Vienberg, S.; Softic, S.; Deng, L.; Bry, L.; Gordon, J.I.; Kahn, C.R. Interactions between gut microbiota, host genetics and diet modulate the predisposition to obesity and metabolic syndrome. *Cell Metab.* **2015**, *22*, 516–530. [CrossRef] [PubMed]
15. Sonnenburg, E.D.; Smits, S.A.; Tikhonov, M.; Higginbottom, S.K.; Wingreen, N.S.; Sonnenburg, J.L. Diet-induced extinctions in the gut microbiota compound over generations. *Nature* **2016**, *529*, 212. [CrossRef] [PubMed]
16. Marchesi, J.R.; Adams, D.H.; Fava, F.; Hermes, G.D.; Hirschfield, G.M.; Hold, G.; Quraishi, M.N.; Kinross, J.; Smidt, H.; Tuohy, K.M. The gut microbiota and host health: A new clinical frontier. *Gut* **2015**, *65*, 330–339. [CrossRef] [PubMed]
17. Sánchez, B.; Delgado, S.; Blanco-Míguez, A.; Lourenço, A.; Gueimonde, M.; Margolles, A. Probiotics, gut microbiota, and their influence on host health and disease. *Mol. Nutr. Food Res.* **2017**, *61*, 1600240. [CrossRef]
18. Bauer, E.; Williams, B.A.; Smidt, H.; Mosenthin, R.; Verstegen, M.W. Influence of dietary components on development of the microbiota in single-stomached species. *Nutr. Res. Rev.* **2006**, *19*, 63–78. [CrossRef]
19. FAO/WHO. *Joint FAO/WHO Expert Consultation on Evaluation of Health and Nutritional Properties of Probiotics in Food including Powder Milk with Live Lactic Acid Bacteria*; FAO/WHO: Cordoba, Argentina, 2001.
20. Martín, R.; Bermúdez-Humarán, L.G.; Langella, P. Searching for the bacterial effector: The example of the multi-skilled commensal bacterium faecalibacterium prausnitzii. *Front. Microbiol.* **2018**, *9*, 346. [CrossRef]
21. Heeney, D.D.; Gareau, M.G.; Marco, M.L. Intestinal lactobacillus in health and disease, a driver or just along for the ride? *Curr. Opin. Biotechnol.* **2018**, *49*, 140–147. [CrossRef]
22. Fochesato, A.; Cuello, D.; Poloni, V.; Galvagno, M.; Dogi, C.; Cavaglieri, L. Aflatoxin B1 adsorption/desorption dynamics in the presence of lactobacillus rhamnosus rc 007 in a gastrointestinal tract simulated model. *J. Appl. Microbiol.* **2018**. [CrossRef]
23. Apás, A.L.; González, S.N.; Arena, M.E. Potential of goat probiotic to bind mutagens. *Anaerobe* **2014**, *28*, 8–12. [CrossRef] [PubMed]
24. Damayanti, E.; Istiqomah, L.; Saragih, J.; Purwoko, T. Characterization of Lactic Acid Bacteria as Poultry Probiotic Candidates with Aflatoxin B1 Binding Activities. In *IOP Conference Series: Earth and Environmental Science*; IOP Publishing: Bristol, UK, 2017; p. 012030.
25. Saladino, F.; Posarelli, E.; Luz, C.; Luciano, F.; Rodriguez-Estrada, M.; Mañes, J.; Meca, G. Influence of probiotic microorganisms on aflatoxins B1 and B2 bioaccessibility evaluated with a simulated gastrointestinal digestion. *J. Food Compos. Anal.* **2018**, *68*, 128–132. [CrossRef]
26. Matsumoto, K.; Takada, T.; Shimizu, K.; Moriyama, K.; Kawakami, K.; Hirano, K.; Kajimoto, O.; Nomoto, K. Effects of a probiotic fermented milk beverage containing lactobacillus casei strain shirota on defecation frequency, intestinal microbiota, and the intestinal environment of healthy individuals with soft stools. *J. Biosci. Bioeng.* **2010**, *110*, 547–552. [CrossRef] [PubMed]
27. Winnie-Pui-Pui, L.; Adilah, Z.N.; Leslie, T.T.L.; Sabran, M.-R. The binding efficiency and interaction of lactobacillus casei shirota toward aflatoxin B1. *Front. Microbiol.* **2018**, *9*, 1503.
28. Mohd Redzwan, S.; Mutalib, M.S.A.; Wang, J.-S.; Ahmad, Z.; Kang, M.-S.; Nasrabadi, E.N.; Jamaluddin, R. Effect of supplementation of fermented milk drink containing probiotic lactobacillus casei shirota on the concentrations of aflatoxin biomarkers among employees of universiti putra malaysia: A randomised, double-blind, cross-over, placebo-controlled study. *Br. J. Nutr.* **2016**, *115*, 39–54. [CrossRef]
29. Wos-Oxley, M.L.; Bleich, A.; Oxley, A.P.; Kahl, S.; Janus, L.M.; Smoczek, A.; Nahrstedt, H.; Pils, M.C.; Taudien, S.; Platzer, M. Comparative evaluation of establishing a human gut microbial community within rodent models. *Gut Microbes* **2012**, *3*, 234–249. [CrossRef]
30. Lun, H.; Yang, W.; Zhao, S.; Jiang, M.; Xu, M.; Liu, F.; Wang, Y. Altered gut microbiota and microbial biomarkers associated with chronic kidney disease. *Microbiol. Open* **2018**. [CrossRef] [PubMed]
31. Li, D.; Chen, H.; Mao, B.; Yang, Q.; Zhao, J.; Gu, Z.; Zhang, H.; Chen, Y.Q.; Chen, W. Microbial biogeography and core microbiota of the rat digestive tract. *Sci. Rep.* **2017**, *7*, 45840. [CrossRef]
32. Nguyen, T.L.A.; Vieira-Silva, S.; Liston, A.; Raes, J. How informative is the mouse for human gut microbiota research? *Dis. Models Mech.* **2015**, *8*, 1–16. [CrossRef] [PubMed]
33. Gwinn, D.C.; Allen, M.S.; Bonvechio, K.I.; Hoyer, M.V.; Beesley, L.S. Evaluating estimators of species richness: The importance of considering statistical error rates. *Methods Ecol. Evol.* **2016**, *7*, 294–302. [CrossRef]

34. Zhang, X.; Zhang, M.; Ho, C.-T.; Guo, X.; Wu, Z.; Weng, P.; Yan, M.; Cao, J. Metagenomics analysis of gut microbiota modulatory effect of green tea polyphenols by high fat diet-induced obesity mice model. *J. Funct. Foods* **2018**, *46*, 268–277. [CrossRef]
35. Gharechahi, J.; Zahiri, H.S.; Noghabi, K.A.; Salekdeh, G.H. In-depth diversity analysis of the bacterial community resident in the camel rumen. *Syst. Appl. Microbiol.* **2015**, *38*, 67–76. [CrossRef] [PubMed]
36. Lozupone, C.; Lladser, M.E.; Knights, D.; Stombaugh, J.; Knight, R. Unifrac: An effective distance metric for microbial community comparison. *ISME J.* **2011**, *5*, 169. [CrossRef]
37. Paliy, O.; Shankar, V. Application of multivariate statistical techniques in microbial ecology. *Mol. Ecol.* **2016**, *25*, 1032–1057. [CrossRef] [PubMed]
38. Dexter, E.; Rollwagen-Bollens, G.; Bollens, S.M. The trouble with stress: A flexible method for the evaluation of nonmetric multidimensional scaling. *Limnol. Oceanogr. Methods* **2018**, *16*, 434–443. [CrossRef]
39. Comunian, R.; Ferrocino, I.; Paba, A.; Daga, E.; Campus, M.; Di Salvo, R.; Cauli, E.; Piras, F.; Zurru, R.; Cocolin, L. Evolution of microbiota during spontaneous and inoculated tonda di cagliari table olives fermentation and impact on sensory characteristics. *LWT-Food Sci. Technol.* **2017**, *84*, 64–72. [CrossRef]
40. Xia, Y.; Sun, J. Statistical models and analysis of microbiome data from mice and humans. In *Mechanisms Underlying Host-Microbiome Interactions in Pathophysiology of Human Diseases*; Springer: Boston, MA, USA, 2018; pp. 303–371.
41. Bicalho, M.; Machado, V.; Higgins, C.; Lima, F.; Bicalho, R. Genetic and functional analysis of the bovine uterine microbiota. Part i: Metritis versus healthy cows. *J. Dairy Sci.* **2017**, *100*, 3850–3862. [CrossRef]
42. Stearns, J.C.; Davidson, C.J.; McKeon, S.; Whelan, F.J.; Fontes, M.E.; Schryvers, A.B.; Bowdish, D.M.; Kellner, J.D.; Surette, M.G. Culture and molecular-based profiles show shifts in bacterial communities of the upper respiratory tract that occur with age. *ISME J.* **2015**, *9*, 1246. [CrossRef]
43. Wang, J.; Tang, L.; Glenn, T.C.; Wang, J.-S. Aflatoxin B1 induced compositional changes in gut microbial communities of male f344 rats. *Toxicol. Sci.* **2015**, *150*, kfv259.
44. Cheng, W.; Lu, J.; Li, B.; Lin, W.; Zhang, Z.; Wei, X.; Sun, C.; Chi, M.; Bi, W.; Yang, B. Effect of functional oligosaccharides and ordinary dietary fiber on intestinal microbiota diversity. *Front. Microbiol.* **2017**, *8*, 1750. [CrossRef] [PubMed]
45. Longo, P.L.; Dabdoub, S.; Kumar, P.; Artese, H.P.C.; Dib, S.A.; Romito, G.A.; Mayer, M.P.A. Glycemic status affects the subgingival microbiome of diabetic patients. *J. Clin. Periodontol.* **2018**. [CrossRef] [PubMed]
46. Oh, Y.H.; Oh, I.J.; Jung, C.; Lee, S.Y.; Lee, J. The effect of protectants and pH changes on the cellular growth and succinic acid yield of mannheimia succiniciproducens LPK7. *J. Microbiol. Biotechnol.* **2010**, *20*, 1677–1680. [PubMed]
47. Zhao, T.; Mu, X.; You, Q. Succinate: An initiator in tumorigenesis and progression. *Oncotarget* **2017**, *8*, 53819. [CrossRef]
48. Gupta, R.A.; Motiwala, M.N.; Dumore, N.G.; Danao, K.R.; Ganjare, A.B. Effect of piperine on inhibition of FFA induced TLR4 mediated inflammation and amelioration of acetic acid induced ulcerative colitis in mice. *J. Ethnopharmacol.* **2015**, *164*, 239–246. [CrossRef] [PubMed]
49. Jacques, P.; Elewaut, D. Joint expedition: Linking gut inflammation to arthritis. *Mucosal Immunol.* **2008**, *1*, 364. [CrossRef]
50. Nurul Adilah, Z.; Liew, W.-P.-P.; Mohd Redzwan, S.; Amin, I. Effect of high protein diet and probiotic lactobacillus casei shirota supplementation in aflatoxin B1-induced rats. *BioMed Res. Int.* **2018**, *2018*, 9568351. [CrossRef]
51. Knipstein, B.; Huang, J.; Barr, E.; Sossenheimer, P.; Dietzen, D.; Egner, P.A.; Groopman, J.D.; Rudnick, D.A. Dietary aflatoxin-induced stunting in a novel rat model: Evidence for toxin-induced liver injury and hepatic growth hormone resistance. *Pediatr. Res.* **2015**, *78*, 120–127. [CrossRef]
52. Pitt, J.M.; Vétizou, M.; Waldschmitt, N.; Kroemer, G.; Chamaillard, M.; Boneca, I.G.; Zitvogel, L. Fine-tuning cancer immunotherapy: Optimizing the gut microbiome. *Cancer Res.* **2016**, *76*, 4602–4607. [CrossRef]
53. Di Cerbo, A.; Palmieri, B.; Aponte, M.; Morales-Medina, J.C.; Iannitti, T. Mechanisms and therapeutic effectiveness of lactobacilli. *J. Clin. Pathol.* **2015**, *69*, 187–203. [CrossRef] [PubMed]
54. Kato-Kataoka, A.; Nishida, K.; Takada, M.; Kawai, M.; Kikuchi-Hayakawa, H.; Suda, K.; Ishikawa, H.; Gondo, Y.; Shimizu, K.; Matsuki, T. Fermented milk containing lactobacillus casei strain shirota preserves the diversity of the gut microbiota and relieves abdominal dysfunction in healthy medical students exposed to academic stress. *Appl. Environ. Microbiol.* **2016**, *82*, 3649–3658. [CrossRef] [PubMed]

55. Spanhaak, S.; Havenaar, R.; Schaafsma, G. The effect of consumption of milk fermented by lactobacillus casei strain shirota on the intestinal microflora and immune parameters in humans. *Eur. J. Clin. Nutr.* **1998**, *52*, 899. [CrossRef] [PubMed]
56. Bonvalet, M.; Daillère, R.; Roberti, M.P.; Rauber, C.; Zitvogel, L. The impact of the intestinal microbiota in therapeutic responses against cancer. In *Oncoimmunology;* Springer: Cham, Swithland, 2018; pp. 447–462.
57. Aguilar-Toalá, J.; Santiago-López, L.; Peres, C.; Peres, C.; Garcia, H.; Vallejo-Cordoba, B.; González-Córdova, A.; Hernández-Mendoza, A. Assessment of multifunctional activity of bioactive peptides derived from fermented milk by specific lactobacillus plantarum strains. *J. Dairy Sci.* **2017**, *100*, 65–75. [CrossRef] [PubMed]
58. Donkor, O.N.; Henriksson, A.; Vasiljevic, T.; Shah, N. A-galactosidase and proteolytic activities of selected probiotic and dairy cultures in fermented soymilk. *Food Chem.* **2007**, *104*, 10–20. [CrossRef]
59. Potula, H.-H.; Richer, L.; Werts, C.; Gomes-Solecki, M. Pre-treatment with lactobacillus plantarum prevents severe pathogenesis in mice infected with leptospira interrogans and may be associated with recruitment of myeloid cells. *PLoS Negl. Trop. Dis.* **2017**, *11*, e0005870. [CrossRef]
60. Nikbakht Nasrabadi, E.; Jamaluddin, R.; Mutalib, A.; Khaza'ai, H.; Khalesi, S.; Mohd Redzwan, S. Reduction of aflatoxin level in aflatoxin-induced rats by the activity of probiotic lactobacillus casei strain shirota. *J. Appl. Microbiol.* **2013**, *114*, 1507–1515. [CrossRef]
61. Qian, G.; Tang, L.; Guo, X.; Wang, F.; Massey, M.E.; Su, J.; Guo, T.L.; Williams, J.H.; Phillips, T.D.; Wang, J.S. Aflatoxin B1 modulates the expression of phenotypic markers and cytokines by splenic lymphocytes of male f344 rats. *J. Appl. Microbiol.* **2014**, *34*, 241–249.
62. Daniel, J.H.; Lewis, L.W.; Redwood, Y.A.; Kieszak, S.; Breiman, R.F.; Flanders, W.D.; Bell, C.; Mwihia, J.; Ogana, G.; Likimani, S. Comprehensive assessment of maize aflatoxin levels in eastern Kenya, 2005–2007. *Environ. Health Perspect.* **2011**, *119*, 1794. [CrossRef]
63. Li, M.; Shu, X.; Xu, H.; Zhang, C.; Yang, L.; Zhang, L.; Ji, G. Integrative analysis of metabolome and gut microbiota in diet-induced hyperlipidemic rats treated with berberine compounds. *J. Transl. Med.* **2016**, *14*, 237. [CrossRef]
64. Ferrand, J.; Patron, K.; Legrand-Frossi, C.; Frippiat, J.-P.; Merlin, C.; Alauzet, C.; Lozniewski, A. Comparison of seven methods for extraction of bacterial DNA from fecal and cecal samples of mice. *J. Microbiol. Methods* **2014**, *105*, 180–185. [CrossRef] [PubMed]
65. Kelly, J.R.; Borre, Y.; O'Brien, C.; Patterson, E.; El Aidy, S.; Deane, J.; Kennedy, P.J.; Beers, S.; Scott, K.; Moloney, G. Transferring the blues: Depression-associated gut microbiota induces neurobehavioural changes in the rat. *J. Psychiatr. Res.* **2016**, *82*, 109–118. [CrossRef]
66. Chan, C.S.; Chan, K.-G.; Tay, Y.-L.; Chua, Y.-H.; Goh, K.M. Diversity of thermophiles in a malaysian hot spring determined using 16s rRNA and shotgun metagenome sequencing. *Front. Microbiol.* **2015**, *6*, 177. [CrossRef]
67. Jesser, K.J.; Noble, R.T. Characterizing the ecology of Vibrio in the Neuse River Estuary, North Carolina using heat shock protein 60 (hsp60) next-generation amplicon sequencing. *Appl. Environ. Microbiol.* **2018**, *84*, e00333-18. [CrossRef] [PubMed]
68. Caporaso, J.G.; Kuczynski, J.; Stombaugh, J.; Bittinger, K.; Bushman, F.D.; Costello, E.K.; Fierer, N.; Pena, A.G.; Goodrich, J.K.; Gordon, J.I.; et al. QIIME allows analysis of high-throughput community sequencing data. *Nat. Methods* **2010**, *7*, 335. [CrossRef] [PubMed]
69. Cole, J.R.; Wang, Q.; Cardenas, E.; Fish, J.; Chai, B.; Farris, R.J.; Kulam-Syed-Mohideen, A.S.; McGarrell, D.M.; Marsh, T.; Garrity, G.M. The ribosomal database project: Improved alignments and new tools for rRNA analysis. *Nucleic Acids Res.* **2009**, *37*, 141–145. [CrossRef]
70. Kraemer, J.G.; Ramette, A.; Aebi, S.; Oppliger, A.; Hilty, M. Influence of pig farming on the human's nasal microbiota: The key role of the airborne microbial communities. *Appl. Environ. Microbiol.* **2018**. [CrossRef] [PubMed]
71. Astudillo-García, C.; Bell, J.J.; Webster, N.S.; Glasl, B.; Jompa, J.; Montoya, J.M.; Taylor, M.W. Evaluating the core microbiota in complex communities: A systematic investigation. *Environ. Microbiol.* **2017**, *19*, 1450–1462. [CrossRef]
72. Afgan, E.; Baker, D.; Batut, B.; Van, M.; Bouvier, D.; Čech, M.; Chilton, J.; Clements, D.; Coraor, N.; Grüning, B.A.; et al. The Galaxy platform for accessible, reproducible and collaborative biomedical analyses: 2018 update. *Nucleic Acids Res.* **2018**, *46*, W537–W544. [CrossRef]

toxins

MDPI

Article

Cytotoxic Properties of HT-2 Toxin in Human Chondrocytes: Could T_3 Inhibit Toxicity of HT-2?

Feng'e Zhang [1], Mikko Juhani Lammi [1,2,*], Wanzhen Shao [1], Pan Zhang [1], Yanan Zhang [1], Haiyan Wei [1] and Xiong Guo [1,*]

1 School of Public Health, Health Science Center of Xi'an Jiaotong University, Key Laboratory of Trace Elements and Endemic Diseases, National Health Commission of the People's Republic of China, Xi'an 710061, China; fenge0929@stu.xjtu.edu.cn (F.Z.); shaowz@stu.xjtu.edu.cn (W.S.); zhangpan891112@stu.xjtu.edu.cn (P.Z.); sahalasanmao@stu.xjtu.edu.cn (Y.Z.); ziyunpiaoxue700@stu.xjtu.edu.cn (H.W.)

2 Department of Integrative Medical Biology, University of Umeå, 90187 Umeå, Sweden

* Correspondence: mikko.lammi@umu.se (M.J.L.); guox@xjtu.edu.cn (X.G.); Tel.: +358-40-587-0601 (M.J.L.)

Received: 27 September 2019; Accepted: 9 November 2019; Published: 15 November 2019

Abstract: Thyroid hormone triiodothyronine (T_3) plays an important role in coordinated endochondral ossification and hypertrophic differentiation of the growth plate, while aberrant thyroid hormone function appears to be related to skeletal malformations, osteoarthritis, and Kashin-Beck disease. The T-2 toxin, present extensively in cereal grains, and one of its main metabolites, HT-2 toxin, are hypothesized to be potential factors associated with hypertrophic chondrocyte-related osteochondropathy, known as the Kashin-Beck disease. In this study, we investigated the effects of T_3 and HT-2 toxin on human chondrocytes. The immortalized human chondrocyte cell line, C-28/I2, was cultured in four different groups: controls, and cultures with T_3, T_3 plus HT-2 and HT-2 alone. Cytotoxicity was assessed using an MTT assay after 24-h-exposure. Quantitative RT-PCR was used to detect gene expression levels of *collagen types II* and *X*, *aggrecan* and *runx2*, and the differences in runx2 were confirmed with immunoblot analysis. T_3 was only slightly cytotoxic, in contrast to the significant, dose-dependent cytotoxicity of HT-2 alone at concentrations $\geq$ 50 nM. T_3, together with HT-2, significantly rescued the cytotoxic effect of HT-2. HT-2 induced significant increases in *aggrecan* and *runx2* gene expression, while the hypertrophic differentiation marker, *type X collagen*, remained unchanged. Thus, T_3 protected against HT-2 induced cytotoxicity, and HT-2 was an inducer of the pre-hypertrophic state of the chondrocytes.

Keywords: triiodothyronine; HT-2 toxin; cytotoxicity; Kashin-Beck disease

Key Contribution: Triiodothyronine partly rescued the chondrocytes from cytotoxicity caused by HT-2. HT-2 toxin appeared to effectively induce the switch of the chondrocytes into pre-hypertrophic state.

---

1. Introduction

Thyroid hormone (triiodothyronine, T_3) is converted to this active form from thyroxine (T_4) by deiodinase 2 (DIO2), and it is known to be an essential regulator in metabolism, growth, and development of the human body, and it is critical for the maturation of the skeletal system [1]. It controls the linear growth of bone by regulating endochondral ossification and promotes chondrocyte maturation and hypertrophic differentiation [2]. It has also been exploited to enhance cartilage formation and improve the functional properties of tissue-engineered neocartilage [3]. Furthermore, T_3 enhances chondrogenesis of mesenchymal stem cells of the umbilical cord [4]. In addition, T_3 regulates the transition between proliferation and terminal differentiation of chondrocytes in the growth plate via the

Wnt/β-catenin signaling pathway [5,6]. Thus, a body of evidence implies that T_3 has significant effects on cartilage and chondrocyte physiology. It is worth mentioning that up-regulated *DIO2* expression has been observed in osteoarthritic human articular cartilage and transgenic mice overexpressing *DIO2* [7]. Moreover, low serum T_3 syndrome led to DIO2 dysfunction in Kashin-Beck disease (KBD) children [8,9].

T-2 and HT-2 toxins are two of the most representative and toxic members of the trichothecenes family, which are widely present in cereal grains and other cereal-based products, and are produced by various fungi species, such as Fusarium [10]. In rats, T-2 and HT-2 toxins were mainly distributed in the skeletal system at significantly higher concentrations than those in other organs [11]. In addition, the HT-2 toxin was shown to be a detectable metabolite of T-2 toxin in human chondrocytes, although it was deduced to be less toxic than T-2 [12]. After ingestion, the T-2 toxin is converted into more than 20 metabolites in animals [13]. The T-2 toxin is a cytotoxic fungal secondary metabolite produced by various species of Fusarium, and it interferes especially with the immune system, can harm fetal tissues, and induces cell death by apoptosis [13]. Furthermore, both the T-2 toxin and HT-2 toxin can result in apoptosis of chondrocytes by increased oxidative stress, which causes a release of *Bax*, *caspase-3*, and *caspase-9* [14]. A number of studies have reported that the T-2 toxin induces chondrocytes' apoptosis, promotes catabolism and intracellular impairment of cartilage, and is a risk factor of KBD [15–17]. However, studies on the direct effects of the HT-2 toxin on cartilage and chondrocytes are still missing.

It is important to clarify the potentially damaging effect of the HT-2 toxin on human chondrocytes to enrich our knowledge of the possible molecular mechanisms of the HT-2 toxin causing cartilage lesions observed in KBD. Furthermore, this study aimed to explore whether T_3 can protect from the chondrocytic injury caused by the HT-2 toxin in vitro, which may contribute to the combined effects both on cartilage and the potential pathogenesis of KBD. The concurrence of the abnormal T_3 level and HT-2 toxin in vivo of KBD prompted this study to explore the effect of T_3 and the HT-2 toxin on C-28/I2 chondrocytes and their combined effects.

2. Results

2.1. Individual Cytotoxicity of T_3 and HT-2 Toxin in Human C-28/I2 Chondrocytes

MTT assay was used to evaluate the cytotoxicity in C-28/I2 chondrocyte cultures treated with T_3 at concentrations ranging from 0 to 1000 nM. T_3 was found to produce no major effect on the cell viability of C-28/I2 chondrocytes, even at 1000 nM concentration, although a statistically significant difference was observed at 50 nM (Figure 1A). In contrast, HT-2 was highly toxic to C-28/I2 cells, especially at concentrations $\geq$ 50 nM (Figure 1B).

2.2. T_3 Protects against HT-2 Toxin-Induced Toxicity

Mixtures of HT-2 toxin and T_3 at different concentration ratios of both were tested following 24-hour-long exposures. In general, HT-2 concentrations $\geq$50 nM significantly decreased the cell viability in comparison to control cultures (Figure 2). However, at equimolar concentrations, it took a 100 nM concentration of HT-2 to result in a significant decrease in the cell viability (Figure 2A). Also, when T_3 was present at higher molar ratios in relation to HT-2, cytotoxicity was obvious at HT-2 toxin concentrations $\geq$50 nM (Figure 2B,C). At the ratio 1:1000, HT-2 concentration did not reach 50 nM concentration, and no decrease in cell viability was observed (Figure 2D).

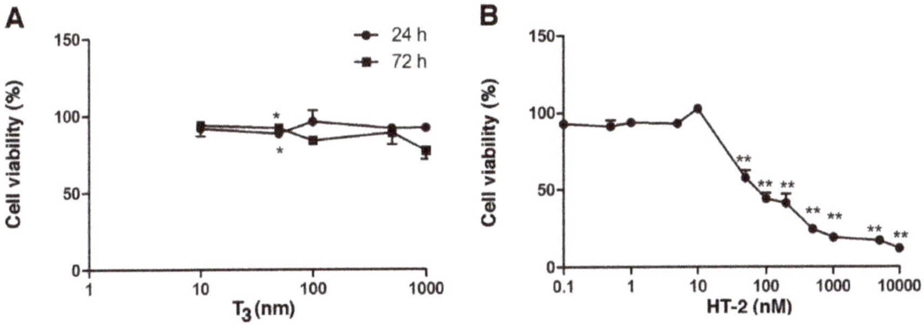

Figure 1. (**A**) Effect of T_3 on viability of human C-28/I2 chondrocytes cultured for 24 and 72 h at T_3 concentrations of 10, 50, 100, 500, and 1000 nM; (**B**) effect of HT-2 on human C-28/I2 chondrocytes cultured for 24 h at 0.1, 0.5, 1, 5, 10, 50, 100, 200, 500 1000, 5000, and 10,000 nM concentrations. The values show means ± SEM of three independent experiments. Cell viability of non-treated cultures in T_3 experiments for 24 and 72 h were 100.0% ± 1.11% and 100.0% ± 10.06%, respectively, and in the HT-2 experiment, 100.0% ± 4.7%. Statistically significant differences against control cultures are indicated with asterisks, * $p < 0.05$ and ** $p < 0.01$.

When the molar concentration of HT-2 toxin was higher than T_3, a decrease in the cell viability due to HT-2 toxin was obvious starting from 50 nM concentrations (Figure 2E–G). However, the addition of T_3 could partially rescue the effect of HT-2 toxin on cell viability (Figure 2E). At high molar ration of HT-2 toxin, T_3 did not have a protective effect on cell viability (Figure 2F,G). The dose-effect plot of all ratios generated by CompuSyn software is shown as the Figure S1.

2.3. Expressions of Extracellular Matrix and Hypertrophy Related-Genes in Chondrocyte Cultures Treated with T_3 and/or HT-2 Toxin

The expression levels of four chondrocyte phenotype-related genes (*aggrecan*, *collagen types II* and X, and *runx2*) were quantified in C-28/I2 chondrocytes treated with 50 nM T_3, 50 nM T_3 plus 50 nM HT-2 toxin, or 50 nM HT-2 for 24 h. Compared with the control group, 50 nM T_3 did not produce any significant changes in the gene expression levels of *collagen types II* and X, *aggrecan*, or *runx2* (Figure 3). The expression level of *aggrecan* was significantly increased in the presence of the HT-2 toxin ($p < 0.05$), and the level of *collagen type II* was 2-fold higher than the control (Figure 3). For the combination treatment of T_3 and HT-2, gene expression patterns were similar to those by the HT-2 toxin alone (Figure 3).

It is well known that runx2 is a crucial transcription factor for chondrocyte maturation, and it induces the expression of *type X collagen* during the maturation process [18]. Thus, it was expected that T_3, which takes part in hypertrophic differentiation, would increase the expression of *runx2* and *collagen type X*. However, neither were affected by T_3 (Figure 3). Surprisingly, the HT-2 toxin significantly increased gene expression of *runx2*, although *type X collagen* expression remained unchanged from control levels. Immunoblot analysis was performed to confirm the induction of runx2 at the protein level. Indeed, immunoblotting confirmed the induced expression of runx2 produced by HT-2 (Figure 4). A slight, but not significant, increase in runx2 level was also observed for the T_3 treatment. In conclusion, chondrocytes apparently reached the pre-hypertrophic stage in the presence of HT-2, while T_3 could not promote this in the relatively short, 24-h-long time of the experiment. The indication that HT-2 would be such a strong inducer of runx2 expression was surprising.

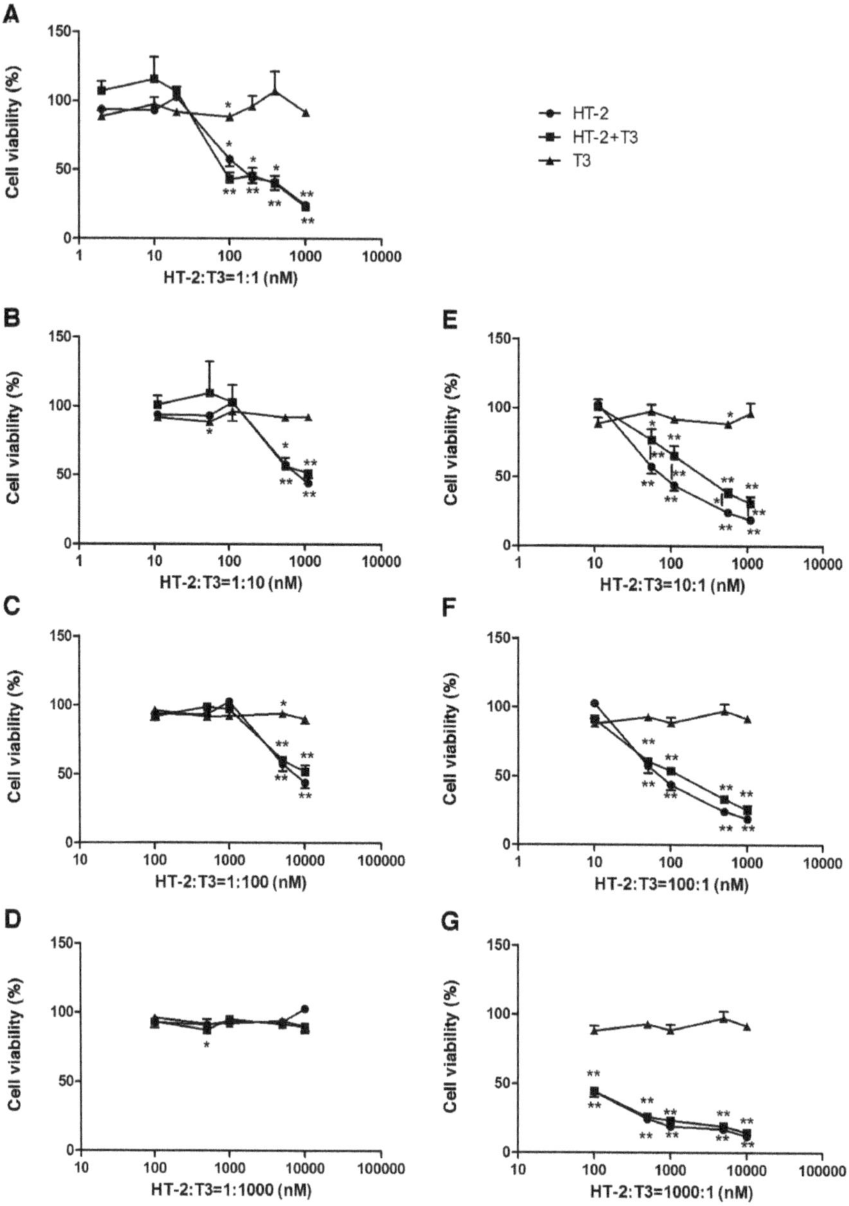

Figure 2. Cytotoxicity of T_3 and the HT-2 toxin. The ratios of HT-2:T_3 were (**A**) 1:1, (**B**) 1:10, (**C**) 1:100, (**D**) 1:1000, (**E**) 10:1, (**F**) 100:1, and (**G**) 1000:1. The values are shown as means ± SEM of three independent experiments. The cell viability in the non-treated control cultures were (**A**) 100.0% ± 4.5%, (**B**) 100.0% ± 3.7%, (**C**) 100.0% ± 5.0%, (**D**) 100.0% ± 4.1%, (**E**) 100.0% ± 0.4%, (**F**) 100.0% ± 1.3%, and (**G**) 100.0% ± 5.4%. Statistically significant differences against control cultures are marked with asterisks, * $p < 0.05$ and ** $p < 0.01$. The statistically significant differences observed between the HT-2 toxin and the mixture of the HT-2 toxin and T_3 are also marked in (**E**–**G**). The amounts of T_3 and HT-2 toxin for each mixture are provided in Table 1.

Table 1. The contents of the HT-2 toxin and T_3 mixtures.

Ratios	Components	Concentrations (nM)
1:1	HT-2	1, 5, 10, 50, 100, 200, 500
	T_3	1, 5, 10, 50, 100, 200, 500
	HT-2:T_3	1:1, 5:5, 10:10, 50:50, 100:100, 200:200, 500:500
1:10	HT-2	1, 5, 10, 50, 100
	T3	10, 50, 100, 500, 1000
	HT-2:T_3	1:10, 5:50, 10:100, 50:500, 100:1000
1:100	HT-2	1, 5, 10, 50, 100
	T_3	100, 500, 10, 50, 100, 200, 500
	HT-2:T_3	1:100, 5:500, 10:1000, 50:5000, 100:10,000
1:1000	HT-2	0.1, 0.5, 1, 5, 10
	T_3	100, 500, 1000, 5000, 10,000
	HT-2:T_3	0.1:100, 0.5:500, 1:1000, 5:5000, 10:10,000
10:1	HT-2	10, 50, 100, 500, 1000
	T_3	1, 5, 10, 50, 100
	HT-2:T_3	10:1, 50:5, 100:10, 500:50, 1000:100
100:1	HT-2	10, 5,0 100, 500, 1000
	T_3	0.1, 0.5, 1, 5, 10
	HT-2:T_3	10:0.1, 50:0.5, 100:1, 500:5, 1000:10
1000:1	HT-2	100, 500, 1000, 5000, 10,000
	T_3	0.1, 0.5, 1, 5, 10
	HT-2:T_3	100:0.1, 500:0.5, 1000:1, 5000:5, 10,000:10

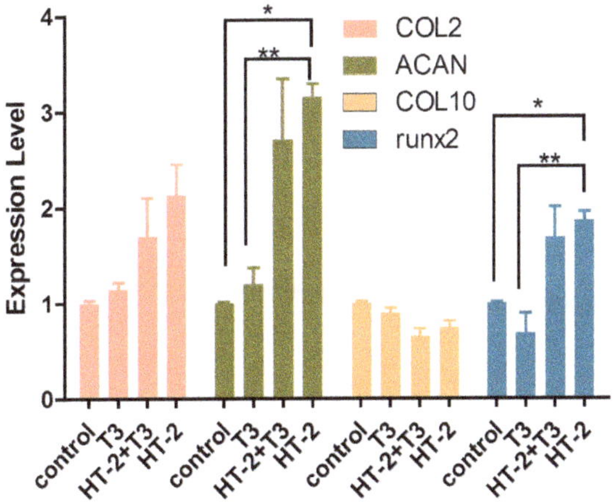

Figure 3. Gene expression levels of *collagen types II* and *X*, *aggrecan* and *runx2*, in C-28/I2 chondrocytes in control cultures and those treated with 50 nM T_3 alone, 50 nM T_3 plus 50 nM HT-2 toxin, and 50 nM HT-2 alone for 24 h. The fold changes are shown as mean ± SEM from three independent experiments. Statistically significant differences against control cultures are marked with asterisks, * $p < 0.05$ and ** $p < 0.01$.

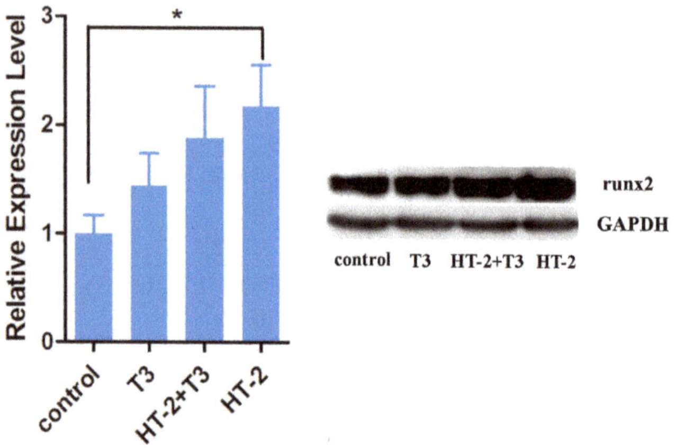

Figure 4. Protein expression levels of runx2 in C-28/I2 chondrocytes in control cultures and those treated with 50 nM T_3 alone, 50 nM T_3 plus 50 nM HT-2 toxin, and 50 nM HT-2 alone for 24 h. The fold changes are shown as mean ± SEM from four independent experiments. Statistically significant differences against control cultures are marked with asterisks, * $p < 0.05$.

3. Discussion

It is well known that T_3 has an important role in growth plate maturation and development [1,2] and that inhibition of the T_3 response by dominant-negative nuclear receptors promotes defects in cartilage maturation, ossification, and bone mineralization [19]. The regulation of T_3 is particularly important during growth, which is the time when aberrations in endochondral ossification and growth occur in KBD [20]. Mycotoxins T-2 and its metabolite HT-2 have been shown to accumulate especially in the skeletal tissues [11], and they have been considered as possible factors for the KBD.

In this study, the cytotoxicities of T_3 and the HT-2 toxin alone were first examined. At most, a very weak T_3-mediated cytotoxicity in C-28/I2 chondrocytes was noticed, even at a non-physiologically high dose following 24-h of exposure. Also, a longer, 72-h-treatment, changed the response only minimally. In contrast, the HT-2 toxin had a cytotoxic effect on human chondrocytes at a 50 nM concentration after 24-h-exposure. In growth plate chondrocytes, long-term exposure to T_3 inhibits cellular proliferation, which obviously is also related to hypertrophic differentiation [1].

When HT-2 toxin and T_3 were administered at equal concentrations, the concentration to induce a statistically significant decrease in cell viability was shifted from 50 nM to 100 nM, indicating a protective effect of T_3 on cytotoxicity induced by the HT-2 toxin. This led us to investigate how different molar ratios of the HT-2 toxin and T_3 affect chondrocyte viability. When the ratio of HT-2:T_3 was 10:1, HT-2 toxin concentrations ≥50 nM caused a significantly reduced cell viability, which was partly rescued by T_3. At ratios 100:1 and 1000:1, there were no obvious combined effects on cell viability.

Therefore, although T_3 helped to reduce the cytotoxicity produced by the HT-2 toxin to human chondrocytes, it was most effective at an HT-2 toxin concentration range of 50–100 nM. However, the mechanism of the protective effect of T_3 to chondrocyte death still remains unknown. In sheep growth plate chondrocytes, it has been shown that T_3 is linked to chondrocyte proliferative capacity by targeted *FGFR3* to regulate telomerase reverse transcriptase expression and telomerase activity [21]. Also, the bone morphogenetic protein pathway has been implicated to be essential for the function of T_3 in chondrogenesis [22].

To study the HT-2 and T_3 effects on gene expression, we selected 50 nM T_3 and 50 nM HT-2, since the 50 nM concentration of HT-2 was the lowest concentration that decreased the cell viability of cultured chondrocytes. It was also noticed that the HT-2 toxin induced an increase in gene expression of *aggrecan* and *runx2* and a trend for increased expression of *type II collagen*. The expression of *type X collagen*, a marker for hypertrophic chondrocytes [23], remained stable. Therefore, the cellular stage after HT-2 exposure can be considered to be pre-hypertrophic [18]. The increased level of runx2 at the protein level confirmed the mRNA result.

As mentioned previously, such a strong response in *aggrecan* and *runx2* by HT-2 in comparison to the T_3 effect was surprising, since T_3 is known to induce hypertrophic differentiation. In tissue engineering applications, T_3 has been shown to increase the expression and synthesis of type II collagen [24], and improve articular cartilage surface architecture [25]. As the metabolite of T-2 toxin, it would be reasonable to assume that the HT-2 toxin will share similarity with the T-2 toxin, which leads to cartilage destruction by the degradation of the extracellular matrix [26,27]. In another study, the T-2 toxin promoted *aggrecanase-2* mRNA expression [28]. The *ROS-NFκB-HIF-2α* pathway was shown to be essential for the catabolic effects of the T-2 toxin [29]. However, in this cell culture model, it was not possible to confirm the possible anabolic or catabolic effects of HT-2 or T_3 at the protein level due to the limited contents of extracellular matrix molecules secreted into the medium during the exposure time.

4. Conclusions

In conclusion, the HT-2 toxin led to significant cell death of human chondrocytes at rather low concentrations (threshold above 50 nM). Supplementation of T_3 in cell culture medium decreased the cytotoxic effects of the HT-2 toxin only when it was applied in molar ratio 1:10, while other molar combinations failed to produce protective effects. The decrease in cell viability caused by the HT-2 toxin may be partly related to the finding that the cells appeared to shift quickly into a pre-hypertrophic state, indicated by an increased expression of *aggrecan* and *runx2*, and partly *collagen type II*. However, the major part of the HT-2 toxin effects is most likely due to its toxicity. Thus, further studies on the exact mechanism underlying the combined effect of T_3 and HT-2 toxin on chondrocytes are warranted to provide a better understanding of the mechanism of HT-2 toxin cytotoxicity.

5. Materials and Methods

5.1. Chondrocyte Culture

The immortalized human chondrocyte cell line C28/I2 was a kind gift from Dr. Mary B. Goldring (Hospital for Special Surgery, New York, NY, USA). Chondrocytes were cultured in Dulbecco's modified Eagle's medium (DMEM/F12; Hyclone, Logan, UT, USA), supplemented with 10% fetal bovine serum (FBS; Zhejiang Tianhang Biological Technology Stock Co., Huzhou, China), 100 U/mL penicillin/100 μg/mL streptomycin (Hyclone) at 37 °C and 5% CO_2. During the culture period, the cells were passaged at subconfluency by sequential digestion in trypsin/EDTA (Hyclone; Sigma, St Louis, MO, USA), and the medium was replaced every 2 days [30]. Three to four independent experiments were performed.

5.2. MTT Cytotoxicity Assay

Human chondrocytes C-28/I2 were seeded in 96-well plates at a density of 6.5×10^3 cells/well. After incubation for 24 h, the culture medium was replaced to fresh medium (DMEM/F12 with 10% FBS and 1% penicillin and streptomycin) containing several mixture concentrations of T_3 and/or HT-2 toxin (Table 1), then treated for another 24 or 72 h. At the end of the intervention, the medium with T_3 and/or HT-2 toxin was removed and replaced with fresh medium, and 20 μL aliquots of 5 mg/mL MTT stock solution (Amresco, Solon, OH, USA) were added into each well. After 4 h incubation in the presence of MTT to allow time for formazan formation, the medium was removed, and 150 μL dimethylsulfoxide was used to dissolve the formazan crystals from the wells. Optical densities of the samples were measured with a multi-plate reader (Infinite M200; Tecan Group, Männedorf, Switzerland) at a wavelength of 490 nm. The control groups included blank controls and normal controls. The blank control was fresh medium without the cells, and the normal control referred to the medium from the cell without T_3 or the HT-2 toxin.

5.3. RNA Isolation and Quantitative Real-Time RT-PCR

Total RNA was isolated from the chondrocytes according to the manufacturer's protocols using Trizol reagent (Invitrogen, Carlsbad, CA, USA). Reverse-transcription was performed using PrimeScript™ RT Master Mix Kit (Takara, Kusatsu, Shiga, Japan). Real-time PCR reactions were conducted in the Real-Time PCR Detection System (Bio-Rad, Hercules, CA, USA) using TB Green Premix Ex Taq™ II Kit (Takara), using the following parameters: 95 °C for 5 s, then 60 °C for 30 s, and 72 °C for 30 s, 40 cycles. The fold changes of relative gene expression were calculated with the $2^{(-\Delta\Delta Ct)}$ method [31] using *GAPDH* as the reference gene. The primer sequences used in this study are shown in Table 2.

Table 2. Specific primers for quantitative RT-PCR.

Genes	Forward Primer	Reverse Primer
COL2A1	AGACTGGCGAGACTTGCGTCTA	ATCTCGGACGTTGGCAGTGTTG
ACAN	CTGAACGACAGGACCATCGAA	CGTGCCAGATCATCACCACA
COL10A1	GACTCATGTTTGGGTAGGCCTGTA	CCCTGAAGCCTGATCCAGGTA
Runx2	AGCTTCTGTCTGTGCCTTCTGG	GGAGTGGACGAGGCAAGAGTTT
GAPDH	GCACCGTCAAGGCTGAGAAC	TGGTGAAGACGCCAGTGGA

5.4. Immunoblot Analysis

The total protein was extracted from the cultured chondrocytes according to the manufacturer's protocols using an RIPA buffer (Beyotime, Shanghai, China). After denaturation, 30 μg of total protein was electrophoresed for immunoblot analysis. The blots were probed with primary antibodies directed against runx2 (Abcam, Cambridge, UK) overnight at 4 °C. GAPDH polyclonal antibody (Bioworld, Minneapolis, MN, USA) was used as a housekeeping reference. Peroxidase-conjugated goat anti-rabbit IgG (Thermo Fisher Scientific, Waltham, MA, USA) or goat anti-mouse IgG (Bioss, Shanghai, China) antibodies were used to visualize proteins using Western blotting chemiluminescence luminol reagent on a GeneGnome XRQ Western Blotting Analysis System (Syngene, Frederick, MD, USA). Working concentrations for each antibody were determined empirically based on the recommended stock solutions. Image J was used to quantify the band intensities of proteins of interest in the experimental and control groups.

5.5. Statistical Analysis

All experiments were performed three to four times. Parametric statistical analyses were selected to compare the effect of T3 and/or HT-2 toxin on C-28/I2 chondrocytes. One-way analysis of variance (ANOVA) was used to analyze the general difference, and the LSD-*t* (equal variances assumed) or Dunnett's T3-test (equal variances not assumed) post-hoc tests were used for further pairwise comparison with SPSS 13.0 (SPSS Inc., Chicago, IL, USA). The difference was considered statistically significant when the *p*-value was less than 0.05.

Supplementary Materials: The following are available online at http://www.mdpi.com/2072-6651/11/11/667/s1, Figure S1: The dose-effect plot for Figure 2 generated by CompuSyn software.

Author Contributions: Conceptualization, M.J.L. and X.G.; methodology, F.Z., M.J.L. and, X.G.; software, F.Z.; resources, W.S. and P.Z.; data curation, Y.Z. and H.W.; writing—original draft preparation, F.Z.; writing—review and editing, M.J.L., W.S., P.Z., Y.Z., H.W. and X.G.; supervision, M.J.L. and X.G.; project administration, X.G.; funding acquisition, X.G.

Funding: This research was funded by the National Natural Science Foundation of China, grant numbers 81620108026 and 81472924.

Acknowledgments: We thank Mary B. Goldring for donating the immortalized human chondrocyte cell line C-28/I2. We thank Daniel Marcellino, Umeå University for checking the language of the manuscript.

Conflicts of Interest: The authors declare no conflict of interest. The funders had no role in the design of the study; in the collection, analyses, or interpretation of data; in the writing of the manuscript, or in the decision to publish the results.

References

1. Robson, H.; Siebler, T.; Stevens, D.A.; Shalet, S.M.; Williams, G.R. Thyroid hormone acts directly on growth plate chondrocytes to promote hypertrophic differentiation and inhibit clonal expansion and cell proliferation. *Endocrinology* **2000**, *141*, 3887–3897. [CrossRef] [PubMed]
2. Bassett, J.H.D.; Williams, G.R. The molecular actions of thyroid hormone in bone. *Trends Endocrinol. Metab.* **2003**, *14*, 356–364. [CrossRef]
3. Lee, J.K.; Gegg, C.A.; Hu, J.C.; Reddi, A.H.; Athanasiou, K.A. Thyroid hormone enhance the biomechanical functionality of scaffold-free neocartilage. *Arthritis Res. Ther.* **2015**, *17*, 28. [CrossRef] [PubMed]
4. Fernandez-Pernas, P.; Fafian-Labora, J.; Lesende-Rodriguez, I.; Mateos, J.; de la Fuente, A.; Fuentes, I.; de Toro Santos, J.; Blanco Garcia, F.; Arufe, M.C. 3,3′,5-triiodo-L-thyronine increases in vitro chondrogenesis of mesenchymal stem cells from umbilical cord stroma through SRC2. *J. Cell. Biochem.* **2016**, *117*, 2097–2108. [CrossRef] [PubMed]
5. Wang, L.; Shao, Y.Y.; Ballock, R.T. Thyroid hormone interacts with the Wnt/β-catenin signaling pathway in the terminal differentiation of growth plate chondrocytes. *J. Bone Miner. Res.* **2007**, *22*, 1988–1995. [CrossRef] [PubMed]
6. Ray, R.D.; Asling, C.W.; Walker, D.G.; Simpson, M.E.; Li, C.H.; Evans, H.M. Growth and differentiation of the skeleton in thyreoidectomized-hypophysectomized rats treated with thyroxin, growth hormone, and combination. *J. Bone Jt. Surg. Am.* **1954**, *36*, 94–103. [CrossRef]
7. Nagase, H.; Nagasawa, Y.; Tachida, Y.; Sakakibara, S.; Okutsu, J.; Suematsu, N.; Arita, S.; Shimada, K. Deiodinase 2 upregulation demonstrated in osteoarthritis patients cartilage causes cartilage destruction in tissue-specific transgenic rats. *Osteoarthr. Cartil.* **2013**, *21*, 514–523. [CrossRef]
8. Xiong, Y.M.; Song, R.X.; Jiao, X.H.; Du, X.L.; Liu, J.F.; Liu, X.; Chen, Q. PMS13-Study on mechanism of type 2 deiodinase gene and Erk signal transduction in Kashin-Beck disease. *Value Health* **2014**, *17*, A43. [CrossRef]
9. Wen, Y.; Zhang, F.; Li, C.; He, S.; Tan, W.; Lei, Y.; Zhang, Q.; Yu, H.; Zheng, J.; Guo, X. Gene expression analysis suggests bone development-related genes GDF5 and DIO2 are involved in the development of Kashin-Beck disease in children rather than adults. *PLoS ONE* **2014**, *9*, e103618. [CrossRef]
10. Van der Fels-Klerx, H.J. Occurrence data of trichothecene mycotoxins T-2 toxin and HT-2 toxin in food and feed. *EFSA Support. Publ.* **2010**, *7*, 1–43. [CrossRef]
11. Yu, F.F.; Lin, X.L.; Yang, L.; Liu, H.; Wang, X.; Fang, H.; Lammi, M.J.; Guo, X. Comparison of T-2 toxin and HT-2 toxin distributed in the skeletal system with that in other tissues of rats by acute toxicity test. *Biomed. Environ. Sci* **2017**, *30*, 851–854. [CrossRef] [PubMed]
12. Yu, F.F.; Lin, X.L.; Liu, H.; Yang, L.; Goldring, M.B.; Lammi, M.J.; Guo, X. Selenium promotes metabolic conversion of T-2 toxin to HT-2 toxin in cultured human chondrocytes. *J. Trace Elem. Med. Biol.* **2017**, *44*, 218–224. [CrossRef]
13. Li, Y.; Wang, Z.; Beier, R.C.; Shen, J.; de Smet, D.; de Saeger, S.; Zhang, S. T-2 toxin, a trichothecene mycotoxin: Review of toxicity, metabolism, and analytical methods. *J. Agric. Food Chem.* **2011**, *59*, 3441–3453. [CrossRef] [PubMed]
14. Yu, F.F.; Lin, X.L.; Wang, X.; Ping, Z.G.; Guo, X. Comparison of apoptosis and autophagy in human chondrocytes induced by the T-2 and HT-2 toxins. *Toxins* **2019**, *11*, 260. [CrossRef] [PubMed]
15. Liu, J.; Wang, L.; Guo, X.; Pang, Q.; Wu, S.; Wu, C.; Xu, P.; Bai, Y. The role of mitochondria in T-2 toxin-induced human chondrocytes apoptosis. *PLoS ONE* **2014**, *9*, e108394. [CrossRef]
16. Chang, Y.; Wang, X.; Sun, Z.; Jin, Z.; Chen, M.; Wang, X.; Lammi, M.J.; Guo, X. Inflammatory cytokine of IL-1β is involved in T-2 toxin-triggered chondrocyte injury and metabolism imbalance by the activation of Wnt/β-catenin signaling. *Mol. Immunol.* **2017**, *91*, 195–201. [CrossRef]

17. Li, D.; Han, J.; Guo, X.; Qu, C.; Yu, F.; Wu, X. The effects of T-2 toxin on the prevalence and development of Kashin-Beck disease in China: A meta-analysis and systematic review. *Toxicol. Res.* **2016**, *5*, 731–751. [CrossRef]
18. Bruderer, M.; Richards, R.G.; Alini, M.; Stoddart, M.J. Role and regulation of RUNX2 in osteogenesis. *Eur. Cell Mater.* **2014**, *28*, 269–286. [CrossRef]
19. Desjardin, C.; Charles, C.; Benoist-Lasselin, C.; Riviere, J.; Gilles, M.; Chassande, O.; Morgenthaler, C.; Laloe, D.; Lecardonnel, J.; Flamant, F.; et al. Chondrocytes play a major role in the stimulation of bone growth by thyroid hormone. *Endocrinology* **2014**, *155*, 3123–3135. [CrossRef]
20. Guo, X.; Ma, W.J.; Zhang, F.; Ren, F.L.; Qu, C.J.; Lammi, M.J. Recent advances in the research of an endemic osteochondropathy in China: Kashin-Beck disease. *Osteoarthr. Cartil.* **2014**, *22*, 1774–1783. [CrossRef]
21. Smith, L.B.; Belanger, J.M.; Oberbauer, A.M. Fibroblast growth factor receptor 3 effects on proliferation and telomerase activity in sheep growth plate chondrocytes. *J. Anim. Sci. Biotechnol.* **2012**, *3*, 39. [CrossRef]
22. Karl, A.; Olbrich, N.; Pfeifer, C.; Berner, A.; Zellner, J.; Kujat, R.; Angele, P.; Nerlich, M.; Mueller, M.B. Thyroid hormone-induced hypertrophy in mesenchymal stem cell chondrogenesis is mediated by bone morphogenetic protein-4. *Tissue Eng. A* **2014**, *20*, 178–188. [CrossRef] [PubMed]
23. Von der Mark, K.; Kirsch, T.; Nerlich, A.; Kuss, A.; Weseloh, G.; Glückert, K.; Stöss, H. Type X collagen synthesis in human osteoarthritic cartilage. Indication of chondrocyte hypertrophy. *Arthritis Rheumatol.* **1992**, *35*, 806–811. [CrossRef] [PubMed]
24. Whitney, G.A.; Kean, T.J.; Fernandes, R.J.; Waldman, S.; Tse, M.Y.; Pang, S.C.; Mansour, J.M.; Dennis, J.E. Thyroxine increases collagen type II expression and accumulation in scaffold-free tissue-engineered articular cartilage. *Tissue Eng. A* **2018**, *24*, 369–381. [CrossRef] [PubMed]
25. Jia, P.T.; Zhang, X.L.; Zuo, H.N.; Lu, X.; Gai, P.Z. A study on role of triiodothyronine (T3) hormone on the improvement of articular cartilage surface architecture. *Exp. Toxicol. Pathol.* **2017**, *69*, 625–629. [CrossRef] [PubMed]
26. Chen, J.; Chu, Y.; Cao, J.; Wang, W.; Liu, J.; Wang, J. Effects of T-2 toxin and selenium on chondrocyte expression of matrix metalloproteinases (MMP-1, MMP-13), α2-macroglobulin (α2M) and TIMPs. *Toxicol. Vitro* **2011**, *25*, 492–499. [CrossRef] [PubMed]
27. Li, Y.; Zou, N.; Wang, J.; Wang, K.W.; Li, F.Y.; Chen, F.X.; Sun, B.Y.; Sun, D.J. TGF-β1/Smad3 signaling pathway mediates T-2 toxin-induced decrease of type II collagen in cultured rat chondrocytes. *Toxins* **2017**, *9*, 359. [CrossRef]
28. Li, S.Y.; Cao, J.L.; Shi, Z.L.; Chen, J.H.; Zhang, Z.T.; Hughes, C.E.; Caterson, B. Promotion of the articular cartilage proteoglycan degradation by T-2 toxin and selenium protective effect. *J. Zhejiang Univ. Sci. B* **2008**, *9*, 22–33. [CrossRef]
29. Tian, J.; Yan, J.; Wang, W.; Zhong, N.; Tian, L.; Sun, J.; Min, Z.; Ma, J.; Lu, S. T-2 toxin enhances catabolic activity of hypertrophic chondrocytes through ROS-NF-κB-HIF-2α pathway. *Toxicol. Vitro* **2012**, *26*, 1106–1113. [CrossRef]
30. Goldring, M.B. Immortalization of human articular chondrocytes for generation of stable, differentiated cell lines. *Methods Mol. Med.* **2004**, *100*, 23–36. [CrossRef]
31. Livak, K.J.; Schmittgen, T.D. Analysis of relative gene expression data using real-time quantitative PCR and the 2(-delta delta C(T)) method. *Methods* **2001**, *25*, 402–408. [CrossRef]

toxins

MDPI

Article

Comprehensive Evaluation of the Efficiency of Yeast Cell Wall Extract to Adsorb Ochratoxin A and Mitigate Accumulation of the Toxin in Broiler Chickens

Suvi Vartiainen [1,*], Alexandros Yiannikouris [2], Juha Apajalahti [1] and Colm A. Moran [3]

1 Alimetrics Research Ltd., 02920 Espoo, Finland; j.apajalahti@alimetrics.com
2 Alltech Inc., 3031 Catnip Hill Road, Nicholasville, KY 40356, USA; ayiannikouris@Alltech.com
3 Alltech SARL, Rue Charles Amand, 14500 Vire, France; cmoran@alltech.com
* Correspondence: suvi.vartiainen@alimetrics.com; Tel.: +358-405-715-147

Received: 28 October 2019; Accepted: 31 December 2019; Published: 7 January 2020

Abstract: Ochratoxin A (OTA) is a common mycotoxin contaminant in animal feed. When absorbed from the gastrointestinal tract, OTA has a propensity for pathological effects on animal health and deposition in animal tissues. In this study, the potential of yeast cell wall extracts (YCWE) to adsorb OTA was evaluated using an in vitro method in which consecutive animal digestion events were simulated. Low pH markedly increased OTA binding to YCWE, which was reversed with a pH increased to 6.5. Overall, in vitro analysis revealed that 30% of OTA was adsorbed to YCWE. Additional computational molecular modelling revealed that change in pH alters the OTA charge and modulates the interaction with the YCWE β-D-glucans. The effectiveness of YCWE was tested in a 14-day broiler chicken trial. Birds were subjected to five dietary treatments; with and without OTA, and OTA combined with YCWE at three dosages. At the end of the trial, liver OTA deposition was evaluated. Data showed a decrease of up to 30% in OTA deposits in the liver of broilers fed both OTA and YCWE. In the case of OTA, a tight correlation between the mitigation efficacy of YCWE between in vitro and in vivo model could be observed.

Keywords: ochratoxin A; mitigation; mycotoxin binding; yeast cell wall extracts

Key Contribution: Parallel mechanistic experiments conducted in vitro and in silico to measure the OTA sequestration efficacy of YCWE detected a tight correlation with in vivo mitigation of the liver deposition of OTA by the product. This suggests that the methods applied were able to model the in vivo situation and can reliably be used for initial product testing.

---

1. Introduction

Ochratoxin A (OTA), a mycotoxin produced by toxigenic species of *Aspergillus* and *Penicillium* fungi, is a common contaminant in cereals, fruits, and nuts intended for human and animal consumption. For both these fungal species, moisture and temperature are key factors for growth and toxin production. Thus, OTA can be produced during plant growth, harvest, and storage [1,2]. The European Commission provides maximum guidance levels for OTA in animal feeds. For broiler chickens, the OTA concentration in complete feed and in individual cereal ingredients used for feed formulation should not exceed 0.1 and 0.25 mg/kg, respectively [3]. Nevertheless, the presence of OTA at a chronic concentration, whilst not necessarily posing a health issue, could be disadvantageous to bird performance and as such contribute to a negative economic output in a broiler operation. In this context, the use of appropriate mitigation programs is often recommended. Toxin adsorbents are frequently supplemented to animal diets to prevent the deleterious effect of mycotoxins, among them specific yeast cell wall extracts have shown promising results [4–6].

Several experiments were carried out to study the effects of OTA on production parameters in animal husbandry. Studies have shown that administration of diets contaminated with OTA reduces feed intake and body weight gain in broiler chickens in a dose-dependent manner and negatively affects weight gain in swine [7]. OTA has been shown to exert toxicity by inhibition of mitochondrial function, increased oxidative stress, and inhibition of protein synthesis [8]. At a molecular level, OTA pathology includes damaged membrane lipids, DNA mutations, and nitrosylated proteins [8]. In both mammalian and avian animals, sub-acute exposure to OTA has nephrotoxic, immunosuppressive, and teratogenic effects [9]. Carcinogenic effects of OTA have been demonstrated in mice and rats; while in humans, renal and testicular cancer have been associated with OTA exposure [9].

To date, absorption of OTA has been studied mainly in mice and rats. The results for rats indicate that the major sites of OTA absorption are the duodenum and proximal jejunum, but the toxin is also absorbed from the stomach [10]. Studies of OTA absorption show that the toxin can be quickly detected in peripheral blood, with the maximum concentration in blood following oral administration of OTA being reached after 20 min in chickens, 1 h in rabbits, and 10 h in pigs [11]. Absorbed OTA binds to blood proteins, such as albumin, and distributes throughout the animal. The half-life of OTA in blood after oral administration depends greatly on animal species, e.g., it is 6.7 h in quail, 39 h in mice, 120 h in rats, and 510 h in Rhesus monkeys (*Macaca mulatta*) [12]. OTA is mainly detoxified into ochratoxin α (OTα) by animal tissues and by intestinal anaerobic bacteria. Other metabolites of OTA are formed in the liver by cytochrome P450 and these metabolites differ from one animal species to another [13]. OTA and OTα are excreted in faeces, whereas other OTA metabolites, together with OTA and OTα, are found in urine [14].

Mycotoxin adsorbents or sequestrants are used in animal husbandry due to the common occurrence of mycotoxins in feedstuffs. The purpose of the mycotoxin adsorbents is to bind to the toxin in the digestive tract of the animal, after which the adsorbent-toxin complex is transported intact through the gastro-intestinal tract of the animal and excreted. In poultry, adsorbents such as yeast cell walls, esterified glucomannan, and aluminosilicate have been tested [15]. For the toxin adsorbent to be functional, it is essential that the digestive processes of the animal do not alter its properties. In order to analyse the effects of digestion, toxin, and adsorbent have been subjected to digestion treatments—such as low pH—in in vitro conditions, and the results compared with a control without digestion treatment [16,17].

Yeast cell wall extract (YCWE) has been studied with emphasis on its toxin adsorbent properties [18]. The YCWE has been shown efficacious in sequestering mycotoxins in in vitro and decreasing the adverse effects of mycotoxins in vivo conditions [15,16]. In the current study, the adherence of YCWE to OTA were examined both in vitro and in silico. The aim was to obtain accurate information on the interaction between OTA and YCWE during digestion treatments and on the effect of low pH on OTA-YCWE complex formation. Unlike previous studies, the effectiveness of YCWE in decreasing the OTA bioavailability was subsequently assessed in vivo in broiler chickens, at a dose that did not exceed the recommendation for commercial broiler feeds presented in the European Union guidance [3]. In accordance with the EFSA dossier preparation instructions for Substances for the Reduction of Mycotoxin Contamination (SMRC) [19], the efficacy of YCWE in reducing bioavailability of OTA was determined with analysis of OTA deposited in broiler liver tissue.

2. Results

2.1. In Vitro Evaluation of the Influence of Simulated Digestive Conditions on OTA Sequestration

When radiolabelled OTA was incubated with YCWE at pH 6.5, there was a significant decrease in the level of free OTA compared to the control treatment without YCWE. The level of free OTA decreased by 17.1 ± 0.5% (SE) with a YCWE dose of 5 mg/mL and by 28.4 ± 0.6% with a YCWE dose of 15 mg/mL. Subjecting the YCWE solution to further digestion treatments—i.e., low pH—and a 2-step pepsin and pancreatin enzymatic treatment, did not alter the binding properties of YCWE to OTA measured at pH 6.5, as shown in Figure 1. This suggests that the YCWE product tested was not susceptible to the digestive treatments.

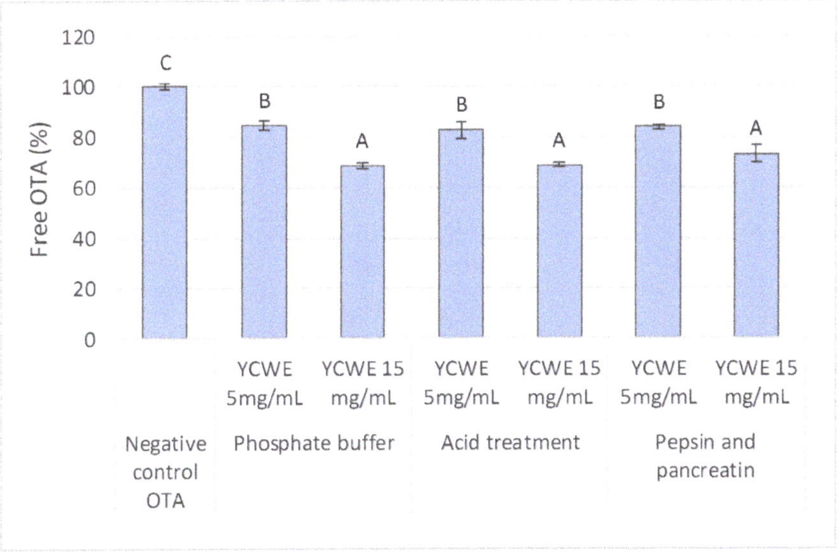

Figure 1. Percentage of free ochratoxin A (OTA) measured in the supernatant after pH adjustment to 6.5 following reaction in a two-step digestive simulation (acidic and two-step pepsin and pancreatin enzymatic treatment) with yeast cell wall extract (YCWE) used at 5.0 and 15.0 mg/mL inclusion level. Error bars indicate standard error. Different letters above bars indicate significant differences between treatments ($p < 0.05$).

2.2. In Vitro OTA Sequestration by YCWE

Evaluation of the effect of pH in each digestion phase on YCWE sequestering activity toward OTA revealed a major decrease in the level of free [^{3}H]-OTA activity at pH 2.5, implying that the binding efficacy was increased in an acidic gastric environment (Figure 2). Further analysis revealed that the decrease in free [^{3}H]-OTA level depended only on the pH lowering step and was reversible, as the level of free toxin increased following pH neutralization to 6.5. None of the treatments with digestive enzymes had any additional effect on the detected [^{3}H]-OTA activity.

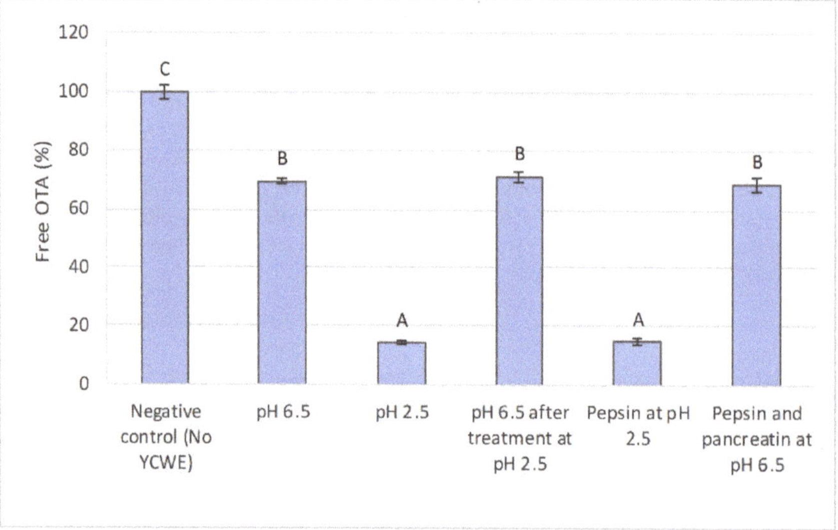

Figure 2. Percentage of free ochratoxin A (OTA) measured after the interaction with yeast cell wall extract (YCWE), at each individual digestion phases and evaluation of the influence of pH on sequestration. The YCWE inclusion level was 15 mg/mL. Error bars indicate standard error. Different letters above bars indicate significant differences between treatments ($p < 0.05$).

2.3. *In Silico Assessment of the Sequestration Properties Investigated by Molecular Mechanics*

Molecular mechanics modelling and docking were performed under vacuum and demonstrated that, because OTA possesses five rotatable bonds mainly located around the amide bond connecting the dihydroisocoumarin moiety to L-phenylalanine, it could adapt to a larger set of docking sites with little energetic penalties of 3 kcal/mol of amplitude. In the docking experiment performed, parallel positioning of these two moieties (Figure S1A1,A2) gave the lowest binding energy and thus accounting for the highest affinity of interaction (Table S1), whereas an orthogonal positioning of the two moieties was less favourable. Nevertheless, the extension of the interaction to the entire chain of β-D-glucans demonstrated that OTA can be positioned in several adjacent binding sites along the β-(1,3)-carbohydrate chain (Figure 3) forming up to three hydrogen bonds. The presence of side chains of β-(1,6)-D-glucans provided increased stability of interaction, with the majority of the most favourable poses centered around the β-(1,3)/β-(1,6)-D-glucans pocket (Figure 4), especially in the case of a compact side chain conformation (Figure 4B1,B2). The OTA molecule has a five hydrogen bond acceptor count and three donor count, and the strongest acidic pKa was of 3.17. Under the conditions investigated in vitro and in vivo, the uncharged form of OTA represented 82.50% of the OTA population at pH 2.5 whereas at pH 6.5, 96.45% of the OTA population consists of a single charged deprotonated molecule on the carboxylic moiety, with a charge of −1.03. An increase of pH to 8.5 would produce a second charge on the hydroxyl group of the coumarin moiety. The β-D glucan carbohydrate has its strongest acidic pKa for a value of 11.22, making this a fully uncharged molecule for values of pH under pH 9.0. The changes in protonation of the OTA molecule were evaluated in terms of docking interaction, but both states exhibited somewhat comparable binding affinities (Table S1). The orientation of the L-phenylalanine moiety was further influenced by the presence of side chains of β-(1,6)-D-glucans which could involve further π-stacking interactions than protonation changes.

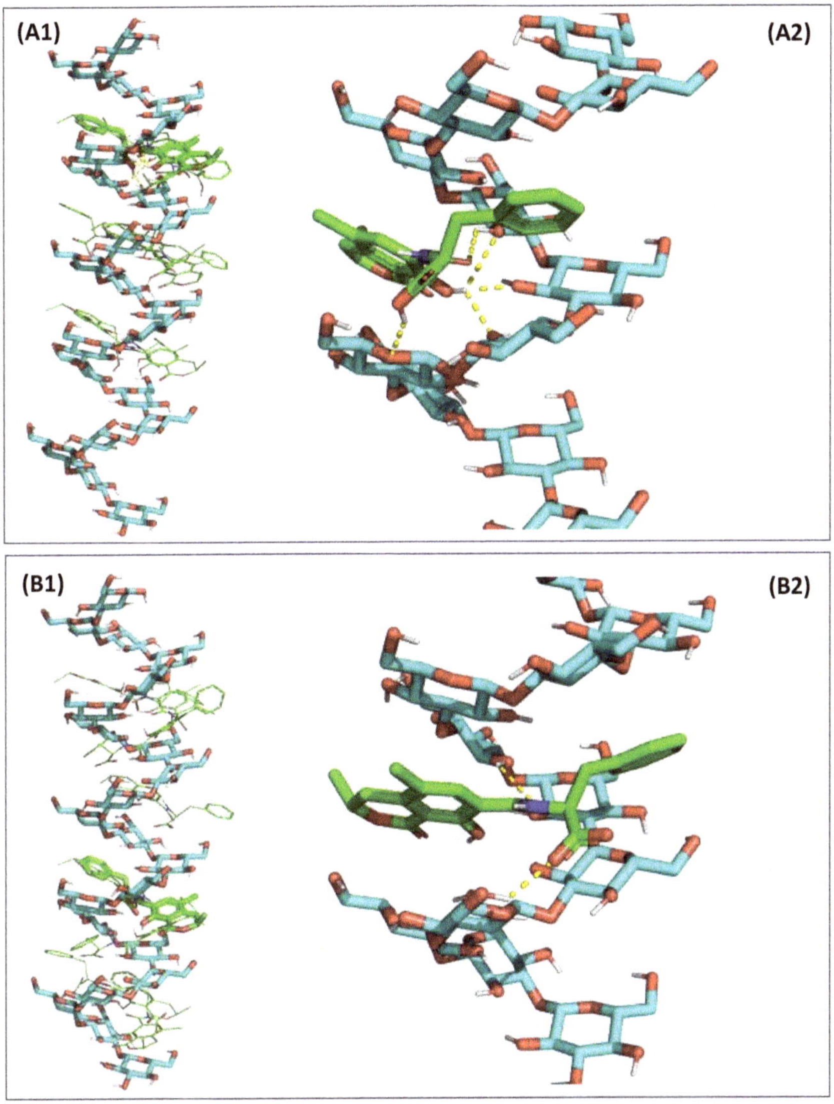

Figure 3. Computer generated views of the energy-minimized 9 states (**A1**,**B1**) of ochratoxin A (OTA) docking into β-(1,3)-D-glucans chain alone with (**A2**) corresponding to the most energy favorable OTA docking with no charge (corresponding to charge state at pH 3.0) and (**B2**) corresponding to the most energy favorable OTA docking with a partial charge equal to −1 (corresponding to charge state at pH 6.5).

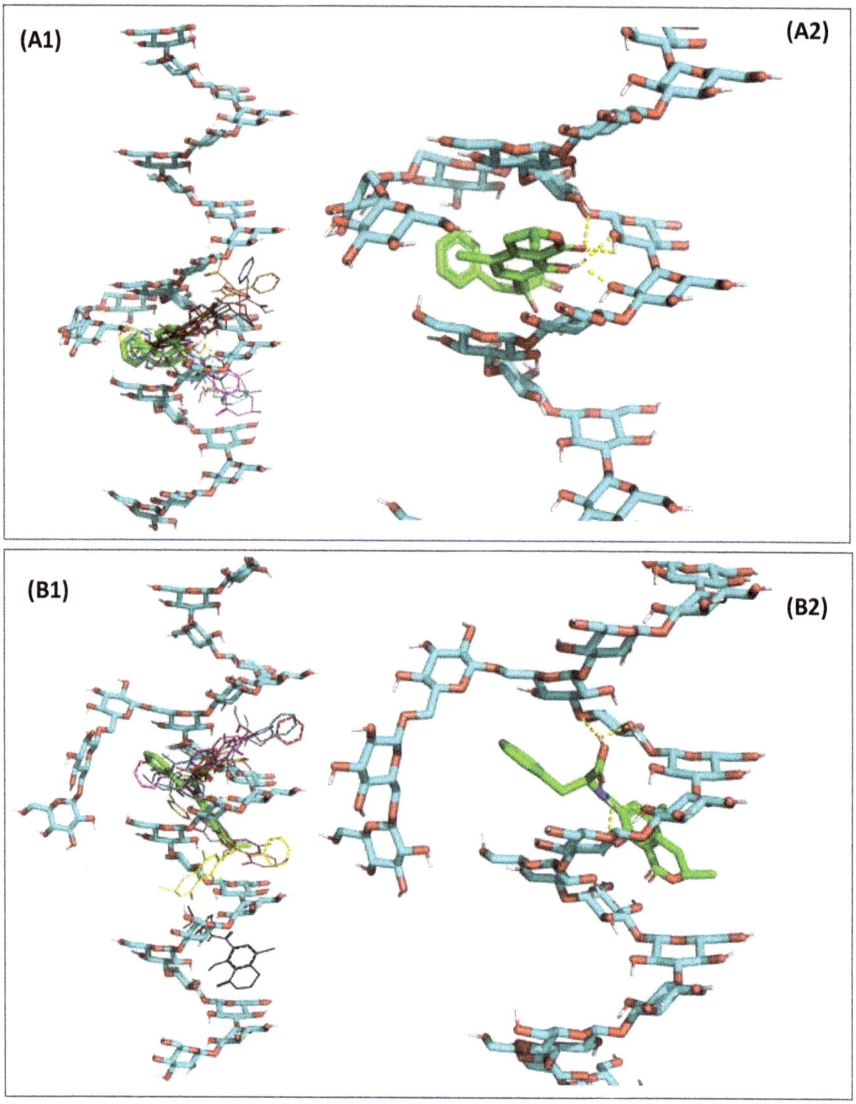

Figure 4. Computer generated views of the energy-minimized 9 states (**A1**,**B1**) of ochratoxin A (OTA) docking into β-(1,3)-D-glucans either branched with the first conformation of β-(1,6)-D-glucans (**A2**, most energy favorable OTA docking position) and the second conformation of β-(1,6)-D-glucans (**B2**, most energy favorable OTA docking).

2.4. *In Silico Assessment of the Sequestration Properties Investigated by Molecular Dynamics*

To understand the chemical interaction of OTA and glucans further, we carried out molecular dynamics simulation to understand the stability of the interaction in a solvated system using the best pose of OTA in the β-(1,3)-D-glucan chain as determined with the molecular mechanics investigations. To study the impact of pH, if it is possible to introduce ions in the solvent box environment it is only useful for the extreme ends of the pH scale due to the limited size of the solvent box and ion to water molecule ratio. A better approach was to evaluate the strength of interaction by calculating all relevant pKa values for the molecules of interest and assign their dominant protonation state at the two pH studied herein. In this context, if β-(1,3)-D-glucans have a very high pKa and do not exhibit any charges under the conditions tested, OTA was studied either fully protonated or singly deprotonated corresponding to the protonation stages at pH 2.5 and 6.5, respectively. In this context, after neutralization and a short minimization step, a molecular dynamics simulation was carried out. The results showed that under simulation conditions, the β-(1,3)-D-glucans structure was affected, and the positioning of the OTA could then move outside the β-(1,3)-D-glucans binding pocket, which was particularly the case at pH 6.5. Two models were tested with and without constraints on the glucan chain to work with two degrees of conformational changes of the carbohydrate. In a non-constrained receptor setting, the interaction between the β-(1,3)-D-glucans and the fully protonated OTA exhibited a higher incidence of neutral interaction (Lennard-Jones potential energy) than a singly unprotonated OTA, with energy values of −114.7 and −47.4 kJ/mol respectively, whereas coulombic potential energy accounting for ionic interactions was, as expected, more important for the singly deprotonated OTA state, −47.5 and −104.4 kJ/mol (Table 1). In this context, the total potential energy of interactions favoured the protonated OTA stage and the observed increased stability at pH 2.5 compared to pH 6.5. In a restraint β-(1,3)-D-glucan conformation, if Coulombic energy was of the same order of magnitude for the two stages of protonation of OTA, neutral stability interactions were increased for the singly deprotonated OTA, increasing the overall total stability of the complex at pH 6.5. For both β-(1,3)-D-glucan conformations, average hydrogen bonds for unprotonated OTA was around 3, whereas it varied between 1 and 2 for the protonated OTA. Interaction with water was more pronounced with the deprotonated OTA, inducing a higher degree of competition between the glucan receptor and the solvent environment. The computer generated views at pH 2.5 (Figure 5) and at pH 6.5 (Figure 6) showed that in acidic condition, both unconstrainted and constrained β-(1,3)-D-glucan conformations tended to have their helical shape preserved and could maintain the protonated OTA in the docking site. Under neutral pH 6.5 conditions, the β-(1,3)-D-glucan structure was heavily affected and the position of OTA tended to move outside of the binding pocket site, the binding of the deprotonated OTA molecule becoming more of a surface interaction, prone to higher interaction with water molecule of the solvent box.

Table 1. Interaction energy measured as short-range Coulombic potential energy (ionic interaction), short-range Lennard-Jones potential energy (neutral molecules interaction) and total energy (kJ/mol) after molecular dynamic simulation, in a two conformation of β-(1,3)-D-glucans unconstrained or constrained using a force constant of 1000 kJ/mol/nm^2, in a solvent box (water) when interacting with two protonated stages of ochratoxin A (OTA).

pH	OTA State	Energy	(kJ/mol)	Average H-Bond G3-OTA	Average H-Bond OTA-Water
		Constrained Receptor			
pH 2.5	Protonated OTA and glucan chain Energy	Coulombic Energy	−47.5541 ± 3.0	2.218	3.861
		Lennard-Jones energy	−114.6890 ± 3.9		
		Total	−162.2431		
pH 6.5	Singly deprotonated OTA and glucan chain energy	Coulombic Energy	−104.4470 ± 4.6	3.010	5.624
		Lennard-Jones energy	−47.3817 ± 4.4		
		Total	−151.8287		
		Unconstrainted Receptor			
pH 2.5	Protonated OTA and glucan chain Energy	Coulombic Energy	−58.1255 ± 2.4	0.911	4.316
		Lennard-Jones energy	−87.1747 ± 2.9		
		Total	−145.3002		
pH 6.5	Singly deprotonated OTA and glucan chain energy	Coulombic Energy	−101.9410 ± 9.2	2.891	6.604
		Lennard-Jones energy	−80.0512 ± 6.7		
		Total	−181.9922		

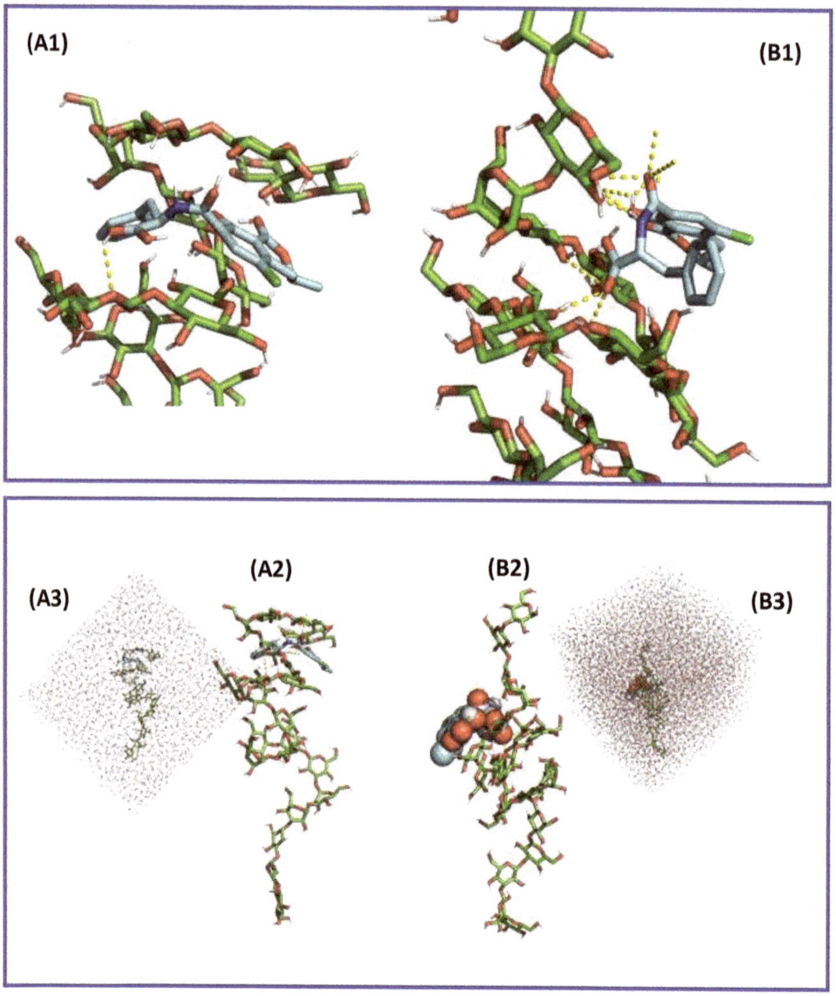

Figure 5. Computer generated views of the molecular interaction following a molecular dynamic simulation in a solvent box containing 8172 molecules of water, with a singly deprotonated molecule of ochratoxin A accounting for its state at a pH of 2.5 and when docked according to its highest affinity pose into an unconstrained (**A1**, interaction site detail, **A2**, full molecules displayed, **A3**, full molecule within solvent box displayed) and constrained (**B1**, interaction site detail, **B2**, full molecules displayed, **B3**, full molecule within solvent box displayed) conformation of β-(1,3)-D-glucans chain. The generated views corresponded to a 10-ns molecular dynamic simulation equilibrated at 310 K.

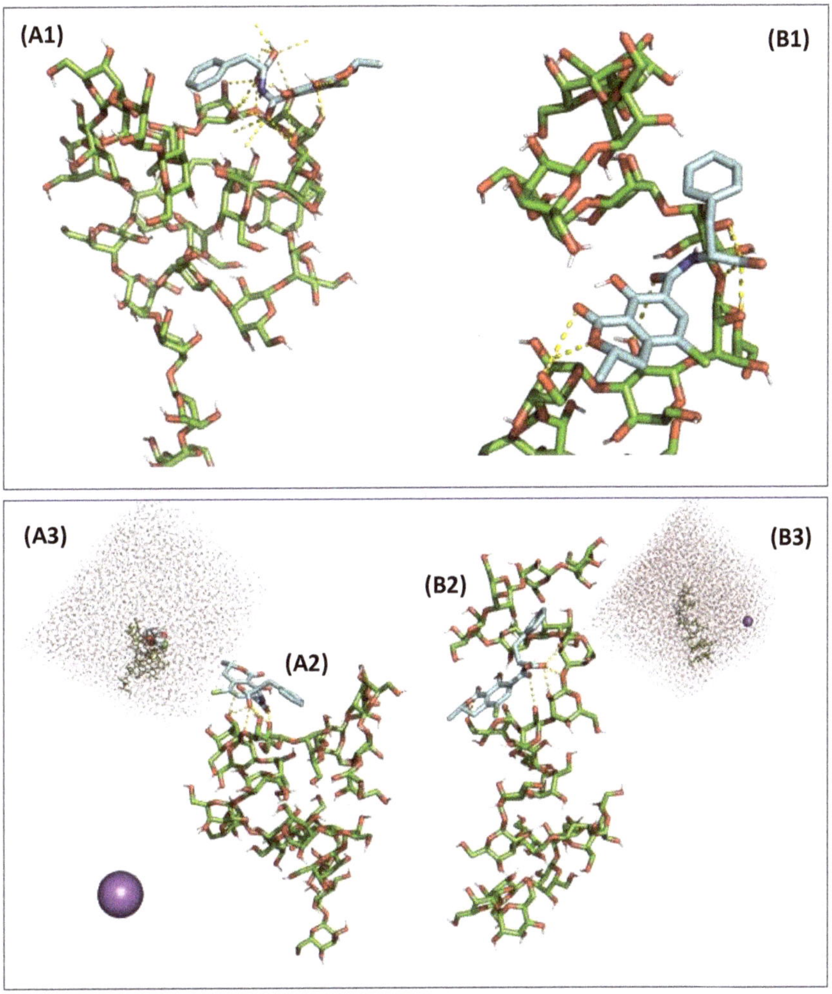

Figure 6. Computer generated views of the molecular interaction following a molecular dynamic simulation in a solvent box containing 8171 molecules of water and 1 Na^+ ion, with a singly deprotonated molecule of ochratoxin A accounting for its state at a pH of 6.5 and when docked according to its highest affinity pose into an unconstrained (**A1**, interaction site detail, **A2**, full molecules displayed, **A3**, full molecule within solvent box displayed) and constrained (**B1**, interaction site detail, **B2**, full molecules displayed, **B3**, full molecule within solvent box displayed) conformation of β-(1,3)-D-glucans chain. The generated views corresponded to a 10-ns molecular dynamic simulation equilibrated at 310 K.

2.5. In Vivo Broiler Chicken Feeding Trial

Feeding broilers with OTA at the maximum concentration recommended under European Commission guidance did not affect any of the broiler performance parameters measured (Table 2), e.g., no differences were observed in body weight, feed consumption (not shown), or mortality. Moreover, FCR was unaffected by OTA and YCWE addition (Table 2). Thus, administration of OTA and YCWE to broilers for 14 days was well tolerated by the birds.

Table 2. Broiler chicken performance in the 21-day feeding trial with ochratoxin A (OTA) and yeast cell wall (YCWE) added to the diet ($p < 0.05$), FCR = feed conversion ratio.

Diet	Body Weight (g)		Mortality (%)	FCR Day 1–21
	Day 1	Day 21		
Control	45.9 ± 0.7	856 ± 33	2.1 ± 2.1	1.62 ± 0.12
+ OTA	46.5 ± 0.6	841 ± 37	4.2 ± 4.2	1.48 ± 0.03
+ OTA + YCWE 2.0 kg/T	45.0 ± 0.6	782 ± 22	6.3 ± 3.0	1.73 ± 0.15
+ OTA + YCWE 4.0 kg/T	45.6 ± 0.5	832 ± 22	2.1 ± 2.1	1.49 ± 0.05
+ OTA + YCWE 8.0 kg/T	46.0 ± 0.9	832 ± 45	2.1 ± 2.1	1.50 ± 0.04

2.6. Analysis of OTA Deposits in Broiler Livers

Feeding broiler chickens the maximum recommended concentration of OTA led to toxin deposition in the liver (Figure 7). The toxin deposition rate was highest in birds fed OTA alone, while adding YCWE to the diet lowered the level of OTA in the liver. In broilers fed the control diet without OTA, the level of OTA was negligible. Adding YCWE to the diet at doses of 4.0 and 8.0 kg/T significantly reduced deposition of OTA in the liver compared with birds on diets without YCWE addition. When the datasets from the in vitro trial at pH 6.5 and the feeding trial were compared, it was observed that in both experiments YCWE addition decreased OTA by a similar fraction from the maximum detected level (Figures 2 and 7).

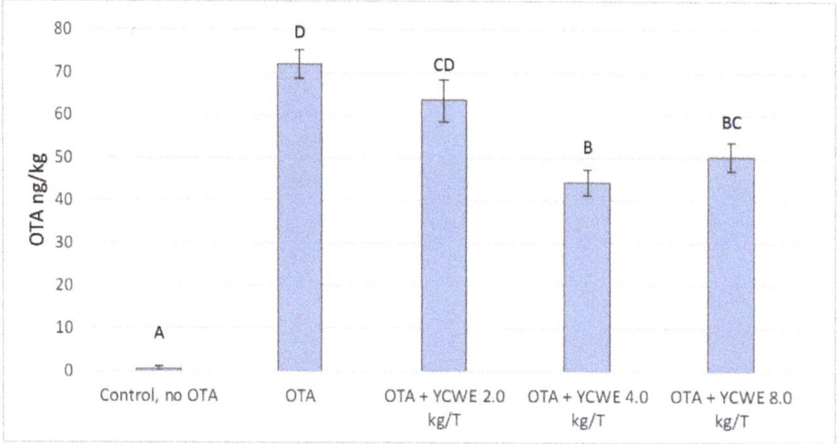

Figure 7. Deposition of ochratoxin A (OTA) in the liver of broiler chickens expressed in ng/kg following the dietary administration of yeast cell wall extract (YCWE) at varying inclusion rates. Error bars indicate standard error of the mean. Different letters above bars indicate significant differences between treatments ($p < 0.05$).

3. Discussion

Functional feed additives, such as toxin adsorbents, must remain active throughout the digestive tract of the animal and as such evaluating their integrity and susceptibility to the digestive environmental condition is necessary. Therefore, the YCWE product tested in this study was subjected to chemical, enzymatic, and physical digestion treatments simulating in vitro broiler chicken digestion. Tests of the toxin sequestration properties of YCWE after each digestion step revealed no significant changes in the level of radioactive OTA bound to YCWE, indicating that YCWE functionality and activity are preserved in the gastro-intestinal tract of broilers. Measuring changes in radioactivity is a highly sensitive method for assessing alterations in the concentration of radiolabelled compound (tritium-labelled OTA was selected as a signal molecule when assaying in vitro product efficacy). The method allowed analysis of the experimental samples directly after one centrifugation step, thus avoiding more laborious extraction procedures, isolation, and detection methods.

Analysis of the adsorption of OTA to YCWE during simulated consecutive digestion steps revealed a substantial increase in adherence at low pH. At pH 2.5, more than 80% of OTA was found to have bound to YCWE, whereas the enzymatic digestion treatments tested (pepsin, pancreatin) had no effect on binding performance. However, when the pH was re-adjusted to 6.5, OTA release from YCWE was observed. In broiler chickens, it has been shown that through reverse peristalsis digesta can also occasionally move from distal to proximal digestive tract. Thus, it is possible that digesta moves back from neutral duodenum to acidic gizzard [20]. Although our model did not specifically mimic such reverse peristalsis, we showed that when changing pH from neutral to acidic, and again to neutral, OTA binding was reversible, which is to say it becomes bound and is then released again. Thus, our model enables also predicting such a situation. This observation shows similarities with results obtained by Oh et al. [17], where low pH in combination with YCWE was found to decrease the toxicity of OTA in cultured macrophages. Oh et al. [17] suggest that the mechanism of decreased toxicity involved conformational changes in OTA at pH below 5.0, which in turn affected hydrogen bonding and van der Waals forces between OTA and YCWE. The increased adherence of OTA to YCWE at pH 2.5 and the detachment of OTA at pH 6.5 observed in the present study may support the mechanism suggested by Oh et al. [17]. However, it appears from our in silico studies that the changes in OTA conformation tended to happen independently of pH, due to several degrees of liberty from the presence of seven rotatable bonds around the amide bond. The observed changes in affinity could then be attributed rather to protonation level of the molecule than OTA conformational changes. The OTA molecule has a carboxylic acid group with pKa1 at 4.4 [21] and, according to our result, has a strong acidic pKa of 3.17. This functional group increasingly occurs in protonated form at pH lower than the pKa1 and protonation affects the molecule, making it electrochemically uncharged and decreasing its polarity. When pH is increased up to pH 6.5, OTA has a theoretical charge of −1.03 involving a deprotonation of the carboxyl group. If changes in the molecular structure due to deprotonation are minimal compared to protonated form (Figure S1), the glucan conformational structure can be dramatically affected, as demonstrated by the molecular dynamics simulation using two protonation states of OTA (Figures 5 and 6, Table 1), as well as the stability of interaction that involves in its majority, the carboxylic group of OTA in the formation of hydrogen bonds. All these factors may have an effect on OTA adherence to YCWE and demonstrated that the changes in β-(1,3)-D-glucan organization could transform the docking occurring at pH 2.5 into a surface interaction at pH 6.5. Moreover, the deprotonated form of OTA was more prone at interacting with the solvent environment, with an increased amount of H-bond formed, that directly competed with the capacity of the molecule at binding to the YCWE.

In the broiler trial, no acute OTA toxicity occurred in the birds, since all measured growth parameters, including mortality, were similar between the treatment groups. The dose of OTA fed to the broiler chickens was 0.1 mg/kg of feed, which is the maximum recommended level in commercial broiler feed in the European Union. In earlier studies, decreased body weight gain has been reported for broilers fed OTA at a dose of 4 mg/kg [22] or 0.5–0.25 mg/kg [23,24]. However, literature data on body weight changes are not conclusive, as no change in body weight gain was observed in a study by Politis et al. [25] in which 0.5 mg/kg of OTA was fed to broilers for 42 days. Therefore, the finding that the low dose of OTA applied in the present study did not change broiler performance parameters was expected and is in line with the previous research. However, these findings apply to a single mycotoxin and it is hypothesised that when several toxins are present at the same time, even if their levels are within the statutory or guidance limits, there may be synergistic forms of toxicity, as demonstrated by the impact of OTA in conjunction with the presence of penicillic acid (*Penicillium* spp. mycotoxin) in a macrophage culture assay [26] and negative effects on animal performance. In such cases, toxin binders may significantly improve the performance of production animals.

Analysis of the liver of broilers fed an OTA-containing diet for 14 days showed clear accumulation of OTA in liver tissues. It is thus evident that OTA is deposited in broiler liver tissues even when the dose of toxin is present in feed below the guidance level of the European Commission. However, the concentration of OTA in liver samples (0.072 ± 0.003 μg/kg) was low relative to the maximum recommended level of 2–10 μg/kg in products intended for human consumption in the European Union and Canada [27]. Several-fold higher OTA concentrations than were found in the present study have been detected in broiler products and chicken eggs in Pakistan, where 41% of broiler products have been found to be contaminated with OTA and the OTA concentration in broiler liver is as high as 3.56 μg/kg [28]. As the concentration of OTA in broiler chicken tissues is a result of toxin concentration in feed [29,30] it is clear that OTA concentrations exceeding 0.1 mg/kg are present in broiler feeds in some geographical regions.

When the broiler chickens in the present study were fed both YCWE and OTA, the OTA deposits in the liver decreased significantly. This decrease in OTA deposition was dependent on the dose of YCWE. The optimal YCWE dose tested was 4.0 kg/T, because the concentration of OTA detected in broiler liver was found the lowest with this dose. Lowered OTA deposition in the liver has also been reported in previous studies in which broiler chickens were fed OTA-contaminated feed together with toxin-deactivating products such as *Trichosporon mycotoxinivorans* [29,30] plant extracts [31], and yeast products [32]. However, in all those studies the concentration of OTA in broiler feed was at least five-fold higher than in the present study. Thus, a novel finding in the present study is that OTA deposition can be reduced using YCWE at chronic level of exposure of OTA. A low level can still be potentially damaging, e.g., in a study by Pozzo et al. [33], an OTA level of 0.1 mg/kg feed did not induce clinical signs but was shown to induce mild histological pathology in immune organs.

In the present study, a clear correlation was observed between results from in vitro and in vivo studies. The relative decrease in free OTA in the adsorption models used herein was comparable to the reduction in OTA concentration found in broiler livers. Dose dependence was observed both in vitro and in vivo, as an increase in the YCWE dosage decreased the measured OTA concentration. Previous studies have revealed a specific dose dependency in the fraction of OTA deposited in the liver, e.g., in a study by Hanif et al. [29] using mycotoxin deactivators, the effect of the deactivators was greater when the OTA dosage in broiler feed was increased. In the present study, there was an indication of a similar effect with the increase in YCWE inclusion from 2.0 to 4.0 kg/T but no difference was observed with a further increase of the level inclusion up to 8.0 kg/T. At 4.0 kg/T, the highest measured OTA concentration in the feed, OTA deposition in the liver was the lowest observed in the study, apart from the control. Thus, addition of YCWE to animal feed has the potential to decrease OTA deposition in the liver.

4. Conclusions

Overall, this work provides a methodological and practical insight to the demonstration of the binding properties of YCWE, showing an ability to chemically interact with OTA, dependent on the digestive physiological conditions and pH. This was demonstrated in vitro and by both biochemical and computational mechanistic/dynamic experiments. As reported here, changes in pH can induce conformational changes not only of the OTA molecule but also of the β-D-glucans, the bioactive component of YCWE, affecting the geometry of the binding site and consequently the affinity of interaction. A complementary in vivo study demonstrated that YCWE, when fed to broiler chickens at different inclusion levels, could tightly correlate these in vitro/in silico observations and mitigate the impact of OTA by significantly reducing accumulation in liver tissue. Collectively, these results showed that YCWE could sequester OTA and prevent its deposition in liver, which in turn can protect the animal from a mycotoxin challenge when present at low and chronic levels in the diet.

Mycotoxins, including OTA, are highly prevalent in animal feed. A three-year survey by Rodrigues et al. [34] found that up to 93% of feed samples were contaminated with OTA, while other mycotoxins, such as aflatoxin and fumonisin, were similarly common. As a consequence, correct harvest and storage methods are essential in controlling mycotoxin contamination of feedstuffs [35]. However, as this study indicates, including mycotoxin adsorbents or deactivators provides further assurance of good animal health and diminished toxin presence in human foodstuffs.

5. Materials and Methods

5.1. In Vitro Assessment of OTA Sequestration by YCWE

Yeast cell wall extract (YCWE) (Mycosorb A+®, Alltech Inc., Nicholasville, KY, USA) used in the study was added to 50 mM Na-phosphate buffer (pH 6.5) in silyated test vials (Supelco, Sigma-Aldrich, Saint Louis, MO, USA) in a final reaction volume of 10 mL. Buffer alone was used as a control. A mixture of tritium ([^{3}H])-labelled OTA (Moravek Biochemicals, Inc., Brea, CA, USA) and non-radiolabeled OTA (AppliChem GmbH, Darmstad, Germany) was prepared in Na-phosphate buffer to give a final OTA concentration of 20 ng/mL and [^{3}H] activity of 0.08 µCi/mL. The OTA solution was added to test treatment vials (see treatment condition below) for a final YCWE concentration of 5 and 15 mg/mL. Reaction vials were mixed and incubated at +37 °C for 2 h on a rotary shaker (GFL, Burgwedel, Germany). After incubation, the vials were centrifuged for 10 min at 3000× *g*. The [^{3}H] activity of unbound [^{3}H]-OTA was analysed by taking a 50 µL sample of the supernatant, adding it to 3.5 mL of scintillation cocktail (OptiPhase SuperMix, Perkin Elmer, Waltham, MA, USA) and measuring the [^{3}H] activity using a scintillation counter (Microbeta 1450, Perkin Elmer, Waltham, MA, USA).

5.2. In Vitro Digestive Simulation Conditions and OTA Sequestration Activity of YCWE

In the first in vitro model experiment, YCWE at two final concentrations (5 and 15 mg/mL) was subjected to three successive environmental conditions before the resultant adsorption efficacy was calculated based on the measure of the amount of free OTA remaining in the supernatant: (1) a 50 mM Na-phosphate buffer environment maintained at pH 6.5, considered as the control treatment; (2) a simulated gastric environment initiated by adjusting the pH to 2.5 with 1 M HCl and reacting with YCWE for 3 h at +37 °C, which represented the acid alone gastric digestion treatment; (3) a simulated enzymatic digestion treatment in an initial conditioning step through the addition of pepsin (Sigma-Aldrich, Saint Louis, MO, USA) at 7.5 mg/mL under the same environmental conditions as with (2), followed by a second step of pH adjustment to 6.5 with 1 M NaOH and addition of 2.5 mg/mL of pancreatin (Sigma-Aldrich, Saint Louis, MO, USA), representing the concomitant digestive enzymatic treatment. YCWE was incubated during the two successive enzymatic digestion steps at +37 °C for 3 h on a rotary shaker. After incubation in the pH was adjusted to 6.5 and the free OTA was measured.

In the second in vitro model experiment, the adsorption efficacy of YCWE (15 mg/mL) was evaluated based on the amount of free OTA remaining in the supernatant after each stage of digestive simulation: (1) starting stage, Na phosphate buffer maintained, pH 6.5; (2) first intermediate stage, after the acid gastric digestion treatment at pH 2.5; (3) second intermediate stage, after acid gastric digestion and neutralisation at pH 6.5; (4) third intermediate stage, after the one-step enzymatic (pepsin) treatment at pH 2.5; (5) final stage, after the two-step enzymatic (pepsin followed by pancreatin) treatment at pH 6.5.

In both experiments, a mixture of OTA (final concentration 20 ng/mL, [^{3}H] activity 0.08 µCi/mL) was added to the digested YCWE and non-digested control. The activity of unbound [^{3}H] OTA was measured in five replicates following the above described assessment of OTA sequestration by YCWE. The pH adjustments between digestive phases were monitored, and the indicated values represent the actual pH measurements.

5.3. *In Silico Assessment of the Sequestration Properties Investigated by Means of Molecular Mechanics and Dynamics*

Molecular mechanics investigations were carried out using several open-source programs: (1) Constructs of the β-(1,3)-D-glucan chain branched with a side chain of β-(1,6)-D-glucan previously generated on a Silicon Graphics computer with the Accelrys package (formerly Accelrys, now Biova Dassault Systemes, San Diego, CA, USA) in CFF91 force-field with steepest descent minimization [36]. This structural assembly was considered in the present study as the receptor, with three distinct conformations being investigated, a β-(1,3)-D-glucan chain alone, and two different β-(1,6)-D-glucan branched β-(1,3)-D-glucan chain conformations, as modelled in previous work; (2) OTA three-dimensional structure was downloaded from Chemspider compound repository under the permalink record 390954 (Royal Society of Chemistry, Burlington, VT, USA, http://www.chemspider.com/Chemical-Structure.390954.html) with OTA considered as the ligand in our study; (3) Molecular docking experiments were run on AutoDock Vina (The Scripps Research Institute, La Jolla, CA, USA, [37]). Before starting the docking process, all molecules were added with their polar hydrogens and were evaluated for their rotatable bonds. Seven degrees of liberty were found on the particular OTA molecule. The receptor conformation was constrained to the previously minimized conformation [38]. A grid box with a spacing of 60.0 Å in every x, y, z direction was parameterized and centered on a site of interaction at the proximity of the β-(1,3)- and β-(1,6)-D-glucans branching but also including in the grid box dimension adjacent binding sites over the entire single helical chain length consisting of 36 glucopyrannose +/− 3 side chain residues. PDB extension files were converted into pdbqt files before performing docking using Autodock Vina (v1.5.6, The Scripps Research Institute, La Jolla, CA, USA), an empirical scoring function that calculates affinity. The docking experiment was performed under C++ generic programming in a Microsoft Windows® (10 Pro, 1809, Microsoft Corporation, Redmond, WA, USA) environment and produced a maximum number of nine binding modes with a maximum energy range of 3 kcal/mol, and for which an affinity (kcal/mol) and distances from the best modes were measured.

Molecular dynamics were investigated using several open-source programs: (1) doGlycans (v1.0, Open Source program under GNU General Public License, v3.0, Free Software Foundation Inc, Boston, MA, USA), a tool to prepare carbohydrate structures under an Optimized Potentials for Liquid Simulations for All Atoms (OPLS-AA) modified force-field and related topology files for simulation [39] was used under Python 3 script and the Conda management system (Anaconda Inc., Austin, TX, USA) applied to the β-D-glucans receptor; (2) TopolGen (v1.1, Open Source Program under GNU General Public License, v3.0, Free Software Foundation Inc., Boston, MA, USA), a Perl script, and LigParGen (Open Source Program,http://zarbi.chem.yale.edu/ligpargen/) were used to produced GROMACS-formatted topology from the above generated PDB files docking experiment, compatible with an OPLS-AA force-field for OTA [40–42]; (3) GROMACS 2019.1 (GROMACS, Open Source Program under GNU General Public License, v3.0, Free Software Foundation Inc., Boston, MA, USA, www.gromacs.org, [43]) molecular dynamics simulation package was used to simulate receptor-ligand complex over 10 ns in a neutralized solvated system (water) at 37 °C and to study the initiation of the interaction energy at different charge states corresponding to a pH simulation performed at pH 3.0 and 6.5 to match our in vitro evaluations [44,45]. OTA was restrained using a force constant of 1000 kJ mol^{-1} nm^{-2} while the constrained and unconstrained structure of β-D-glucans were evaluated. Interaction energy was evaluated according to ionic coulomb energy potential and Lennard-Jones neutral molecule interaction potential energy expressed in kJ/mol.

PyMOL (The PyMOL Molecular Graphics System, v2.2.3 Schrödinger, LLC., New York, NY, USA) was used for visualization of the 3D molecular structures for all stages of molecular mechanics and molecular dynamics simulations. The chemical properties of OTA were calculated using the Chemicalize Chemoinformatic platform (ChemAxon, Cambridge, MA, USA, http://www.chemaxon.com) for the calculation of pKa of the molecules and chemical properties at different pH values.

5.4. *In Vivo Dietary Treatments*

The trial was conducted with a basal diet (Table 3) that was used as a negative control and also to generate the mycotoxin challenge dietary treatments. For these latter treatments, pure OTA (Sigma-Aldrich, Saint Louis, MO, USA) was dissolved in ethanol and mixed into a small amount of broiler feed. This mixture was step-wise mixed into larger batch of feed and eventually to final OTA challenge diet. The different doses of YCWE were added to small batches of broiler feed which were then mixed into final dietary treatments.

Table 3. Composition of the basal diet fed to broiler chickens for 21 days.

Ingredient	%
Wheat	60.31
Soybean meal	31.60
Rapeseed oil	4.0
Monocalcium phosphate	1.70
Limestone	1.30
NaCl	0.40
Mineral premix [1]	0.20
Vitamin premix [2]	0.20
Methionine	0.10
Lysine	0.09
Threonine	0.10
Total	100.00

[1] Containing: calcium 296.8 g/kg; iron 12.5 g/kg; copper 4 g/kg; manganese 25 g/kg; zinc 32.5 g/kg; iodine 0.225 g/kg; selenium 0.1 g/kg. [2] Containing: calcium 331.3 g/kg, vitamin A 6,000,000 IU, vitamin D3 2,250,000 IU; vitamin E 30,000; tocopherol 27,270 mg/kg; vitamin K3 1505 mg/kg; vitamin B1 1257.3 mg/kg; vitamin B2 3000 mg/kg; vitamin B6 2009.7 mg/kg; vitamin B12 12.5 mg/kg; biotin 75 mg/kg; folic acid 504 mg/kg; niacin 20,072 mg/kg; and pantothenic acid 7506.8 mg/kg.

5.5. *Animal Trial*

The feeding trial was conducted in the research facility of Alimetrics Ltd. in Southern Finland, in accordance with EU Directive 2010/63/EU. Following the standard operating procedures of Alimetrics Ltd., ethical approval or animal trial permit was not required as the substance under investigation is an approved feed ingredient in the EU and the level of Ochratoxin A included in the diets were below EU guidance levels (European Commission, 2006, [3]). 240 newly hatched male Ross 508 broiler chicks were randomly allocated to five feeding treatments divided between 40 pens (8 pens per treatment, 6 birds per pen). Temperature and lighting programs followed the Aviagen recommendations for Ross broilers (Aviagen Group, Huntsville, AL, USA). For the first 7 days, all birds were fed a basal diet (Table 4). From day 8 onwards, the birds on the control diet continued a basal diet while the other treatment groups received a targeted 0.090 mg/kg OTA-contaminated diet added to three varying amounts of YCWE (2.0, 4.0, 8.0 kg/T). The birds were individually weighed on days 1 and 21. Feed conversion ratio (FCR) was corrected for mortality by including the weight of deceased birds in the calculation. FCR was calculated over the period 1–21 days.

Table 4. Amounts of ochratoxin A (OTA) and yeast cell wall (YCWE) added to the experimental diets.

Diet	Target Dose of OTA (mg/kg)	Analysed Dose of OTA (mg/kg) [1]
Control	0.0	<0.001
+ OTA	0.090	0.110
+ OTA + YCWE 2.0 kg/T	0.090	0.099
+ OTA + YCWE 4.0 kg/T	0.090	0.140
+ OTA + YCWE 8.0 kg/T	0.090	0.110

[1] OTA analysis performed at NutriControl (Veghel, The Netherlands). The reported repeatability and reproducibility of the analysis was 20% and 25%, respectively.

5.6. Mycotoxin Analysis of Dietary Treatments

Confirmation of the levels of OTA in final feed via analysis (Table 4). Basal diets were also analysed for their content in aflatoxin B1 and B2, deoxynivalenol, nivalenol, zearalenone, fumonisins B1 and B2, T-2 toxin, and HT-2 toxin by means of LC-MSMS (Nutricontrol, Veghel, The Netherlands). Considering the measurement uncertainty announced by Nutricontrol, we can conclude that the content of OTA in the diets did not significantly differ from each other.

5.7. OTA Analysis of Liver Tissues

Livers were collected from four broilers per pen. The livers were combined in pairs, resulting in two analytical samples per pen. The tissues were ground and stored at −20 °C until analysis. OTA analysis was performed by extracting 5.0 g of ground liver with 25 mL of 1% $NaHCO_3$: methanol (30:70, v/v). After centrifugation, 10.0 mL of the supernatant was mixed with an equal volume of PBS and applied onto an OchraTest WB immunoaffinity column (Vicam, Milford, MA, USA). The effluent was filtered through a 0.45 µm syringe filter and analysed by high pressure liquid chromatography equipped with a fluorescent detector (HPLC Prominence, Shimadzu, Kyoto, Japan). The HPLC separation was performed by means of a Phenomenex Luna C18(2) 3 µm, 150 × 4.60 mm column equipped with a Gemini C18, 4 × 3 mm SecurityGuard pre-column (Phenomenex Inc., Torrance, CA, USA) at a flow rate of 0.8 mL/min. Injection volume was set to 40 µL and column oven temperature 30 °C. Fluorescence detection was carried out at an excitation wavelength of 333 nm and emission wavelength of 460 nm. The limit of detection measured from standard deviation of background signal was 0.4 ng/kg and the limit of quantification was 2 ng/kg.

5.8. Data Analysis

Statistically significant differences between mean values of the parameters tested were analyzed with ANOVA using Tukey's honestly significant difference (HSD) post-hoc test in the SPSS statistical software package (IBM, version 22, Armonk, NY, USA).

Supplementary Materials: The following are available online at http://www.mdpi.com/2072-6651/12/1/37/s1, Figure S1: Computer generated views of the aligned energy-minimized nine states of ochratoxin A (OTA) docking into β-(1,3)-d-glucans chain alone (A) with A1 corresponding to OTA with no charge (corresponding to charge state at pH 3.0) and A2 with a partial charge equal to −1 (corresponding to charge state at pH 6.5); into β-(1,3)-d-glucans branched with β-(1,6)-d-glucans conformation 1 (B); and conformation 2 (C). In these views, only the OTA is represented to account for conformational changes of the ligand molecule; Table S1: Energy values describing the affinity of interaction between ochratoxin A (OTA) and three different β-D-glucans conformations found in yeast cell wall extract.

Author Contributions: Conceptualization, S.V., A.Y., J.A., and C.A.M.; Methodology, S.V., and A.Y.; Validation, S.V., and A.Y.; Formal analysis, S.V., and A.Y.; Investigation, S.V. and A.Y.; Resources, A.Y., J.A., and C.A.M.; Data curation, S.V.; Writing—original draft preparation, S.V.; Writing—review and editing, S.V., A.Y., J.A., and C.A.M.; Visualization, A.Y.; Supervision, J.A., and C.A.M.; Project administration, A.Y., J.A., and C.A.M.; Funding acquisition, C.A.M. All authors have read and agreed to the published version of the manuscript.

Funding: The work was financially supported by Alltech SARL, Vire, France. Alltech also provided the test products used in the study.

Conflicts of Interest: The authors C.A.M. and A.Y. are employees of Alltech which produces and markets Mycosorb A+®, the commercial product used in this study.

References

1. Ramos, A.; Labernia, N.; Marín, S.; Sanchis, V.; Magan, N. Effect of water activity and temperature on growth and ochratoxin production by three strains of Aspergillus ochraceus on a barley extract medium and on barley grains. *Int. J. Food Microbiol.* **1998**, *44*, 133–140. [CrossRef]
2. Cairns-Fuller, V.; Aldred, D.; Magan, N. Water, temperature and gas composition interactions affect growth and ochratoxin A production by isolates of Penicillium verrucosum on wheat grain. *J. Appl. Microbiol.* **2005**, *99*, 1215–1221. [CrossRef] [PubMed]

3. European Commission. Commission Recommendation 2006/576/EC of 17 August 2006 on the presence of deoxynivalenol, zearalenone, ochratoxin A, T-2 and HT-2 and fumonisins in products intended for animal feeding. *Off. J. Eur. Union L* **2006**, *229*, 7–9.
4. Swamy, H.V.L.N.; Smith, T.K.; Karrow, N.A.; Boermans, H.J. Effects of Feeding Blends of Grains Naturally Contaminated with Fusarium. *Poult. Sci.* **2004**, *83*, 533–543. [CrossRef] [PubMed]
5. Moran, C.A.; Apajalahti, J.; Yiannikouris, A.; Ojanpera, S.; Kettunen, H. Effects of low dietary aflatoxin B1 on broiler liver concentration without and with Mycosorb® toxin binder. *J. Appl. Anim. Nutr.* **2013**, *2*. [CrossRef]
6. Moran, C.A.; Kettunen, H.; Yiannikouris, A.; Ojanpera, S.; Pennala, E.; Helander, I.M.; Apajalahti, J. A dairy cow model to assess aflatoxin transmission from feed into milk—Evaluating efficacy of the mycotoxin binder Mycosorb®. *J. Appl. Anim. Nutr.* **2013**, *2*. [CrossRef]
7. Battacone, G.; Nudda, A.; Pulina, G. Effects of ochratoxin a on livestock production. *Toxins* **2010**, *2*, 1796–1824. [CrossRef]
8. Tao, Y.; Xie, S.; Xu, F.; Liu, A.; Wang, Y.; Chen, D.; Pan, Y.; Huang, L.; Peng, D.; Wang, X.; et al. Ochratoxin A: Toxicity, oxidative stress and metabolism. *Food Chem. Toxicol.* **2018**, *112*, 320–331. [CrossRef]
9. Pfohl-Leszkowicz, A.; Manderville, R.A. Ochratoxin A: An overview on toxicity and carcinogenicity in animals and humans. *Mol. Nutr. Food Res.* **2007**, *51*, 61–99. [CrossRef]
10. Kumagai, S.; Aibara, K. Intestinal absorption and secretion of ochratoxin A in the rat. *Toxicol. Appl. Pharm.* **1982**, *64*, 94–102. [CrossRef]
11. Galtier, P.; Alvinerie, M.; Charpenteau, J.L. The pharmacokinetic profiles of ochratoxin A in pigs, rabbits and chickens. *Food Cosmet. Toxicol.* **1981**, *19*, 735–738. [CrossRef]
12. Hagelberg, S.; Hult, K.; Fuchs, R. Toxicokinetics of ochratoxin A in several species and its plasma-binding properties. *J. Appl. Toxicol.* **1989**, *9*, 91–96. [CrossRef] [PubMed]
13. Vettorazzi, A.; González-Peñas, E.; de Cerain, A.L. Ochratoxin A kinetics: A review of analytical methods and studies in rat model. *Food Chem. Toxicol.* **2014**, *72*, 273–288. [CrossRef] [PubMed]
14. Galtier, P.; Charpenteau, J.; Alvinerie, M.; Labouche, C. The pharmacokinetic profile of ochratoxin A in the rat after oral and intravenous administration. *Drug Metab. Dispos.* **1979**, *7*, 429–434.
15. Vila-Donat, P.; Marín, S.; Sanchis, V.; Ramos, A.J. A review of the mycotoxin adsorbing agents, with an emphasis on their multi-binding capacity, for animal feed decontamination. *Food Chem. Toxicol.* **2018**, *114*, 246–259. [CrossRef]
16. Yiannikouris, A.; Kettunen, H.; Apajalahti, J.; Pennala, E.; Moran, C.A. Comparison of the sequestering properties of yeast cell wall extract and hydrated sodium calcium aluminosilicate in three in vitro models accounting for the animal physiological bioavailability of zearalenone. *Food Addit. Contam.-Part A* **2013**, *30*, 1641–1650. [CrossRef]
17. Oh, S.Y.; Quinton, V.M.; Boermans, H.J.; Swamy, H.V.L.N.; Karrow, N.A. In vitro exposure of Penicillium mycotoxins with or without a modified yeast cell wall extract (mYCWE) on bovine macrophages (BoMacs). *Mycotoxin Res.* **2015**, *31*, 167–175. [CrossRef]
18. Yiannikouris, A.; François, J.; Poughon, L.; Dussap, C.G.; Bertin, G.; Jeminet, G.; Jouany, J.P. Alkali extraction of β-d-glucans from Saccharomyces cerevisiae cell wall and study of their adsorptive properties toward zearalenone. *J. Agric. Food Chem.* **2004**, *52*, 3666–3673. [CrossRef]
19. European Food Safety Authority (EFSA). Guidance for the preparation of dossiers for technological additives. *EFSA J.* **2012**, *10*, 2528. [CrossRef]
20. Sacranie, A.; Svihus, B.; Denstadli, V.; Moen, B.; Iji, P.A.; Choct, M. The effect of insoluble fiber and intermittent feeding on gizzard development, gut motility, and performance of broiler chickens. *Poult. Sci.* **2012**, *91*, 693–700. [CrossRef]
21. Bazin, I.; Faucet-Marquis, V.; Monje, M.-C.; El Khoury, M.; Marty, J.-L.; Pfohl-Leszkowicz, A.; Bazin, I.; Faucet-Marquis, V.; Monje, M.-C.; El Khoury, M.; et al. Impact of pH on the Stability and the Cross-Reactivity of Ochratoxin A and Citrinin. *Toxins* **2013**, *5*, 2324–2340. [CrossRef] [PubMed]
22. Rotter, R.G.; Frohlich, A.A.; Marquardt, R.R. Influence of dietary charcoal on ochratoxin A toxicity in Leghorn chicks. *Can. J. Vet. Res.* **1989**, *53*, 449–453. [PubMed]
23. García, A.R.; Avila, E.; Rosiles, R.; Petrone, V.M. Evaluation of Two mycotoxin binders to reduce toxicity of broiler diets containing ochratoxin A and T-2 toxin contaminated grain. *Avian Dis.* **2003**, *47*, 691–699. [CrossRef]

24. Santin, E.; Paulillo, A.; Nakagui, L.; Alessi, A.; Maiorka, A. Evaluation of yeast cell wall on the performance of broiles fed diets with or without mycotoxins. *Braz. J. Poult. Sci.* **2006**, *8*, 221–225. [CrossRef]
25. Politis, I.; Fegeros, K.; Nitsch, S.; Schatzmayr, G.; Kantas, D. Use of Trichosporon mycotoxinivorans to suppress the effects of ochratoxicosis on the immune system of broiler chicks. *Br. Poult. Sci.* **2005**, *46*, 58–65. [CrossRef]
26. Oh, S.Y.; Cedergreen, N.; Yiannikouris, A.; Swamy, H.V.L.N.; Karrow, N.A. Assessing interactions of binary mixtures of Penicillium mycotoxins (PMs) by using a bovine macrophage cell line (BoMacs). *Toxicol. Appl. Pharm.* **2017**, *318*, 33–40. [CrossRef]
27. Haighton, L.A.; Lynch, B.S.; Magnuson, B.A.; Nestmann, E.R. A reassessment of risk associated with dietary intake of ochratoxin A based on a lifetime exposure model. *Crit. Rev. Toxicol.* **2012**, *42*, 147–168. [CrossRef]
28. Iqbal, S.Z.; Nisar, S.; Asi, M.R.; Jinap, S. Natural incidence of aflatoxins, ochratoxin A and zearalenone in chicken meat and eggs. *Food Control* **2014**, *43*, 98–103. [CrossRef]
29. Hanif, N.Q.; Muhammad, G.; Muhammad, K.; Tahira, I.; Raja, G.K. Reduction of ochratoxin A in broiler serum and tissues by Trichosporon mycotoxinivorans. *Res. Vet. Sci.* **2012**, *93*, 795–797. [CrossRef]
30. Joo, Y.D.; Kang, C.W.; An, B.K.; Ahn, J.S.; Borutova, R. Effects of ochratoxin a and preventive action of a mycotoxin-deactivation product in broiler chickens. *Vet. Ir. Zootech.* **2013**, *61*, 22–29.
31. Stoev, S.D.; Stefanov, M.; Denev, S.; Radic, B.; Domijan, A.M.; Peraica, M. Experimental mycotoxicosis in chickens induced by ochratoxin A and penicillic acid and intervention with natural plant extracts. *Vet. Res. Commun.* **2004**, *28*, 727–746. [CrossRef] [PubMed]
32. Pfohl-Leszkowicz, A.; Hadjeba-Medjdoub, K.; Ballet, N.; Schrickx, J.; Fink-Gremmels, J. Assessment and characterisation of yeast-based products intended to mitigate ochratoxin exposure using in vitro and in vivo models. *Food Addit. Contam.-Part A Chem. Anal. Control. Expo. Risk Assess.* **2015**, *32*, 604–616. [CrossRef] [PubMed]
33. Pozzo, L.; Cavallarin, L.; Antoniazzi, S.; Guerre, P.; Biasibetti, E.; Capucchio, M.T.; Schiavone, A. Feeding a diet contaminated with ochratoxin A for broiler chickens at the maximum level recommended by the EU for poultry feeds (0.1 mg/kg). 2. Effects on meat quality, oxidative stress, residues and histological traits. *J. Anim. Physiol. Anim. Nutr.* **2013**, *97*, 23–31. [CrossRef] [PubMed]
34. Rodrigues, I.; Naehrer, K.; Rodrigues, I.; Naehrer, K. A Three-Year Survey on the Worldwide Occurrence of Mycotoxins in Feedstuffs and Feed. *Toxins* **2012**, *4*, 663–675. [CrossRef]
35. Peng, W.-X.; Marchal, J.L.M.; van der Poel, A.F.B. Strategies to prevent and reduce mycotoxins for compound feed manufacturing. *Anim. Feed Sci. Technol.* **2018**, *237*, 129–153. [CrossRef]
36. Yiannikouris, A.; André, G.; Buleon, A.; Jeminet, G.; Canet, I.; François, J.; Bertin, G.; Jouany, J.-P. Comprehensive Conformational Study of Key Interactions Involved in Zearalenone Complexation with beta-d-Glucans. *Biomacromolecules* **2004**, *7*, 2176–2185. [CrossRef]
37. Trott, O.; Olson, A.J. AutoDock Vina: Improving the speed and accuracy of docking with a new scoring function, efficient optimization and multithreading, J. *Comput. Chem.* **2010**, *31*, 455–461. [CrossRef]
38. Yiannikouris, A.; André, G.; Poughon, L.; François, J.; Dussap, C.-G.; Jeminet, G.; Bertin, G.; Jouany, J.-P. Chemical and Conformational Study of the Interactions Involved in Mycotoxin Complexation with beta-D-Glucans. *Biomacromolecules* **2006**, *7*, 1147–1155. [CrossRef]
39. Danne, R.; Poojari, C.; Martinez-Seara, H. doGlycans-Tools for Preparing Carbohydrate Structures for Atomistic Simulations of Glycoproteins, Glycolipids, and Carbohydrate Polymers for GROMACS. *J. Chem. Inf. Model.* **2017**, *57*, 2401–2406. [CrossRef]
40. Jorgensen, W.L.; Tirado-Rives, J. Potential energy functions for atomic-level simulations of water and organic and biomolecular systems. *Proc. Natl. Acad. Sci. USA* **2005**, *102*, 6665–6670. [CrossRef]
41. Dodda, L.S.; Vilseck, J.Z.; Tirado-Rives, J.; Jorgensen, W.L.J. 1.14* CM1A-LBCC: Localized Bond-Charge Corrected CM1A Charges for Condensed-Phase Simulations. *Phys. Chem. B* **2017**, *121*, 3864–3870. [CrossRef] [PubMed]
42. Dodda, L.S.; Cabeza de Vaca, I.; Tirado-Rives, J.; Jorgensen, W.L. LigParGen web server: An automatic OPLS-AA parameter generator for organic ligands. *Nucleic Acids Res.* **2017**, *45*, W331–W336. [CrossRef] [PubMed]
43. Abraham, M.J.; Murtola, T.; Schulz, R.; Páll, S.; Smith, J.C.; Hess, B.; Lindahl, E. GROMACS: High Performance Molecular Simulations Through Multi-Level Parallelism from Laptops to Supercomputers. *SoftwareX* **2015**, *1–2*, 19–25. [CrossRef]

44. Berendsen, H.J.C.; van der Spoel, D.; van Drunen, R. GROMACS: A message-passing parallel molecular dynamics implementation. *Comput. Phys. Commun.* **1995**, *91*, 43–56. [CrossRef]
45. Lindahl, E.; Hess, B.; van der Spoel, D. GROMACS 3.0: A package for molecular simulation and trajectory analysis. *Mol. Model. Annu.* **2001**, *7*, 306–317. [CrossRef]

toxins

MDPI

Article

A Novel Modified Hydrated Sodium Calcium Aluminosilicate (HSCAS) Adsorbent Can Effectively Reduce T-2 Toxin-Induced Toxicity in Growth Performance, Nutrient Digestibility, Serum Biochemistry, and Small Intestinal Morphology in Chicks

Jin-Tao Wei [1,2,†], Kun-Tan Wu [1,2,†], Hua Sun [1], Mahmoud Mohamed Khalil [3], Jie-Fan Dai [4], Ying Liu [5], Qiang Liu [6], Ni-Ya Zhang [1], De-Sheng Qi [1] and Lv-Hui Sun [1,2,*]

1 Department of Animal Nutrition and Feed Science, College of Animal Science and Technology, Huazhong Agricultural University, Wuhan 430070, China; jintao001@163.com (J.-T.W.); kuntanwu@webmail.hzau.edu.cn (K.-T.W.); huasun@webmail.hzau.edu.cn (H.S.); zhangniya@mail.hzau.edu.cn (N.-Y.Z.); qds@mail.hzau.edu.cn (D.-S.Q.)
2 Key Laboratory of Animal Embryo Engineering and Molecular Breeding of Hubei Province, Institute of Animal Husbandry and Veterinary Sciences, Hubei Academy of Agricultural Sciences, Wuhan 430064, China
3 Animal Production Department, Faculty of Agriculture, Benha University, Benha 13736, Egypt; mahmoud.khalil@fagr.bu.edu.eg
4 Sichuan Green Food Development Center, Chengdu 610041, China; daijiefan@126.com
5 Tianjin Animal Disease Prevention and Control Center, Tianjin 300402, China; yingliuadpcc@sohu.com
6 Jiangsu Aomai Bio-Technology Co., Ltd., Nanjing 211226, China; liuayang@njau.edu.cn
* Correspondence: lvhuisun@mail.hzau.edu.cn; Tel.: +86-27-87281793
† These authors contributed equally to this work.

Received: 5 March 2019; Accepted: 2 April 2019; Published: 2 April 2019

Abstract: The objective of this study was to evaluate the ability of a modified hydrated sodium calcium aluminosilicate (HSCAS) adsorbent to reduce the toxicity of T-2 toxin in broilers. Ninety-six one-day-old male broilers were randomly allocated into four experimental groups with four replicates of six birds each. The four groups, 1–4, received a basal diet (BD), a BD plus 6.0 mg/kg T-2 toxin, a BD plus 6.0 mg/kg T-2 toxin with 0.05% modified HSCAS adsorbent, and a BD plus 0.05% modified HSCAS adsorbent, respectively, for two weeks. Growth performance, nutrient digestibility, serum biochemistry, and small intestinal histopathology were analyzed. Compared to the control group, dietary supplementation of T-2 toxin decreased ($p < 0.05$) body weight gain, feed intake, and the feed conversion ratio by 11.4–31.8% during the whole experiment. It also decreased ($p < 0.05$) the apparent metabolic rates of crude protein, calcium, and total phosphorus by 14.9–16.1%. The alterations induced by T-2 toxin were mitigated ($p < 0.05$) by the supplementation of the modified HSCAS adsorbent. Meanwhile, dietary modified HSCAS adsorbent supplementation prevented ($p < 0.05$) increased serum aspartate aminotransferase by T-2 toxin at d 14. It also prevented ($p < 0.05$) T-2 toxin-induced morphological changes and damage in the duodenum, jejunum, and ileum of broilers. However, dietary supplementation of the modified HSCAS adsorbent alone did not affect ($p > 0.05$) any of these variables. In conclusion, these findings indicate that the modified HSCAS adsorbent could be used against T-2 toxin-induced toxicity in growth performance, nutrient digestibility, and hepatic and small intestinal injuries in chicks.

Keywords: modified HSCAS; absorption; T-2 toxin; broilers

Key Contribution: This study reveals that the modified HSCAS adsorbent, Amdetox^{TM}, could be used as a promising adsorbent for the counteracting of T-2 toxin in practice.

---

1. Introduction

Trichothecenes are secondary fungal metabolites largely produced by *Fusarium, Trichoderma,* and *Mycothecium* species [1]. T-2 toxin has shown the highest toxicity of the commonly tested type A trichothecenes [1]. T-2 toxin has been detected in grains and animal feed all over the world [2,3]. Previous reports have shown that about 20–70% of European cereal samples, including maize, barley, and wheat, have T-2 toxin [2,3]. T-2 toxin can be quickly absorbed in the intestinal tract, and then causes severe damage to various organs of animals, especially the liver and the digestive system [4,5]. After consumption, T-2 toxin is known to reduce feed intake and weight gain in mice [6], broiler chickens [7], and pigs [8]. Furthermore, many studies have considered T-2 toxin impacts on the relative weight of organs [9], serum biochemistry [10], restrained protein synthesis [1], cell apoptosis [11], and the suppression of immune functions [1]. Therefore, the development of effective strategies to reduce T-2 toxicity has attracted much interest over the past few decades.

Generally, there are several methods to reduce the harmful effects of T-2 toxin, including physical, chemical, and biological procedures. Irradiation provides intense energy to break down T-2 toxin in grains [12], and strong alkaline solutions can inhibit T-2 toxin biological activity [13]. Furthermore, enzymatic treatment can also degrade T-2 toxin, destroying its 12,13-epoxide ring [14]. However, methods to remove T-2 toxin from feed and food can be unstable and expensive and can further affect grain quality [15]. Physical adsorption is more effective and directly detoxifies mycotoxins by inhibiting absorption in the gastrointestinal tract [16], but there is a lack of efficient adsorbent for T-2 toxin and deoxynivalenol (DON) [17]. Previous studies have reported that adsorbents contain aluminosilicates, such as bentonite [18], montmorillonite [19], and zeolite [20], displaying an ability to effectively protect against zearalenone [21], aflatoxin B_1 (AFB_1), and fumonisin B_1 (FB_1) [22] in several farm and experimental animals. Hydrated sodium calcium aluminosilicate (HSCAS) is a material obtained by using natural zeolite ore: It is purified through crushing, screening, and high-temperature treatment, allowing the structure to increase its size, surface area, and adsorption volume [23]. Amdetox^{TM} is an adsorbent that mainly contains HSCAS whose surface is modified by cetylpyridinium chloride and the intercalation of β-glucan. The modified HSCAS adsorbent increases surface area and might be able to increase adsorbing mycotoxins and avoid adsorbing the nutrients in feed. The objective of this study was to determine the ameliorative effects of Amdetox^{TM} detoxification on the toxicity induced by T-2 toxin.

2. Results

2.1. Growth Performance

Growth performance results are presented in Table 1. Nonsignificant differences in initial body weight were observed among the four groups ($p > 0.05$, Table 2). Compared to the control (group 1), dietary T-2 supplementation (group 2) decreased ($p < 0.05$) body weight gain and feed intake by 15.3–31.8% and 12.4–20.6%, respectively, during d 1–7, d 8–14, and d 1–14, while it increased ($p < 0.05$) feed intake by 11.4–15.9% during d 8–14 and d 1–14. Although dietary supplementation of Amdetox^{TM} (group 3) did not alleviate T-2 toxin-induced (group 2) adverse effects on body weight gain and feed intake in d 1–7, dietary supplementation of Amdetox^{TM} (group 3) alleviated T-2 toxin-induced (group 2) adverse effects on body weight gain and feed intake by 38.6–46.6% and 33.0–36.0%, respectively, during d 8–14 and d 1–14. Meanwhile, dietary supplementation of Amdetox^{TM} (group 3) mitigated the reduced feed/gain induced by T-2 toxin (group 2) throughout the experiment. Notably, dietary-supplemented Amdetox^{TM} alone (group 4) did not affect ($p > 0.05$) body weight gain, feed intake, and feed/gain compared to the control (group 1) throughout the experiment. Notably, the variation in growth performance was very low for each treatment, indicating that in the current study, the results from four replicates per treatment might be reliable.

Table 1. Effects of T-2 toxin and Amdetox™ on growth performance of broilers. [1]

Item	Group 1	Group 2	Group 3	Group 4
Initial body weight, g/bird	54.3 ± 0.4	54.4 ± 0.7	54.5 ± 0.7	54.0 ± 0.2
d 1 to 7				
Body weight gain, g/bird	138.9 ± 6.2 ^{a}	117.6 ± 5.4 ^{b}	115.9 ± 8.7 ^{b}	136.2 ± 18.4 ^{a}
Feed intake, g/bird	167.6 ± 3.8 ^{a}	146.9 ± 4.8 ^{b}	149.1 ± 5.3 ^{b}	166.3 ± 1.8 ^{a}
Feed/gain, g/g	1.21 ± 0.05	1.25 ± 0.08	1.29 ± 0.06	1.24 ± 0.17
d 8 to 14				
Body weight gain, g/bird	280.2 ± 17.0 ^{a}	191.1 ± 10.1 ^{c}	232.6 ± 11.9 ^{b}	289.8 ± 22.7 ^{a}
Feed intake, g/bird	385.2 ± 11.9 ^{a}	305.8 ± 10.7 ^{c}	334.4 ± 28.9 ^{b}	376.3 ± 18.8 ^{a}
Feed/gain, g/g	1.38 ± 0.05 ^{b}	1.60 ± 0.07 ^{a}	1.44 ± 0.05 ^{b}	1.30 ± 0.06 ^{b}
d 1 to 14				
Body weight gain, g/bird	419.2 ± 21.7 ^{a}	308.7 ± 8.1 ^{c}	351.3 ± 11.6 ^{b}	426.0 ± 9.1 ^{a}
Feed intake, g/bird	552.8 ± 11.9 ^{a}	452.7 ± 14.5 ^{b}	485.7 ± 30.7 ^{b}	542.9 ± 17.9 ^{a}
Feed/gain, g/g	1.32 ± 0.05 ^{b}	1.47 ± 0.02 ^{a}	1.38 ± 0.05 ^{b}	1.27 ± 0.02 ^{b}

$^{a-c}$ Means within a row lacking a common superscript differ significantly ($p < 0.05$). [1] Results are reported as the mean ± SD, $n = 4$. Group 1 = basal diet; group 2 = basal diet + 6 mg/kg T-2 toxin; group 3 = basal diet + 6 mg/kg T-2 toxin + 0.05% of Amdetox™; group 4 = basal diet + 0.05% of Amdetox™.

2.2. Apparent Metabolic Rate

The nutrient metabolic rate results are shown in Table 2. Although dietary supplementation of T-2 toxin (group 2) did not affect ($p > 0.05$) the apparent metabolic rate of gross energy, it decreased ($p < 0.05$) the apparent metabolic rate of crude protein, calcium, and total phosphorus by 14.9%, 18.0%, and 16.1%, respectively. Notably, the changes in the apparent metabolic rates of crude protein and total phosphorus induced by T-2 toxin were alleviated by dietary supplementation of Amdetox™ (group 3) when compared to the control (group 1). In addition, dietary-supplemented Amdetox™ alone (group 4) did not affect ($p > 0.05$) the apparent metabolic rates of gross energy, crude protein, calcium, and total phosphorus compared to the control (group 1).

Table 2. Effects of T-2 toxin and Amdetox™ on the metabolic rates of gross energy, crude protein, calcium, and total phosphorus of broilers during d 8–14. [1]

Item	Group 1	Group 2	Group 3	Group 4
Gross energy, %	67.1 ± 3.0	64.1 ± 2.8	67.0 ± 3.6	66.1 ± 2.6
Crude protein, %	57.6 ± 2.5 ^{a}	49.0 ± 5.0 ^{b}	52.5 ± 6.9 ^{ab}	55.3 ± 1.7 ^{a}
Calcium, %	40.5 ± 5.2 ^{a}	33.2 ± 4.9 ^{b}	30.6 ± 1.1 ^{b}	34.9 ± 10.9 ^{ab}
Total phosphorus, %	52.7 ± 6.9 ^{a}	44.2 ± 4.8 ^{b}	48.4 ± 8.1 ^{ab}	49.3 ± 7.8 ^{ab}

$^{a-b}$ Means within a row lacking a common superscript differ significantly ($p < 0.05$). [1] Results are reported as the mean ± SD, $n = 4$. Group 1 = basal diet; group 2 = basal diet + 6 mg/kg T-2 toxin; group 3 = basal diet + 6 mg/kg T-2 toxin + 0.05% of Amdetox™; group 4 = basal diet + 0.05% of Amdetox™.

2.3. Serum Biochemistry and Histopathology

Serum biochemistry results are presented in Table 3. After two weeks of experimental treatments, although T-2 toxin (group 2) did not affect ($p > 0.05$) serum alanine aminotransferase (ALT), total protein (TP), and albumin (ALB), it increased ($p < 0.05$) aspartate aminotransferase (AST) (17.7%) relative to the control (group 1). Strikingly, this change was inhibited by dietary supplementation of Amdetox™ (group 3). Dietary-supplemented Amdetox™ alone (group 4) did not affect ($p > 0.05$) these serum biochemistry variables compared to the control (group 1). Additionally, the histological results showed that dietary T-2 toxin supplementation induced intestinal injury (Figure 1). Specifically, compared to the control (group 1), T-2 toxin (group 2) induced severe degeneration, necrosis, and desquamation of the villous epithelial cells; and increased inflammatory cells in the intestinal mucosa, congestion in the intestinal lamina propria, goblet cell hyperplasia in the intestinal gland, and/or edema and thickening in the serosa, with an infiltration of numerous lymphoid cells in the duodenum (Figure 1A), jejunum (Figure 1B), and ileum (Figure 1C). Intriguingly, dietary supplementation of Amdetox™ (group 3) prevented T-2 toxin-induced (group 2) injury in the small intestine. In contrast, intestinal morphology was not affected by the supplementation of Amdetox™ alone (group 4).

Table 3. Effects of T-2 toxin and Amdetox™ on serum biochemistry of broilers at d 14. [1]

Item	Group 1	Group 2	Group 3	Group 4
ALT/(U/L)	2.68 ± 0.12	2.85 ± 0.34	2.47 ± 0.27	2.80 ± 0.19
AST/(U/L)	196.7 ± 6.0 ^{b}	231.5 ± 5.2 ^{a}	203.0 ± 3.4 ^{b}	200.6 ± 7.9 ^{b}
TP/(g/L)	25.7 ± 1.6	27.2 ± 1.2	28.4 ± 1.0	27.4 ± 1.9
ALB/(g/L)	12.7 ± 1.0	13.1 ± 0.8	13.3 ± 0.6	13.7 ± 1.3

$^{a–b}$ Means within a row lacking a common superscript differ significantly ($p < 0.05$). [1] Results are reported as the mean ± SD, $n = 8$. ALT = alanine transaminase; AST = aspartate aminotransferase; TP = total protein; ALB = albumin. Group 1 = basal diet; group 2 = basal diet + 6 mg/kg T-2 toxin; group 3 = basal diet + 6 mg/kg T-2 toxin + 0.05% of Amdetox™; group 4 = basal diet + 0.05% of Amdetox™.

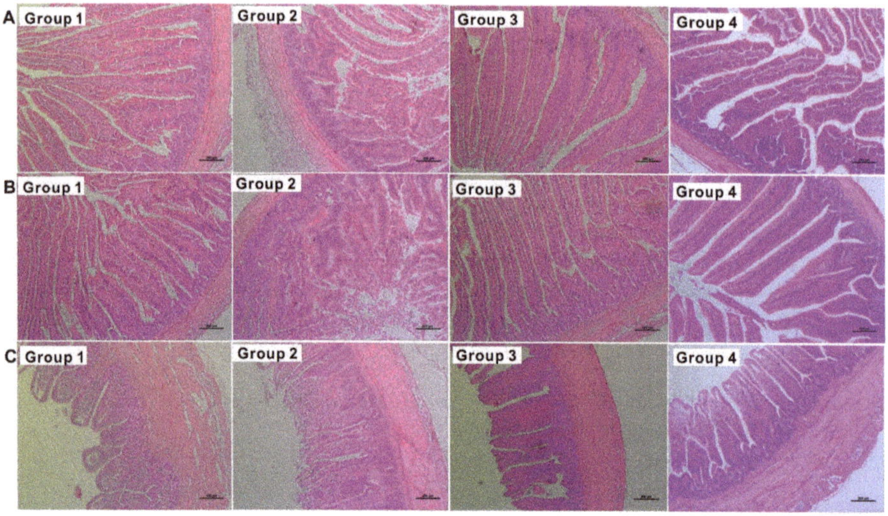

Figure 1. Effects of dietary T-2 toxin and Amdetox™ on histopathology of the (**A**) duodenum, (**B**) jejunum, and (**C**) ileum of chicks. The sections were stained with hematoxylin and eosin. Photomicrographs are shown at 100× magnification. Group 1 = basal diet; group 2 = basal diet + 6 mg/kg T-2 toxin; group 3 = basal diet + 6 mg/kg T-2 toxin + 0.05% of Amdetox™; group 4 = basal diet + 0.05% of Amdetox™.

3. Discussion

The current study demonstrates that the modified HSCAS adsorbent could effectively counteract T-2 toxin-induced adverse effects on broilers. Chick consumption of T-2 toxin reduced body weight, feed intake, and feed conversion, which was in accordance with previous studies [7,24]. The poor growth performance of broilers, induced by T-2 toxin, was further proven to be associated with decreased metabolic rates of crude protein, calcium, and total phosphate in chicks in the current study. These outcomes are similar to previous studies that showed that *Fusarium* toxins can negatively affect nutrient digestibility in chicks [24,25]. Interestingly, the current study showed that dietary supplementation of 0.05% Amdetox^{TM} successfully reduced the negative effect induced by T-2 toxin. Notably, no negative effects in these productive parameters were found between broilers in the experimental group supplemented with Amdetox^{TM} alone and the control group, indicating that Amdetox^{TM} was nontoxic and safe.

The small intestine, including the duodenum, jejunum, and ileum, is the major part where most nutrient digestion and absorption takes place [26]. In this study, the pathological results showed that T-2 toxin caused serious small intestinal detriment in broilers, and these outcomes are in agreement with previous reports that T-2 toxin could induce intestine damage, thus decreasing nutrient utilization efficiency, as described above [27]. Interestingly, T-2 toxin-induced injury in the small intestine was mitigated by Amdetox^{TM} supplementation. Furthermore, the administration of T-2 toxin alone increased AST activity compared to the control group. The activity of serum enzymes such as AST and ALT, and concentrations of serum ALB and TP, have been described as valuable parameters of hepatic function and injury [28]. These outcomes are similar to previous studies that provided evidence that liver injury was induced by T-2 toxins in chicks [29,30]. However, some other reports have shown that T-2 toxin did not affect these parameters in poultry [31], pigs [32], and hamsters [33]. This discrepancy could be attributed to different experimental conditions, including exposure doses, duration, and animal species. The results obtained from the current study show that serum biochemical changes could be ameliorated by Amdetox^{TM} supplementation. Taken together, these results are in agreement with previous studies that reported that growth retardation induced by T-2 toxin was mainly due to induced intestinal and hepatic injury. Dietary Amdetox^{TM} supplementation, however, prevented T-2 toxin-induced poor growth performance, which was associated with the inhibition of intestinal and hepatic injury.

HSCAS adsorbent is a commercial feed additive that has been proven to have an effective ability to adsorb AFB_1 [34,35], while several studies have reported that general HSCAS adsorbents could not effectively adsorb Trichothecenes such as T-2 toxin [36] and DON [37]. Interestingly, artificially modified substances of zeolites [38], glucomannan [39], montmorillonite [40], and diatomaceous earth [30] can enhance the adsorption and detoxification of mycotoxins. Therefore, a modified HSCAS adsorbent product, Amdetox^{TM}, was developed to prevent the harmful effects of T-2 toxin. This HSCAS adsorbent is surface-modified with cetylpyridinium chloride based on natural bentonite and is intercalated with yeast β-glucan. After the special bentonite interlayer cation and water molecules are replaced by modifiers, the spacing between the particles is significantly increased, and the surface of the particles changes from hydrophilic to hydrophobic. Therefore, the modified HSCAS adsorbent has a larger adsorption capacity and lipophilic hydrophobicity, and it could effectively adsorb various mycotoxins in the feed. As expected, the modified HSCAS adsorbent displayed an effective ability to prevent the negative effect of T-2 toxin in broilers. Previous studies have shown that 0.25% adsorbent or 2% polymeric glucomannans could alleviate the harmful effect of 1.0–2.0 mg/kg T-2 toxin [41,42]. An addition of only 0.05% Amdetox^{TM} to a diet could reduce the negative effect induced by 6.0 mg/kg T-2 toxin, indicating that the modified HSCAS adsorbent was quite effective. Meanwhile, consistent with previous studies [19,43], the modified HSCAS adsorbent did not affect nutrient metabolic rates and growth performance in the current study.

4. Conclusions

In summary, these data indicate that the modified HSCAS adsorbent, Amdetox^{TM}, could be used as a promising adsorbent for the detoxification of T-2 toxin in practice.

5. Materials and Methods

5.1. Birds, Treatment, and Growth Performance

Ninety-six one-day-old Cobb-500 male broiler chicks with similar body weights were randomly allocated into four groups with four replicates of six birds/cage. The four groups of birds were allowed free access to water and were fed a corn-soybean-based diet (BD, group 1) formulated to meet the nutritional requirements of broilers (National Research Council (NRC), 1994; Table 4) or BD supplemented with 6.0 mg/kg T-2 toxin (Pribolab Pte. Ltd., Singapore) (group 2), 6.0 mg/kg T-2 toxin with 0.05% of Amdetox^{TM} (Jiangsu Aomai Bio-technology Co., Ltd. Nanjing, China) (group 3), or 0.05% of Amdetox^{TM} (group 4). The T-2 toxin-contaminated diet was made through a stepwise dilution method. Briefly, 150 mg of T-2 toxin was dissolved in 50 mL of ethanol and then mixed with 500 g of corn. The mixed sample was subsequently dried at 65 °C in an oven, which was used to make the T-2 toxin-contaminated diets. The mortality of the birds was monitored daily, whereas feed intake and body weight were measured weekly. The total excreta of each pen were collected during d 8–14 to measure the apparent metabolic rates of gross energy, crude protein, calcium, and total phosphorus of chicks. The experiment lasted for two weeks. At the end of the experiment, eight birds from each treatment group were killed to collect blood and small intestine (duodenum, jejunum, and ileum) for serological and intestinal histological examinations, as previously described [44].

Table 4. Formulation and nutritional content of the basal diet. [1]

Ingredients (%)	Quantity (%)
Corn	54.5
Soybean meal (48%)	30.4
Fish meal (64.5%)	5.6
Soybean oil	5.9
Calcium hydrophosphate	1.2
Limestone	1.0
Salt	0.2
DL-methionine	0.2
Premix [1]	1.0
Approximate composition of the test diets [2]	
Crude protein	23.00
Metabolisable energy, (MJ/kg)	13.38
Lysine	1.40
Methionine	0.58
Methionine + cysteine	0.94
Calcium	1.02
Available phosphorus	0.47

[1] The approximate composition provides the following per-kg diet: Vitamin A, 13800 IU/kg; vitamin D, 3600 IU; vitamin E, 24 IU/kg; vitamin K_3, 3.6 mg; vitamin B_1, 1.5 mg; vitamin B_2, 6.6 mg; vitamin B_6, 3 mg; vitamin B_{12}, 0.015 mg; folate, 0.9 mg; biotin, 0.09 mg; D-pantothenic acid, 9.6 mg; nicotinamide, 36 mg; iron, 96 mg; zinc, 53.9 mg; manganese, 71.4 mg; copper, 12 mg; selenium, 0.3 mg; iodine, 0.42 mg. [2] Calculated value.

5.2. Serum Biochemistry and Histopathology

The serum was prepared by centrifugation of the blood at 1000× *g* at 4 °C for 10 min. The activities of ALT and AST, as well as the concentrations of TP and ALB, in the serum were measured with the use of an automatic biochemistry analyzer (Beckman Synchron CX4 PRO, CA, USA), as previously described [45]. The duodenum, jejunum, and ileum ($n = 4$/group) were removed, fixed in neutral-buffered 10% formalin, embedded in paraffin, sectioned at 5 μm, stained with hematoxylin and eosin (H&E), and examined microscopically for histopathology [46]. Briefly, intestinal tissue was examined for each chick by light microscopy for described lesions: Degeneration, necrosis, and desquamation of the villous epithelial cells; and edema, thickening in the serosa, or both. Sections with no, slight, moderate, or intense presence of lesions were given scores of 0, 1, 2, and 3, respectively [46].

5.3. Apparent Metabolic Rate

The apparent metabolic rates of gross energy, crude protein, calcium, and total phosphorus of chicks were measured and calculated as previously described [47]. Gross energy was analyzed using an adiabatic bomb calorimeter standardized (IKA C2000) with benzoic acid. Calcium, total phosphorus, and crude protein were measured following the permanganate titration method 990.03 (AOAC, 2000), the colorimetric determination method 985.01 (AOAC, 1990), and the Kjeldahl digestion method 984.13 (AOAC, 1990), respectively [48].

5.4. Statistical Analysis

A one-way ANOVA was used to test the main effects of the dietary effect. A Bonferroni *t*-test followed for multiple mean comparisons if there was a main effect. Data are presented as means ± SD, and the significance level was set at $p < 0.05$. The analyses were conducted using the SPSS Statistics 19.0 package (SPSS Inc., IBM, New York, Ny, USA).

5.5. Ethical

This research was approved by Scientific Ethic Committee of Huazhong Agricultural University on 20 March 2017. The project identification code is HZAUCH-2017-008.

Author Contributions: L.-H.S., J.-T.W., and Q.L. conceived and designed the experiments; K.-T.W., J.-T.W. and H.S. performed the experiments; J.-T.W. and K.-T.W. analyzed the data; Q.L., N.-Y.Z., D.-S.Q., J.-F.D., and Y.L. contributed reagents/materials/analysis tools; J.-T.W., K.-T.W., M.M.K. and L.-H.S. wrote the paper.

Funding: This research was funded by the National Key Research and Development Program of China, Project (2018YFD0500601 and 2016YFD0501207); the Open Project of the Key Laboratory of Animal Embryo Engineering and Molecular Breeding of Hubei Province (KLAMEMB-2017-05); the Innovation Group of the Hubei Natural Science Foundation (2018CFA020); and a gift from Jiangsu Aomai Bio-technology Co., Ltd.

Conflicts of Interest: All authors have read and approved the final manuscript and declare that no competing interests exist.

References

1. Wu, Q.; Wang, X.; Nepovimova, E.; Miron, A.; Liu, Q.; Wang, Y.; Su, D.; Yang, H.; Li, L.; Kuca, K. Trichothecenes: Immunomodulatory effects, mechanisms, and anti-cancer potential. *Arch. Toxicol.* **2017**, *91*, 3737–3785. [CrossRef]
2. Gareis, M.; Zimmermann, C.; Schothorst, R.C. Collection of Occurrence Data of *Fusarium* Toxin in Food and Assessment of Dietary Intake by the Population of EU Member States. 2003. Available online: https://ci.nii.ac.jp/naid/20001046845/ (accessed on 2 April 2019).
3. Rasmussen, P.H.; Ghorbani, F.; Berg, T. Deoxynivalenol and other *Fusarium* toxins in wheat and rye flours on the Danish market. *Food Addit. Contam.* **2003**, *20*, 396. [CrossRef] [PubMed]
4. Makowska, K.; Obremski, K.; Gonkowski, S. The impact of T-2 toxin on vasoactive intestinal polypeptide-like immunoreactive (VIP-LI) nerve structures in the wall of the porcine stomach and duodenum. *Toxins* **2018**, *10*, 138. [CrossRef] [PubMed]
5. Makowska, K.; Obremski, K.; Zielonka, L.; Gonkowski, S. The influence of low doses of zearalenone and t-2 toxin on calcitonin gene related peptide-like immunoreactive (CGRP-LI) neurons in the ens of the porcine descending colon. *Toxins* **2017**, *9*, 98. [CrossRef]
6. Zhang, J.; Zhang, H.; Liu, S.; Wu, W.; Zhang, H. Comparison of anorectic potencies of type A trichothecenes T-2 toxin, HT-2 toxin, Diacetoxyscirpenol, and Neosolaniol. *Toxins* **2018**, *10*, 179. [CrossRef] [PubMed]
7. Chi, M.S.; Mirocha, C.J.; Kurtz, H.J.; Weaver, G.; Bates, F.; Shimoda, W. Subacute toxicity of T-2 toxin in broiler chicks. *Poult. Sci.* **1977**, *56*, 306. [CrossRef] [PubMed]
8. Meissonnier, G.M.; Laffitte, J.; Raymond, I.; Benoit, E.; Cossalter, A.M.; Pinton, P.; Bertin, G.; Oswald, I.P.; Galtier, P. Subclinical doses of T-2 toxin impair acquired immune response and liver cytochrome P450 in pigs. *Toxicology* **2008**, *247*, 46–54. [CrossRef]
9. Kubena, L.F.; Edrington, T.S.; Harvey, R.B.; Buckley, S.A.; Phillips, T.D.; Rottinghaus, G.E.; Casper, H.H. Individual and combined effects of fumonisin B_1 present in *Fusarium moniliforme* culture material and T-2 toxin or deoxynivalenol in broiler chicks. *Poult. Sci.* **1997**, *76*, 1239–1247. [CrossRef]
10. Manafi, M.; Mohan, K.; Ali, M.N. Effect of ochratoxin A on coccidiosis-challenged broiler chicks. *World Mycotoxin J.* **2011**, *4*, 177–181. [CrossRef]

11. Wu, J.; Zhou, Y.; Yuan, Z.; Yi, J.; Chen, J.; Wang, N.; Tian, Y. Autophagy and apoptosis interact to modulate T-2 toxin-induced toxicity in liver cells. *Toxins* **2019**, *11*, 179. [CrossRef] [PubMed]
12. Hooshmand, H.; Klopfenstein, C.F. Effects of gamma irradiation on mycotoxin disappearance and amino acid contents of corn, wheat, and soybeans with different moisture contents. *Plant Foods Hum. Nutr.* **1995**, *47*, 227–238. [CrossRef] [PubMed]
13. Faifer, G.C.; Velazco, V.; Godoy, H.M. Adjustment of the conditions required for complete decontamination of T-2 toxin residues with alkaline sodium hypochlorite. *Bull. Environ. Contam. Toxicol.* **1994**, *52*, 102. [CrossRef] [PubMed]
14. Diaz, G.J.; Cortes, A.; Roldan, L. Evaluation of the efficacy of four feed additives against the adverse effects of T-2 toxin in growing broiler chickens. *J. Appl. Poult. Res.* **2005**, *14*, 226–231. [CrossRef]
15. Piva, A.; Galvano, F. Nutritional approaches to reduce the impact of mycotoxins. In *Biotechnology in the Feed Industry*; Nottingham University Press: Nottingham, UK, 1999.
16. Huwig, A.; Freimund, S.; Käppeli, O.; Dutler, H. Mycotoxin detoxication of animal feed by different adsorbents. *Toxicol. Lett.* **2001**, *122*, 179. [CrossRef]
17. Gerez, J.; Buck, L.; Marutani, V.; Calliari, C.; Bracarense, A. Low levels of chito-oligosaccharides are not effective in reducing deoxynivalenol toxicity in swine jejunal explants. *Toxins* **2018**, *10*, 276. [CrossRef] [PubMed]
18. Santurio, J.M.; Mallmann, C.A.; Rosa, A.P.; Appel, G.; Heer, A.; Dageforde, S.; Bottcher, M. Effect of sodium bentonite on the performance and blood variables of broiler chickens intoxicated with aflatoxins. *Br. Poult. Sci.* **1999**, *40*, 115–119. [CrossRef]
19. Desheng, Q.; Fan, L.; Yanhu, Y.; Niya, Z. Adsorption of aflatoxin B_1 on montmorillonite. *Poult. Sci.* **2005**, *84*, 959–961. [CrossRef] [PubMed]
20. Miazzo, R.; Rosa, C.A.; De Queiroz, C.E.; Magnoli, C.; Chiacchiera, S.M.; Palacio, G.; Saenz, M.; Kikot, A.; Basaldella, E.; Dalcero, A. Efficacy of synthetic zeolite to reduce the toxicity of aflatoxin in broiler chicks. *Poult. Sci.* **2000**, *79*, 1–6. [CrossRef]
21. Abbes, S.; Salah-Abbes, J.B.; Ouanes, Z.; Houas, Z.; Othman, O.; Bacha, H.; Abdel-Wahhab, M.A.; Oueslati, R. Preventive role of phyllosilicate clay on the immunological and biochemical toxicity of zearalenone in Balb/c mice. *Int. Immunopharmacol.* **2006**, *6*, 1251–1258. [CrossRef]
22. Mitchell, N.J.; Xue, K.S.; Lin, S.; Marroquin-Cardona, A.; Brown, K.A.; Elmore, S.E.; Tang, L.; Romoser, A.; Gelderblom, W.C.; Wang, J.S.; et al. Calcium montmorillonite clay reduces AFB_1 and FB_1 biomarkers in rats exposed to single and co-exposures of aflatoxin and fumonisin. *J. Appl. Toxicol.* **2014**, *34*, 795–804. [CrossRef]
23. Girish, C.K.; Devegowda, G. Efficacy of Glucomannan-containing Yeast Product (Mycosorb 쪼) and Hydrated Sodium Calcium Aluminosilicate in Preventing the Individual and Combined Toxicity of Aflatoxin and T-2 Toxin in Commercial Broilers. *Asian-Australas. J. Anim. Sci.* **2006**, *19*, 877–883. [CrossRef]
24. Danicke, S.; Matthes, S.; Halle, I.; Ueberschar, K.H.; Doll, S.; Valenta, H. Effects of graded levels of *Fusarium* toxin-contaminated wheat and of a detoxifying agent in broiler diets on performance, nutrient digestibility and blood chemical parameters. *Br. Poult. Sci.* **2003**, *44*, 113–126. [CrossRef]
25. Osborne, D.J.; Huff, W.E.; Hamilton, P.B.; Burmeister, H.R. Comparison of ochratoxin, aflatoxin, and T-2 toxin for their effects on selected parameters related to digestion and evidence for specific metabolism of carotenoids in chickens. *Poult. Sci.* **1982**, *61*, 1646–1652. [CrossRef] [PubMed]
26. Vermeulen, B.; Backer, P.D.; Remon, J.P. Drug administration to poultry. *Adv. Drug Deliv. Rev.* **2002**, *54*, 795–803. [CrossRef]
27. Yang, J.H.; Chen, H.Y.; Han, W.; Zhao, Z.H.; Sun, Z.Z.; Guo, W.B. Influence of T-2 toxin on nutrient apparent digestibility and small intestinal morphology in BALB/c Mice. *Chin. J. Anim. Vet. Sci.* **2015**, *46*, 1584–1592.
28. Sun, L.H.; Lei, M.Y.; Zhang, N.Y.; Zhao, L.; Krumm, C.S.; Qi, D.S. Hepatotoxic effects of mycotoxin combinations in mice. *Food Chem. Toxicol.* **2014**, *74*, 289–293. [CrossRef] [PubMed]
29. Shareef, A.M. Ineffectiveness of different adsorbents in alleviation of oral lesions induced by feeding T-2 toxin in broiler chickens. *Iraqi J. Vet. Sci.* **2007**, *21*, 75–86. [CrossRef]
30. Shivashankar, B.P.; Narayanaswamy, H.D.; Satyanarayana, M.L.; Rao, S.; Rathnamma, D.; Rathnamma, H.K.; Sridhar, N.B. Effect of diatomaceous earth on performance, internalorgans and biochemical alterations in T-2 toxicosis of broiler chickens. *J. Cell Tissue Res.* **2015**, *15*, 4983–4988.
31. Kutasi, J.; Papp, Z.; Jakab, L.; Brydl, E.; Rafai, P. Deactivation of T-2 toxin in broiler ducks by biotransformation. *J. Appl. Poult. Res.* **2012**, *21*, 13–20. [CrossRef]

32. Frankič, T.; Salobir, J.; Rezar, V. The effect of vitamin E supplementation on reduction of lymphocyte DNA damage induced by T-2 toxin and deoxynivalenol in weaned pigs. *Anim. Feed Sci. Technol.* **2008**, *141*, 274–286. [CrossRef]
33. Rajmon, R.; Sedmikova, M.; Jilek, F.; Koubkova, M.; Barta, I.; Smerak, P. Combined effects of repeated low doses of aflatoxin B_1 and T-2 toxin on the Chinese hamster. *Vet. Med.* **2001**, *46*, 301–307. [CrossRef]
34. Chen, S.S.; Li, Y.H.; Lin, M.F. Chronic exposure to the *Fusarium* mycotoxin deoxynivalenol: Impact on performance, immune organ, and intestinal integrity of slow-growing chickens. *Toxins* **2017**, *9*, 334. [CrossRef]
35. Grant, P.G.; Phillips, T.D. Isothermal adsorption of aflatoxin B_1 on HSCAS clay. *J. Agric. Food Chem.* **1998**, *46*, 599–605. [CrossRef]
36. Bailey, R.H.; Kubena, L.F.; Harvey, R.B.; Buckley, S.A.; Rottinghaus, G.E. Efficacy of various inorganic sorbents to reduce the toxicity of aflatoxin and T-2 toxin in broiler chickens. *Poult. Sci.* **1998**, *77*, 1623–1630. [CrossRef]
37. Patterson, R.; Young, L.G. Efficacy of hydrated sodium calcium aluminosilicate, screening and dilution in reducing the effects of mold contaminated corn in pigs. *Can. J. Anim. Sci.* **1993**, *73*, 615–624. [CrossRef]
38. Tomašević-Čanović, M.; Daković, A.; Rottinghaus, G.; Matijašević, S.; Đuričić, M. Surfactant modified zeolites–new efficient adsorbents for mycotoxins. *Microporous Mesoporous Mater.* **2003**, *61*, 173–180. [CrossRef]
39. Reddy, N.B.; Devegowda, G.; Shashidhara, R.G. Ability of modified glucomannan to sequestrate T-2 toxin in the gastrointestinal tract of chicken. *Asian-Australas. J. Anim. Sci.* **2004**, *17*, 259–262. [CrossRef]
40. Lemke, S.L.; Mayura, K.; Reeves, W.R.; Wang, N.; Fickey, C.; Phillips, T.D. Investigation of organophilic montmorillonite clay inclusion in zearalenone-contaminated diets using the mouse uterine weight bioassay. *J. Toxicol. Environ. Health* **2001**, *62*, 243–258. [CrossRef]
41. Fazekas, B.; Tóthné Hajdu, E.; Tanyi, J. Effect of Myco-ad on experimental T-2 toxicosis in broiler chickens. *Magyar Állatorvosok Lapja* **2000**, *122*, 412–416.
42. Meissonnier, G.M.; Raymond, I.; Laffitte, J.; Cossalter, A.M.; Pinton, P.; Benoit, E.; Bertin, G.; Galtier, P.; Oswald, I.P. Dietary glucomannan improves the vaccinal response in pigs exposed to aflatoxin B_1 or T-2 toxin. *World Mycotoxin J.* **2009**, *2*, 161–172. [CrossRef]
43. Abbes, S.; Ouanes, Z.S.J.; Houas, Z.; Oueslati, R.; Bacha, H.; Othman, O. The protective effect of hydrated sodium calcium aluminosilicate against haematological, biochemical and pathological changes induced by Zearalenone in mice. *Toxicon* **2006**, *47*, 567. [CrossRef]
44. Gao, X.; Xiao, Z.H.; Liu, M.; Zhang, N.Y.; Khalil, M.M.; Gu, C.Q.; Qi, D.S.; Sun, L.H. Dietary Silymarin Supplementation Alleviates Zearalenone-Induced Hepatotoxicity and Reproductive Toxicity in Rats. *J. Nutr.* **2018**, *148*, 1209–1216. [CrossRef]
45. Sun, L.H.; Zhang, N.Y.; Zhu, M.K.; Zhao, L.; Zhou, J.C.; Qi, D.S. Prevention of aflatoxin B1 hepatoxicity by dietary selenium is associated with inhibition of cytochrome P450 isozymes and up-regulation of 6 selenoprotein genes in chick liver. *J. Nutr.* **2016**, *146*, 655–661. [CrossRef]
46. Denli, M.; Blandon, J.C.; Guynot, M.E.; Salado, S.; Perez, J.F. Effects of dietary AflaDetox on performance, serum biochemistry, histopathological changes, and aflatoxin residues in broilers exposed to aflatoxin B_1. *Poult. Sci.* **2009**, *88*, 1444–1451. [CrossRef]
47. Namkung, H.; Leeson, S. Effect of phytase enzyme on dietary nitrogen-corrected apparent metabolizable energy and the ileal digestibility of nitrogen and amino acids in broiler chicks. *Poult. Sci.* **1999**, *78*, 1317–1319. [CrossRef]
48. Zhao, L.; Zhang, N.Y.; Pan, Y.X.; Zhu, L.Y.; Batonon-Alavo, D.I.; Ma, L.B.; Khalil, M.M.; Qi, D.S.; Sun, L.H. Efficacy of 2-hydroxy-4-methylthiobutanoic acid compared to DL-Methionine on growth performance, carcass traits, feather growth, and redox status of Cherry Valley ducks. *Poult. Sci.* **2018**, *97*, 3166–3175. [CrossRef]

toxins MDPI

Article

AFM1 Detection in Milk by Fab′ Functionalized Si_3N_4 Asymmetric Mach–Zehnder Interferometric Biosensors

Tatevik Chalyan [1,*,†,‡], Cristina Potrich [2,3,†], Erik Schreuder [4], Floris Falke [4], Laura Pasquardini [2,§], Cecilia Pederzolli [2], Rene Heideman [4] and Lorenzo Pavesi [1]

1 Nanoscience Laboratory, Department of Physics, University of Trento, 38123 Trento, Italy
2 LaBSSAH, Fondazione Bruno Kessler, 38123 Trento, Italy
3 CNR-Consiglio Nazionale delle Ricerche, Istituto di Biofisica, 38123 Trento, Italy
4 LioniX International BV, 7521 AN Enschede, The Netherlands
* Correspondence: tchalyan@b-phot.org
† These authors contributed equally to this work.
‡ Current address: B-PHOT Brussels Photonics, Vrije Universiteit Brussel, 1050 Brussels, Belgium.
§ Current address: Indivenire s.r.l., 38123 Trento, Italy.

Received: 27 May 2019; Accepted: 11 July 2019; Published: 14 July 2019

Abstract: Aflatoxins (AF) are naturally occurring mycotoxins, produced by many species of Aspergillus. Among aflatoxins, Aflatoxin M1 (AFM1) is one of the most frequent and dangerous for human health. The acceptable maximum level of AFM1 in milk according to EU regulation is 50 ppt, equivalent to 152 pM, and 25 ppt, equivalent to 76 pM, for adults and infants, respectively. Here, we study a photonic biosensor based on Si_3N_4 asymmetric Mach–Zehnder Interferometers (aMZI) functionalized with Fab′ for AFM1 detection in milk samples (eluates). The minimum concentration of AFM1 detected by our aMZI sensors is 48 pM (16.8 pg/mL) in purified and concentrated milk samples. Moreover, the real-time detection of the ligand-analyte binding enables the study of the kinetics of the reaction. We measured the kinetic rate constants of the Fab′-AFM1 interaction.

Keywords: lab-on-chip; optical biosensors; Fab′; Aflatoxin M1; asymmetric Mach–Zehnder interferometer; limit of detection; affinity

Key Contribution: An integrated silicon-photonic biosensor based on asymmetric Mach–Zehnder Interferometers (aMZI) functionalized with Fab′ is demonstrated for AFM1 specific detection in milk samples. The system detects down to 48 pM (16.8 pg/mL) of AFM1 in milk as minimum concentration in less than 1.5 h. Moreover, the proposed system can be used out of the laboratory environment. In addition, for the first time we determined the unknown kinetic rate constants of the Fab′-AFM1 interaction.

1. Introduction

Contamination of food and agricultural products by various types of toxigenic molds (fungi) is a serious and global problem in the increasing number of countries. Fungal toxins have been detected in various food commodities and have been recognized to be one of the most dangerous contaminants that affects human and animal health [1]. In particular, mycotoxins produced by several species of fungi are naturally present in nuts, grains, maize, rice, soya [2]. Out of different categories of mycotoxins, aflatoxins produced by toxigenic strains of the fungi *Aspergillus flavus* and *Aspergillus parasiticus* are recognized to be the most toxic/carcinogenic compounds [3,4]. Aflatoxins found in feed are known as aflatoxin B1, B2, G1, and G2. In milk aflatoxin is present as AFB1 metabolite known as Aflatoxin M1 (AFM1). The International Agency for Research on Cancer (IARC) has categorized AFM1 as 2B human carcinogen [5]. Since most of the human species, as well as animals, particularly the nurturing ones, are dependent from milk as a part of complete basal nutrition, AFM1 contamination in milk and its products is of extreme importance and is a serious problem. The European Commission (EC) regulation No. 1881/2006 specifies the maximum level of AFM1 contamination in milk to 50 ppt (50 pg/mL) for adults, and to 25 ppt (25 pg/mL) for infant formulae. However, a long-term consumption of AFM1 at the low levels (ppb) may lead to the development of hepatocellular cancer [6]. In addition, these mycotoxins are thermostable and very resistant to degradation, even after chemical treatments [7]. Therefore, milk contaminated by AFM1 has to be eliminated before entering to the human nutrition.

Methods for fast and effective detection of AFM1 are indeed crucial. However, they have a non-negligible economic impact, being unavailable especially in the poor developing countries, where the level of milk contamination is high. Considering the sensitivity, reproducibility, specificity and cost per unit of test, standard methods such as thin layer chromatography (TLC) [8], High Performance Liquid Chromatography (HPLC) [9,10], immunoassays such as enzyme-linked immunosorbent assay (ELISA) [11,12] have been traditionally identified as more convenient tools for the detection of aflatoxins. These methods are based on fluorescence or electrochemical principles. On the other hand, alternative sensing devices based on optics are getting more and more appealing due to their speed, low cost and performances. Specifically, surface plasmon resonance (SPR) biosensors today are the most popular and commercialized optical biosensors [13]. They are widly used for affinity analyses [14]. They are competitive with HPLC or ELISA. Table 1 shows the comparison of the results from the known AFM1 detection systems with the results reported in this work.

Table 1. Comparison of various methods to detect Aflatoxin M1 (AFM1) in milk.

Method	LOD (ppt)	Detection Time (min)	Reference
TLC	5	4–5	[8]
HPLC	4.5	72	[9,10]
ELISA	4.3	3	[11,12]
ROSA	500	0.15	[15]
Bilayer Lipid Membranes	16	0.5	[16]
Microelectrodes Arrays	8	2	[17]
Electrochemical	10	0.5	[18]
Field Immunoassay	50	3	[19]
DNA-aptasensor	20	4	[20]
SPR	0.6	1	[13]
SPR with gold nanoparticles	18	1	[21]
aMZI	16.8	1.5	This work

Since 1990, the development of the integrated photonics-based optical biosensors gained momentum as a result of the optimization of the microfabrication technologies. Thereafter, label-free optical biosensors have become one of the most attractive biosensing devices thanks to their selectivity and high sensitivity [22]. Moreover, the easy fabrication with standard microelectronic/micromachining processes guarantees a low cost for mass production. These types of devices satisfy the requirements of the portability and, thus, they free the biosensors from the laboratory settings. This is a result of the integration with microfluidics which allows the realization of lab-on-chip devices [23].

Lab-on-a-chip devices got a further impulse after the development of silicon photonics. Silicon photonics takes advantage of the several favorable optical properties of silicon, such as the high refractive index that enables the realization of small optical components or the easy of manufacturing silicon by using complementary metal oxide semiconductor (CMOS) technology [24]. In silicon photonics based biosensors, micro-ring resonators (MRR) based on whispering gallery mode (WGM) cavities and interferometers, such as the Mach–Zehnder interferometer (MZI), are the preferred geometries. The use of a small micro-resonator for biosensing applications made its first appearance only in recent years [25,26]. Different proteins, down to a single molecule level [27], have been detected. In 1993 Heideman et al. [28], demonstrated a biosensor based on MZI using a planar optical waveguide as the sensing element. Biosensor, functionalized with antibodies, successfully detected human chorionic gonadotropin (hCG). Since then many works have been reported on integrated MZI biosensors [29–32].

In search of an economic, portable device to detect AFM1 in milk in less than 1 h and to reach a limit of detection of AFM1 comparable with available commercial systems, the European project SYMPHONY [33] (grant number 610580) has developed a system, based on an integrated photonic sensor, interfaced with a complex microfluidic stage to purify and concentrate the milk samples. The photonic sensor is based on an array of asymmetric Mach–Zehnder interferometers (aMZI). The sensing is performed by measuring the phase shift of the output signal, caused by the binding of the analyte on the functionalized aMZI surface. The binding causes changes on the effective refractive index, n_{eff}, of the optical mode, confined in the waveguide. The change on n_{eff} is converted to the phase shift between the signal from the sensing and the reference arms of the interferometer. In order to have a specific detection of AFM1, a functionalization process, based on antigen-binding fragments (Fab′) is applied to the surface of the sensing arm of an aMZI. The main advantage of using Fab′, with respect to whole antibodies, is the possibility to obtain a higher surface density of the Fab′ fragments which yields a higher biosensor sensitivity as well as a lower limit of detection (LOD_{AFM1}) of AFM1 [34].

In our previous works, we have reported an example of a complete measurement cycle for AFM1 detection in MES buffer as well as AFM1 specificity measurements in comparison with ochratoxin A (OTA) mycotoxin in MES buffer [35]. It has been demonstrated that for a solution which contains 5 nM of AFM1 injected in the Fab′ functionalized sensor the spectral shift is much higher than if we inject a solution with 100 nM of OTA.

Here we focus on AFM1 monitoring at different concentrations in milk samples. First, we report the optical characterization of the sensors such as the bulk sensitivity, S_b, and the LOD. Then, we perform biosensing measurements in milk samples. Finally, we measure the AFM1-Fab′ binding affinity and the dissociation constant in milk. The lowest detectable concentration of AFM1 in milk by our sensor is 48 pM, lower than the EU regulations request.

2. Results

2.1. Experimental Setup

An image of the sensor chip is reported in Figure 1. The devices were fabricated by the single-stripe TriPlex technology [36]. The details of the sensor fabrication process are given in [35].

The sensor design had eight aMZI in a single chip. Each aMZI had two arms realized by spiral waveguides to keep the footprint small. The length of the waveguide in each arm was 6.25 mm. There was a small additional length in one of the two arms, named the reference arm, to obtain an asymmetry. This additional length determines the period of the interference fringes when the input signal wavelength is scanned, i.e., the free spectral range (FSR) of the aMZI. The FSR is set such that it matches the spectral tuning range of the laser source, which was a commercial vertical-cavity surface-emitting laser (VCSEL) emitting at 850 nm. An input waveguide (bright spot on the right in Figure 1) feds two one-to-four channel splitters which distribute the input signal to two groups of four aMZI. In this work, we only use the top set formed by four aMZIs, three of which have an exposed arm. By this we mean that the cladding on top of them is removed to form a sensing window. The sensing window allows the interaction between the evanescent field of the light propagating in the waveguide and the liquid sample of interest. To open the sensing window, the top cladding is locally removed by a photolithography step and BHF wet etch, down to the Si_3N_4 layer. One aMZI (the top one in Figure 1) is left covered to save as a reference for the temperature or laser fluctuations. The signals from the aMZI are then individually sent to the outputs.

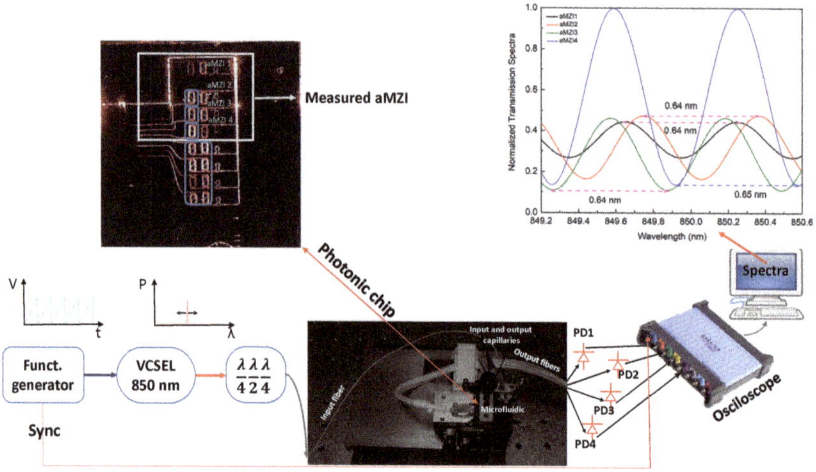

Figure 1. (**top left**) Image of the chip with illuminated Mach–Zehnder Interferometers (aMZI). (**top right**) Normalized transmission spectra of four aMZI. (**bottom**) Schematic of the experimental setup.

In fact, the sensor device was mounted in a miniaturized alignment stage [35] completed with a microfluidic chamber with two inlets. These are connected to a VICI M6 liquid handling pump with capillaries with a diameter of 150 µm which are used for the continuous flow during the sensing measurements. A single mode fiber at 850 nm connects the mentioned light source (VCSEL) and the chip. The polarization of the input light signal is controlled by a two-paddle polarization stages. For the detection, we connected the output fibers to four Si transimpedance amplified photodetectors interfaced to a PicoScope 4824 (an eight channel USB oscilloscope). Wavelength scanning was achieved by current tuning the VCSEL with a periodic current ramp, which also triggers the time scan of the oscilloscope. In this way, a wavelength scan of the four aMZI is performed and the output signals are recorded by the oscilloscope and transferred to a control computer. Figure 1, top right, reports an example of the recorded waveforms from the four aMZI on the same photonic chip. Any variation of the effective indices of the mode travelling in the sensing arm causes a phase shift of the waveforms of the output signals. Therefore, by real-time analysis of the waveforms, a live recording of the phase shifts of the signal light propagating in the four aMZI can be achieved with a VCSEL modulation frequency of 20 Hz, and a data acquisition of 50,000 points per spectrum. The transmission signals of all devices were normalized to the maximum signal of the reference aMZI. Apart from variation of the intensity and relative phase, the FSR of the three aMZI with the sensing arm are the same and equal to 0.64 nm. The FSR of the reference aMZI is slightly different as a result of the presence of the cladding. Knowing the FSR, we can calculate the wavelength shift from the phase shift, considering that 1 rad $\cong \frac{FSR}{2\pi} = 0.1014$ nm. In order to compare results of various sensing methods, it was convenient to report the sensor response in nm and not in radians. To check the repeatability of the sensor production, we characterized more than 60 sensors.

2.2. Surface Preparation

Fab′ were prepared starting from rabbit anti-afltoxin M1 antiserum (Tecna). The functionalization is based on a mixed self assembled monolayer (SAM), a well known method utilized for the covalent immobilization of antibodies [37]. Polyclonal antibodies (IgG) were firstly purified from antiserum components with Amicon Ultra-0.5 10 kDa centrifugal filters (Millipore) to change to the suitable sample buffer (10 mM phosphate buffer, 10 mM ethylenediaminetetraacetic acid (EDTA) pH 7).

IgG were then mixed with immobilized papain (ThermoScientific) pre-activated with cysteine-HCl, following manufacturer's instructions. The digestion of IgG with papain was performed at 37 °C for 6 h. At the end of digestion, three volumes of 10 mM Tris/HCl buffer pH 7.5 (with respect to the starting antibody volume) were added before spinning the reacted antibodies. The obtained supernatant contained the Fab' fragments, the undigested IgG and Fc fragments, which were separated by ion exchange chromatography (Vivapure D Mini, Sartorius). The resulting flow through fraction containing the Fab' fragments was quantified by spectrophotometry (Nanodrop ND-1000 spectrophotometer, Nanodrop Tecnologies, Wilmington, DE, USA) and the quality of Fab was verified by SDS-PAGE (an example is reported in Figure S1).

The desired amount of Fab' was reduced for 2 h with 10 mM DTT just before use. The excess of DTT is then removed with Amicon Ultra-0.5 10 kDa centrifugal filters (Millipore). A general scheme of the surface functionalization is reported in Figure 2.

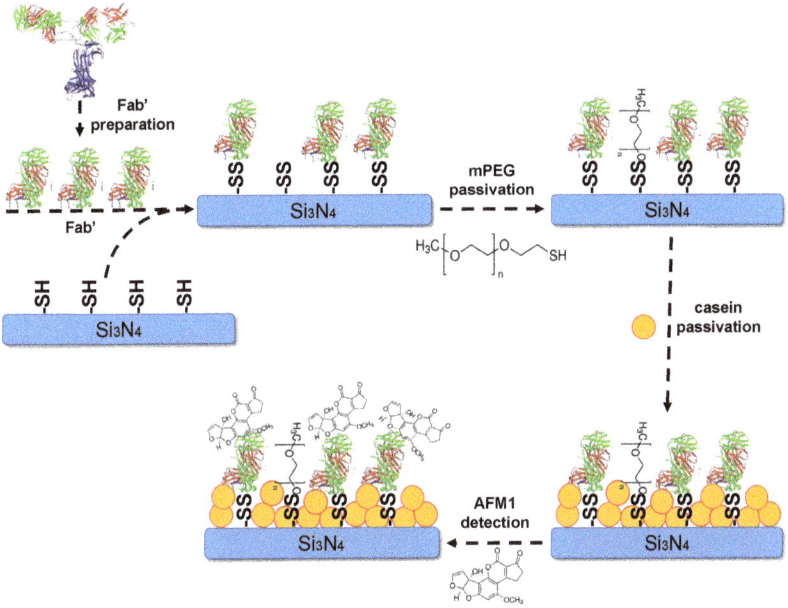

Figure 2. Schematics of the surface functionalization principle. Note, that the molecule sizes are not scaled and are not corresponding to the real proportions.

The Fab' were immobilized on the Si_3N_4 surface of aMZI adapting the protocol described in Yoshimoto et al. for gold surfaces [38], but further characterizations were performed as reported in the Supplementary Material (Figures S2 and S3). Immobilization protocol for Si_3N_4 surface was described in the previous work of our group [39]. An additional passivation step was, indeed, carried out. An optimization of the surface passivation has been already reported [35]. Since in the milk samples there are casein molecules, non-specific adsorption of casein on the Si_3N_4 surface causes a significant fake signal parallel to the one from the Fab'-AFM1 specific binding. Thus, an additional step of casein passivation was carried out. Surfaces were passivated with 0.1 mg/mL of casein for 30 min then extensively rinsed in sample buffer (by using a becker with 150 mL of buffer), moved to a clean well of a 24-wells plate, covered with buffer and kept wet until used. In parallel with aMZI surfaces, Si_3N_4 flat surfaces are functionalized and used to check if the functionalization protocol was correct. At the end of functionalization, flat surfaces were incubated with AFM1-Horseradish Peroxidase (HRP) conjugate (part of Aflatoxin M1 ELISA kit I'screen, Tecna) for 1 h at room temperature on an orbital shaker at 60 rpm. After several washes with buffer (50 mM MES pH 6.6), these surfaces were incubated with the developer solutions (SuperSignal^{TM} ELISA Femto Substrate, ThermoScientific) and measured with a ChemiDoc^{TM} imaging system (BioRad, Figure S4).

2.3. Theoretical Model

The time evolution of the phase shift (sensorgrams) when the toxin is added to the sample follows the molecular binding events. Let us assume that this occurs via a simple 1:1 interaction (i.e., we assume that the ligand has only one binding site). Therefore, the ligand L and the target molecule A bind reversibly in solution to form a binary complex AL via

$$\mathrm{L} + \mathrm{A}[\mathrm{k}_{off}]\mathrm{k}_{on}\mathrm{AL}, \tag{1}$$

where k_{on} is the second-order rate constant for complex association and k_{off} is the first-order rate constant for complex dissociation. The rate of complex formation (whose concentration is [AL]) depends on the free concentration of A and L ([A] and [L] correspondingly) and on the stability of the complex. Since our sensor functionalized by Fab′ for AFM1 detection works by this principle [35], the characteristics of the molecular reaction Equation (1) can be extracted from a fit of the sensorgrams with a kinetic model. For various toxin concentrations, C, the following fit function is used [40]:

$$\mathrm{R}_A(t) = \mathrm{R}_{eq}[1 - \exp(-\mathrm{k}_{obs}t)], \tag{2}$$

where $R_A(t)$ is the sensor response (phase shift) at time t, R_{eq} is the signal level at equilibrium and k_{obs} is the experimentally determined value of the pseudo-first-order rate constant to approach the equilibrium. The latter is given as:

$$\mathrm{k}_{obs} = \mathrm{k}_{on}\mathrm{C} + \mathrm{k}_{off}. \tag{3}$$

The linear fit of k_{obs} vs. C yields k_{on} and k_{off}. Knowing k_{on} and k_{off}, we can compute the complex equilibrium dissociation constant K_D or the molecular affinity K_A:

$$\mathrm{K}_D = \frac{\mathrm{k}_{off}}{\mathrm{k}_{on}} = \frac{1}{\mathrm{K}_A}. \tag{4}$$

3. Discussion

3.1. Bulk Sensitivity and Limit of Detection

We test the performances of our photonic sensors, by characterizing simultaneously the volume (bulk) Sensitivity (S_b) of the three uncovered aMZIs. To calculate this parameter, a real-time monitoring of the phase shift of the aMZI is conducted, when glucose or salt (NaCl) water solutions of various concentrations flow on the sensor. Flowing pure deionized water provides the reference and the baseline. Let us define, the bulk sensitivity of the aMZIs as:

$$\mathrm{S}_b = \frac{\partial \phi_0}{\partial \mathrm{n}_s}, \tag{5}$$

where ϕ_0 is the phase and n_s is the cladding refractive index.

Figure 3a shows the wavelength shifts in nm when the cladding refractive index is changed. The plot refers to the simultaneous measure of the four aMZI. Note, that the results of the measurements reported in this figure correspond to ona photonic chip. The injection of the glucose or salt solutions causes a significant shift, which is similar for the three uncovered aMZIs on the chip. Since aMZI4 is covered, the change of the flowing liquid do not lead to any wavelength shift. The 0% value on the plot refers to the injection of pure water from the same reservoir of the flowing glucose or salt solutions. The observed small shift is caused by the temperature difference between the solution injected from the valve and that flowing continuously inside the tubings. In the further analyses this shift is considered as a baseline.

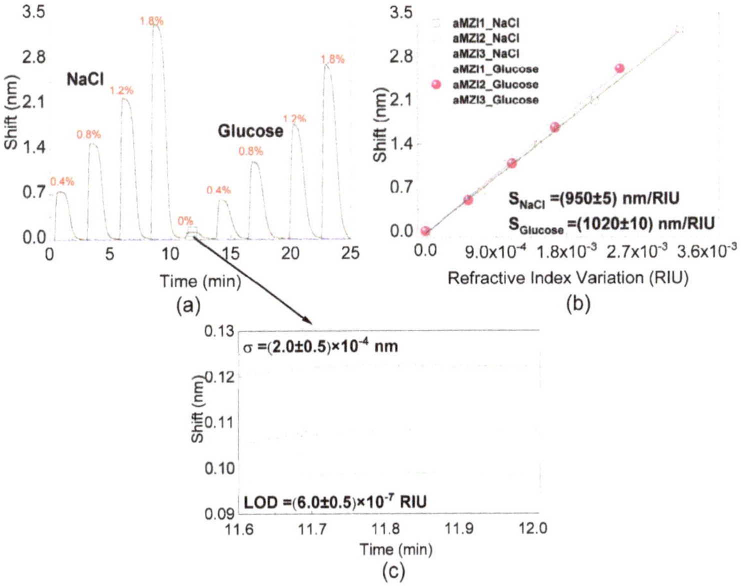

Figure 3. (**a**) Sensorgrams of four aMZI on the same chip for variation in the cladding refractive index, obtained by injections of glucose and salt water solutions at different concentrations (glucose and NaCl concentrations are in $\%w/v$ labelled on the plot). (**b**) Wavelength shift linear fit where the slope is the sensitivity. (**c**) The shift taken in 24 s corresponding to the time interval 11.6 ÷ 12.0 min in the sensorgram. This interval is marked inside the black square.

Figure 3b shows the dependence of the shift versus the refractive index of the solution, i.e., the slope of this plot is the bulk sensitivity. The refractive index variation is given by refractive index units (RIU). We find a sensitivity of (950 ± 5) nm/RIU and (1020 ± 10) nm/RIU, respectively, for NaCl and glucose water solutions for all the three exposed sensors. The small difference between these sensitivities can be a result of the density difference. In fact, there are more molecules of salt than of glucose in a solution with the same concentration when we measure the concentration in percentage of weight per volume. The measurement of both the glucose and salt solutions shows that for non-biological solutions the sensitivity is almost the same.

The minimum concentration that can be distinguished with a certain confidence level defines the limit of detection (LOD) of the biosensor [41]. Knowing S_b, LOD can be calculated as:

$$\mathrm{LOD} = \frac{k\sigma}{S_b}, \tag{6}$$

where σ is the standard deviation of repeated measurements of blank solutions. The use of k = 3 sets the confidence level to 99.7%.

By measuring an average standard deviation of the signal $\sigma = (2.0 \pm 0.5) \times 10^{-4}$ nm within a time interval of 24 s (see Figure 3c), we calculate a LOD $\cong (6.0 \pm 0.5) \times 10^{-7}$ RIU.

In order to verify the reproducibility of the sensor fabrication, we repeat the volumetric sensing measurements for more than 60 different sensors. The sensitivity and LOD histograms are reported in Figure 4. An $\approx$ 10% spread for the mean value of the sensitivity is observed which is an indication of the repeatability of the sensor fabrication and testing. A mean value for $S_b \approx (1250 \pm 150)$ nm/RIU is achieved, while a mean value of LOD $\approx (1.2 \pm 0.3) \times 10^{-6}$ RIU is calculated. These values are comparable with other sensors reported in the literature [35].

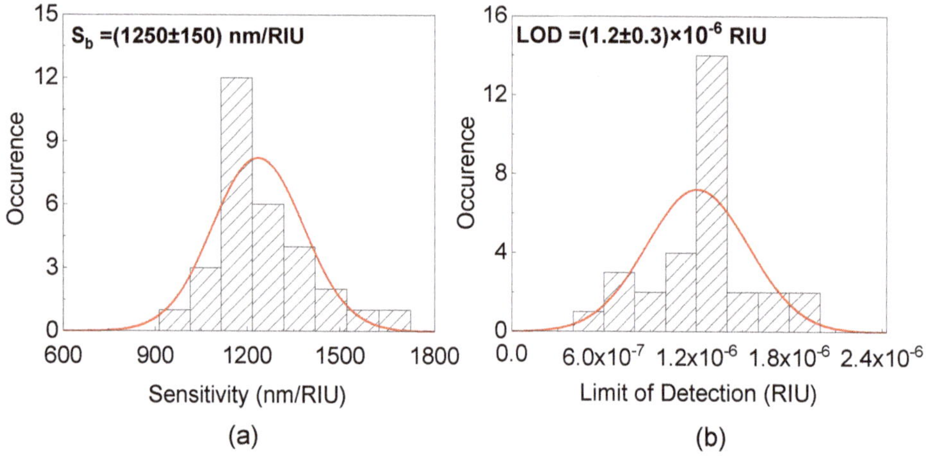

Figure 4. Histograms of the bulk sensitivity (S_b) and of the limit of detection (LOD) for 60 aMZI chips: (**a**) The histogram for the bulk sensitivity obtained by volumetric sensing measurements. The mean value is (1250 $\pm$ 150) nm/RIU, the best measured sensitivity is (1600 $\pm$ 100) nm/RIU. Bin size is 100 nm/RIU. (**b**) The histogram for the LOD with 2 $\times 10^{-7}$ RIU bin size. The minimum LOD is (5.0 $\pm$ 1.0) $\times$ 10^{-7} RIU, the mean value is LOD = (1.2 $\pm$ 0.3) $\times$ 10^{-6} RIU.

3.2. AFM1 Detection

Sensing experiments are performed on filtered and concentrated samples where the toxins are concentrated by a factor of 20 in the eluate with the concentration module of the *SYMPHONY* setup. The AFM1 concentrations in the samples are first determined with the ELISA assay. For each concentration, we use freshly functionalized sensor. This is done in order to avoid surface functionality degradation after the regeneration process.

For the first demonstration of AFM1 specific detection two eluates with 0.09 nM and 2 nM AFM1 concentrations, respectively (see Figure 5a) are used. A flow rate of 15 μL/min and an injected sample volume of 30 μL are used. Note that in the prepared samples still some proteins and, in particular, casein remain causing a non-specific signal. The non-specific adsorption of milk component even on passivated surfaces is a known phenomenon [21]. A clear difference between the measured signals is observed due to the different AFM1 concentrations. After getting confidence that the sensor distinguishes the AFM1 presence in the real milk samples, for the second set of the tests a wider variety of AFM1 concentrations is used. To achieve a faster detection, the flow rate is increased up to 20 μL/min. In this way, the measurement duration is reduced to 90 s. This time the first test of milk is performed on a sample free from AFM1 (blank sample) used as the reference for the sensor. Next, we inject milk samples containing 0.96 nM, 1.3 nM, 1.5 nM and 2.2 nM AFM1, respectively. We observe a wavelength shift which increases with the concentration (see Figure 5b).

In the second set of measurements, a higher signal for the blank sample than for the 0.09 nM AFM1 measurement of the first set is observed. Thus we infer that the 0.09 nM AFM1 concentration is not distinguishable for the sensor and that the signal for this concentration is due to the non-specific adsorption of other milk components. Likewise for the signal for the blank eluate, the signal is considered as a baseline with respect to the other measurements. Note, that the difference of non-specific signal levels in these two cases is caused by the different flow rates and the different buffers. In other words, eluates deriving from the concentrator module can vary in terms of milk components content and this variability is measured by the photonic sensor. Therefore, we set the LOD of the aMZI sensor to the AFM1 concentration of 0.96 nM. Taking into account the concentration factor of 20 times, this corresponds to an AFM1 concentration of 48 pM in the original milk sample. This estimate assumes that no AFM1 loss occurs in the concentration stage.

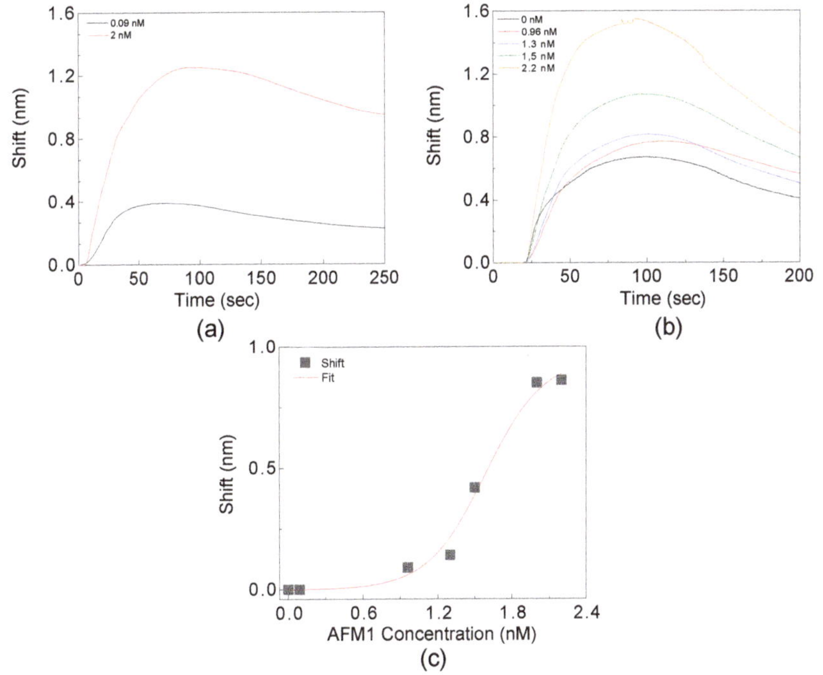

Figure 5. Aflatoxin M1 (AFM1) detection in the milk samples. Sensorgrams for concentrated milk samples with different AFM1 concentrations. (**a**) The first demonstration of AFM1 detection in milk. (**b**) The second set of tests of AFM1 detection. The black line is the response to the blank eluate. (**c**) The calibration function for the aMZI based sensor is extracted from the logistic fit of the shift values for different AFM1 concentrations (C).

By referring the signals to the baselines and by plotting the dependence of the maximum shift at t = 90 s versus the AFM1 concentration, we can build the calibration curve of the sensor (see Figure 5c). In the figure, the error bars show the variation of the shift in a time range t = 90 $\pm$ 5 s. We fit the data with the following logistic function:

$$R(C) = \frac{L}{(1 + e^{-k(C - C_0)})}. \quad (7)$$

where R is the maximum shift and C is the AFM1 concentration, respectively.

From the fit we obtain the values for $L = 0.95 \pm 0.07$; $C_0 = 1.6 \pm 0.06$ and $k = 4.3 \pm 0.9$ yielding to the following callibration function for the sensor:

$$R(C) = \frac{1}{1.05(1 + 975e^{-4.3C})}. \quad (8)$$

A clear differences in the signal levels and kinetics (see Figure 6a) are observed between the reference sample and the ones with AFM1. This difference indicates that a specific interaction between AFM1 and Fab′ takes place, as expected. To further characterize the kinetics of the sensor response, we performed an exponential fit of the association region of the sensorgrams with Equation (2). From the fit of the curves in the 40 $\div$ 90 s interval (see Figure 6b), where the association occurs, we obtain a linear dependence of the rate constants vs the AFM1 concentration (Figure 6c). From the linear fit, we extract k_{on} = (1.3 ± 0.5) × 10^7 $M^{-1}s^{-1}$ and k_{off} = (6.5 ± 0.5) × $10^{-3}s^{-1}$. From these values, we deduce K_D = (0.5 ± 0.2) × 10^{-10} M and K_A = (2 ± 1.5) × 10^9 M^{-1}. These values are comparable to the values for aptamer-AFM1 binding [42], while no data exists for the AFM1-Fab′ binding either in buffer or in real samples. The affinity value is comparable with the known affinity of this family of toxins which is in the range of 10^9–10^{11} M^{-1} values [43].

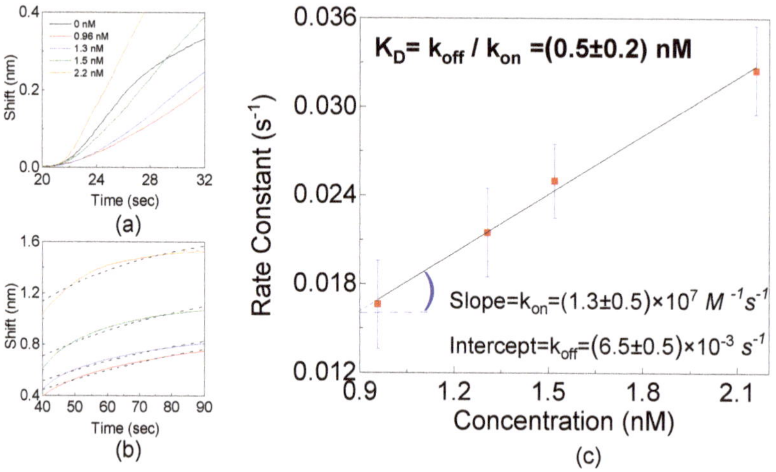

Figure 6. (**a**) The initial slopes of the sensor response for different concentrations of AFM1 in eluates. The black curve corresponds to the blank eluate. It shows a different behavior and a different kinetics supporting the fact that for the other curves the specific binding of AFM1 molecules is taking place. (**b**) The exponential fit (dashed lines) of the sensor response (continuous lines) in the 40 ÷ 90 s interval. (**c**) The dependence of the pseudo-first-order rate constant on the AFM1 concentrations. Slope and intercept of the linear fit correspond to k_{on} and k_{off}.

4. Conclusions

In this work we demonstrated an asymmetric Mach–Zehnder Interferometric biosensor which, when functionalized with Fab′, is able to detect specifically AFM1 in concentrated and filtered milk samples down to ≈48 pM. This LOD is comparable with other state-of-the-art devices (see Table 1). The aMZI described here shows an improved response time compared to the ones reported in the literature [44]. In addition, with respect to SPR sensors, the aMZI biosensor is more compact, easy to operate and cheaper.

Owing to the setup capabilities the kinetic of the AFM1-Fab′ reaction has been characterized as well. Affinity constants of K_A = (2 ± 1.5) × 10^9 M^{-1} in milk are measured which are comparable with the affinities of the same family of antibodies-AFM1 interaction.

This work opens new perspectives for integrated photonic biosensors as viable solutions for lab-on-chip devices for food safety analyses.

5. Materials and Methods

Milk Sample Preparation

Fresh whole milk was spiked with AFM1 in order to prepare samples to be processed for the detection of AFM1 with the biosensor [33]. We collected 400 mL of milk in glass bottles pretreated with 3% BSA; then milk was spiked with different concentrations of AFM1 and incubated at 40 °C for 1 h before placing at 4 °C until used.

After defatting and pre-concentration/purification treatments, eluted fractions containing AFM1 (quantified with Aflatoxin M1 ELISA kit I'screen, Tecna) and control fractions prepared starting from milk without Aflatoxin, were tested with aMZI biosensors.

Supplementary Materials: The following are available online at http://www.mdpi.com/2072-6651/11/7/409/s1, Figure S1: SDS-PAGE of total digest before separation by ion exchange chromatography (lane 2) and after separation: flow through fraction (lane 3), wash fraction (lane 4), eluted fraction (lane 5). Lane 1 and 6: LMW-SDS markers (GE Healthcare Life Science). SDS-PAGE was performed using precast minigels with density gradients ranging 10–15% (GE Healthcare Life Science). A semiautomatic horizontal unit (PhastSystem by Pharmacia) was used. The gel was stained with Coomassie brilliant blue, Figure S2: Chemiluminescence signal of Fab'-functionalized surfaces kept at 4 C until measured. Error bars represent the standard deviations, Figure S3: Optimization of surface passivation with casein. Upper panel: PEG-treated surfaces, without Fab'. Lower panel: Surfaces functionalized with Fab' and a first step of passivation with PEG. NP: non-passivated surface, Figure S4: Chemiluminescence signal of 3 Si3N4 flat surfaces functionalized with Fab' (1–3) or with all steps of the functionalization protocol except Fab' (4–6). Surfaces were inserted in wells of a 96 wells black microplate for handling. No signal is visible were Fab' are missing (wells 4–6).

Author Contributions: T.C. carried out the measurements, analyzed the data. C.P. (Cristina Potrich) functionalized the sensors and prepared the solutions. L.P. (Laura Pasquardini) optimized the sensor functionalization protcol. F.F. and E.S. fabricated the aMZI devices. T.C., C.P. (Cristina Potrich) and L.P. (Lorenzo Pavesi) wrote the paper. T.C., C.P. (Cristina Potrich), L.P. (Laura Pasquardini) and L.P. (Lorenzo Pavesi) reviewed the paper. L.P. (Lorenzo Pavesi), R.H. and C.P. (Cecilia Pederzolli) led the project. All authors discussed the results and commented on the manuscript.

Funding: This work is supported by the FP7 EU project Symphony. Grant agreement no: 610580 (http://www.symphony-project.eu/).

Conflicts of Interest: The authors declare no conflict of interest.

Abbreviations

The following abbreviations are used in this manuscript:

AFM1	Aflatoxin M1
AFB1	Aflatoxin B1
aMZI	Asymmetric Mach–Zehnder interferometer
CMOS	Complementary metal oxide semiconductor
ELISA	Enzyme-linked immunosorbent assay
FSR	Free spectral range
HPLC	High performance liquid chromatography
hCG	Human chorionic Gonadotropin
HRP	Horseradish Peroxidase
LOD	Limit Of detection
MES	2-(*N*-Morpholino)EthaneSulfonic acid
MZI	Mach–Zehnder interferometer
MRR	Micro ring resonator
OTA	Ochratoxin A
PDMS	Polydimethylsiloxane
RIU	Refractive Index Unit
SPR	Surface plasmon resonance
TLC	Thin layer chromatography
VCSEL	Vertical-cavity surface-emitting laser
WGM	Whispering gallery mode

References

1. CAST. *Mycotoxins: Economic and Health Risks;* Council for Agricultural Science and Technology: Ames, IA, USA, 1989.
2. Bhat, R. Mycotoxins in Food and Feed: Present Status and Future Concerns. *Compr. Rev. Food Sci. Food Saf.* **2010**, *9*, 57–81. [CrossRef]

3. Groopman, J.D.; Rai, R.V.; Karim, A.A. Aflatoxin Exposure in Human Populations: Measurements and Relationship to Cancer. *CRC Crit. Rev. Toxicol.* **1988**, *19*, 113–145. [CrossRef] [PubMed]
4. Wild, C.; Yun, Y. Mycotoxins and human disease: A largely ignored global health issue. *Carcinogenesis* **2010**, *31*, 71–82. [CrossRef] [PubMed]
5. IARC. *List of Classifications*; International Agency for Research on Cancer: World Health Organization, Lyon, France, 2012; Volume 56.
6. Henry, S.H.; Bosch, F.X.; Bowers, J.C. Aflatoxin, Hepatitis and Worldwide Liver Cancer Risks. In *Mycotoxins and Food Safety. Advances in Experimental Medicine and Biolog*; Springer: Boston, MA, USA, 2002; Volume 504, pp. 229–233.
7. Polzhofer, K.P. Thermal stability of aflatoxin M1. *Z. Lebensm. Unters. Forsch* **1977**, *164*, 80–81. [CrossRef] [PubMed]
8. Bijl, J.; Peteghem, C.V. Rapid extraction and sample clean-up for the fluorescence densitometric determination of aflatoxin M1 in milk and milk powder. *Anal. Chim. Acta* **1985**, *170*, 149–152. [CrossRef]
9. Behfar, A.; Khorasgani, Z.N.; Alemzadeh, Z.; Goudarzi, M.; Ebrahimi, R.; Tarhani, N. Determination of Aflatoxin M1 Levels in Produced Pasteurized Milk in Ahvaz City by Using HPLC. *Jundishapur J. Nat. Pharm. Prod.* **2012**, *7*, 80–84. [CrossRef]
10. Markaki, P.; Melissari, E. Occurrence of aflatoxin M1 in commercial pasteurized milk determined with ELISA and HPLC. *Food Addit. Contam.* **1997**, *14*, 451–456. [CrossRef] [PubMed]
11. Biancardi, A. Determination of aflatoxin M1 residues in milk. A comparative assessment of ELISA and IAC-HPLC methods. *Ind. Aliment.* **1997**, *36*, 870–876.
12. Abouzied, M.; Bentley, P.; Klein, F.; Rice, J. *A Sensitive ELISA for the Detection and Quantitation of Aflatoxin M1 (AFM1) in Milk and Dairy Products*; Neogen Corporation: Lansing, MI, USA, 2015.
13. Wang, Y.; Dostalek, J.; Knoll, W. Long range surface plasmon enhanced fluorescence spectroscopy for the detection of Aflatoxin M1 in milk. *Biosens. Bioelectron.* **2009**, *24*, 2264–2267. [CrossRef]
14. Xu, F.; Zhen, G.; Yu, F.; Kuennemann, E.; Textor, M.; Knoll, W. Combined Affinity and Catalytic Biosensor: In Situ Enzymatic Activity Monitoring of Surface-Bound Enzymes. *J. Am. Chem. Soc.* **2005**, *127*, 1308–13085. [CrossRef]
15. Salter, R.S.; Douglas, D.; Tess, M.; Markovsky, R.J.; Saul, S.J. *Collaborative Study of the Charm ROSA Safe Level Aflatoxin M1 Quantitative (SLAFMQ) Lateral Flow Test for Raw Bovine Milk*; Charm Sciences, Inc.: Lawrence, MA, USA, 2018.
16. Tothill, I.E. Biosensors and nanomaterials and their application for mycotoxin determination. *World Mycotoxin J.* **2011**, *4*, 361–374. [CrossRef]
17. Parker, C.O.; Lanyon, H.; Manning, M.; Arrigan, D.W.M.; Tothill, I.E. Electrochemical Immunochip Sensor for Aflatoxin M1 Detection. *Anal. Chem.* **2009**, *81*, 5291–5298. [CrossRef] [PubMed]
18. Paniel, N.; Radoi, A.; Marty, J.L. Development of an electrochemical biosensor for the detection of Aflatoxin M1 in milk. *Sensors* **2010**, *10*, 9439–9448. [CrossRef] [PubMed]
19. Sibanda, L.; Saeger, S.; Peteghem, C.V. Development of a portable field immunoassay for the detection of Aflatoxin M in milk. *Int. J. Food Microbiol.* **1999**, *48*, 203–209. [CrossRef]
20. Istamboulie, G.; Paniel, N.; Zara, L.; Granados, L.R.; Barthelmebs, L.; Noguer, T. Development of an impedimetric aptasensor for the determination of aflatoxin M1 in milk. *Talanta* **2016**, *146*, 464–469. [CrossRef] [PubMed]
21. Karczmarczyk, A.; Dubiak-Szepietowska, M.; Vorobii, M.; Rodriguez-Emmeneggerd, C.; Dostálek, J.; Feller, K.H. Sensitive and rapid detection of aflatoxin M1 in milk utilizing enhanced SPR and p(HEMA) brushes. *Biosens. Bioelectron.* **2016**, *81*, 159–165. [CrossRef] [PubMed]
22. Nirschl, M.; Reuter, F.; Voros, J. Review of Transducer Principles for Label-Free Biomolecular Interaction Analysis. *Biosensors* **2011**, *1*, 70–92. [CrossRef]
23. Lafleur, J.P.; Jonsson, A.; Senkbeil, S.; Kutter, J.P. Recent advances in lab-on-a-chip for biosensing applications. *Biosens. Bioelectron.* **2016**, *76*, 213–233. [CrossRef]
24. Lockwood, D.; Pavesi, L. *Silicon Photonics II: Components and Integration Applications*, 2nd ed.; Springer: Berlin, Germany, 2011.
25. Zhu, H.; White, I.M.; Suter, J.D.; Dale, P.S.; Fan, X. Analysis of biomolecule detection with optofluidic ring resonator sensors. *Opt. Express* **2007**, *15*, 9139–9146. [CrossRef]

26. Zlatanovic, S.; Mirkarimi, L.W.; Sigalas, M.M.; Bynum, M.A.; Chow, E.; Robotti, K.M.; Burr, G.W.; Esener, S.; Grot, A. Photonic crystal microcavity sensor for ultracompact monitoring of reaction kinetics and protein concentration. *Sens. Actuators B Chem.* **2009**, *141*, 13–19. [CrossRef]
27. Baaske, M.D.; Foreman, M.R.; Vollmer, F. Single-molecule nucleic acid interactions monitored on a label-free microcavity biosensor platform. *Nat. Nanotechnol.* **2014**, *9*, 933–939. [CrossRef] [PubMed]
28. Heideman, R.G.; Kooyman, R.P.H.; Greve, J. Performance of a highly sensitive optical waveguide Mach–Zehnder interferometer immunosensor. *Sens. Actuators B Chem.* **1993**, *10*, 209–217. [CrossRef]
29. Heideman, R.G.; Lambeck, P.V. Remote opto-chemical sensing with extreme sensitivity: Design, fabrication and performance of a pigtailed integrated optical phase-modulated Mach–Zehnder interferometer system. *Sens. Actuators B Chem.* **1999**, *61*, 100–127. [CrossRef]
30. Liu, Q.; Tu, X.; Kim, K.W.; Kee, J.S.; Shin, Y.; Han, K.; Yoon, Y.J.; Lo, G.Q.; Park, M.K. Highly sensitive Mach–Zehnder interferometer biosensor based on silicon nitride slot waveguide. *Sens. Actuators B Chem.* **2013**, *188*, 681–688. [CrossRef]
31. Duval, D.; Gonzalez-Guerrero, A.B.; Dante, S.; Lechuga, L.M. Interferometric waveguide biosensor based on Si-technology for point-of-care diagnostic. In Proceedings of the Silicon Photonics and Photonic Integrated Circuits III, Brussels, Belgium, 16–19 April 2012; Volume 8431, p. 84310P.
32. Misiakos, K.; Raptis, I.; Salapatas, A.; Makarona, E.; Botsialas, A.; Hoekman, M.; Stoffer, R.; Jobst, G. Broad-band Mach–Zehnder interferometers as high performance refractive index sensors: Theory and monolithic implementation. *Opt. Express* **2014**, *22*, 8856–8870. [CrossRef] [PubMed]
33. SYMPHONY. Available online: http://www.symphony-project.eu (accessed on 12 July 2019).
34. Chalyan, T. Aptamer- and Fab′- functionalized microring resonators for Aflatoxin M1 detection. *IEEE J. Sel. Top. Quantum Electron.* **2017**, *23*, 1–8. [CrossRef]
35. Chalyan, T.; Pasquardini, L.; Falke, F.; Zanetti, M.; Guider, R.; Gandolfi, D.; Schreuder, E.; Pederzolli, C.; Heideman, R.G.; Pavesi, L. Biosensors based on Si_3N_4 Asymmetric Mach–Zehnder Interferometers. In Proceedings of the SPIE Optical Sensing and Detection IV, Brussels, Belgium, 3–7 April 2016; Volume 9899, p. 98991S.
36. Worhoff, K. TriPleX: A versatile dielectric photonic platform. *Adv. Opt. Technol.* **2015**, *4*, 189–207. [CrossRef]
37. Roy, D.; Park, J.W. Spatially nanoscale-controlled functional surfaces toward efficient bioactive platforms. *J. Mater. Chem. B* **2015**, *3*, 5135–5149. [CrossRef]
38. Yoshimoto, K.; Nishio, M.; Sugasawa, H.; Nagasaki, Y. Direct Observation of Adsorption-Induced Inactivation of Antibody Fragments Surrounded by Mixed-PEG Layer on a Gold Surface. *J. Am. Chem. Soc.* **2010**, *132*, 7982–7989. [CrossRef] [PubMed]
39. Chalyan, T.; Guider, R.; Pasquardini, L.; Zanetti, M.; Falke, F.; Schreuder, E.; Heideman, R.G.; Pederzolli, C.; Pavesi, L. Asymmetric Mach–Zehnder Interferometer Based Biosensors for Aflatoxin M1 Detection. *Biosensors* **2016**, *1*, 1. [CrossRef]
40. Chalyan, T.; Besselink, G.A.J.; Heideman, R.G.; Pavesi, L. Use of microring resonators for biospecific interaction analysis. In Proceedings of the SPIE Optical Sensing, Imaging, and Photon Counting: Nanostructured Devices and Applications 2017, San Diego, CA, USA, 6–10 August 2017; Volume 10353, p. 103530Q.
41. Stone, D.C; Ellis, J. *Stats Tutorial-Instrumental Analysis and Calibration;* Department of Chemistry, University of Toronto: Toronto, ON, Canada, 2011.
42. Malhotra, S.; Pandey, A.K.; Rajput, Y.S.; Sharma, R. Selection of aptamers for aflatoxin M1 and their characterization. *J. Mol. Recognit.* **2014**, *27*, 493–500. [CrossRef] [PubMed]
43. Anti-Aflatoxin Antibody [1C6] (ab685). Available online: http://www.abcam.com/aflatoxin-antibody-1c6-ab685.html (accessed on 12 July 2019).
44. Matabaro, E.; Ishimwe, N.; Uwimbabazi, E.; Lee, B.H. Current Immunoassay Methods for the Rapid detection of Aflatoxin in Milk and Dairy Products. *Compr. Rev. Food Sci. Food Saf.* **2017**, *16*, 808–820. [CrossRef]

MDPI
St. Alban-Anlage 66
4052 Basel
Switzerland
Tel. +41 61 683 77 34
Fax +41 61 302 89 18
www.mdpi.com

Toxins Editorial Office
E-mail: toxins@mdpi.com
www.mdpi.com/journal/toxins

www.ingramcontent.com/pod-product-compliance
Lightning Source LLC
LaVergne TN
LVHW070404100526
838202LV00014B/1390
* 9 7 8 3 0 3 9 2 8 7 0 4 8 *